NURTURING MASSAGE FOR PREGNANCY:

A PRACTICAL GUIDE TO BODYWORK FOR THE PERINATAL CYCLE

Leslie Stager, RN, LMT

Continuing Education Instructor
Oregon School of Massage
Portland, Oregon

Lippincott Williams & Wilkins
a Wolters Kluwer business

Philadelphia · Baltimore · New York · London
Buenos Aires · Hong Kong · Sydney · Tokyo

Acquisitions Editor: John Goucher
Developmental Editor: David Payne
Managing Editor: Linda G. Francis
Marketing Manager: Zhan Caplan
Project Manager: Nicole Walz
Design Coordinator: Stephen Druding
Cover Designer: Karen Quigley
Production Services: Cadmus Communications, a Cenveo company

351 West Camden Street   530 Walnut Street
Baltimore, MD 21201   Philadelphia, PA 19106

Printed in China

Library of Congress Cataloging-in-Publication Data

Stager, Leslie.
  Nurturing massage for pregnancy: a practical guide to bodywork for the perinatal cycle / Leslie Stager.
     p. ; cm.
  Includes bibliographical references and index.
  ISBN-13: 978-0-7817-6753-8 (alk. paper)
  ISBN-10: 0-7817-6753-9
  1. Massage. 2. Pregnancy. I. Title.
  [DNLM: 1. Massage—methods. 2. Pregnancy. WB 537 S779n 2010]
  RA780.5.S65 2010
  618.2—dc22
                              2008031194

DISCLAIMER

Care has been taken to confirm the accuracy of the information present and to describe generally accepted practices. However, the authors, editors, and publisher are not responsible for errors or omissions or for any consequences from application of the information in this book and make no warranty, expressed or implied, with respect to the currency, completeness, or accuracy of the contents of the publication. Application of this information in a particular situation remains the professional responsibility of the practitioner; the clinical treatments described and recommended may not be considered absolute and universal recommendations.

The authors, editors, and publisher have exerted every effort to ensure that drug selection and dosage set forth in this text are in accordance with the current recommendations and practice at the time of publication. However, in view of ongoing research, changes in government regulations, and the constant flow of information relating to drug therapy and drug reactions, the reader is urged to check the package insert for each drug for any change in indications and dosage and for added warnings and precautions. This is particularly important when the recommended agent is a new or infrequently employed drug.

Some drugs and medical devices presented in this publication have Food and Drug Administration (FDA) clearance for limited use in restricted research settings. It is the responsibility of the healthcare provider to ascertain the FDA status of each drug or device planned for use in their clinical practice.

The publishers have made every effort to trace the copyright holders for borrowed material. If they have inadvertently overlooked any, they will be pleased to make the necessary arrangements at the first opportunity.

To purchase additional copies of this book, call our customer service department at **(800) 638-3030** or fax orders to **(301) 223-2320**. International customers should call **(301) 223-2300**.

Visit Lippincott Williams & Wilkins on the Internet: http://www.lww.com. Lippincott Williams & Wilkins customer service representatives are available from 8:30 am to 6:00 pm, EST.

10 9 8 7 6 5 4 3 2 1

FOREWORD I

I met Leslie Stager in 1992. We were two lone pregnancy massage therapists in Portland, Oregon, looking to establish a referral network. Over the years our careers developed and grew. Leslie has focused on writing and teaching. I am so happy she has written this book. Now people who can't take her classes can still learn from the master. As a midwife, therapeutic bodyworker, and teacher of perinatal bodywork, I have longed for a comprehensive textbook and reference guide that I could use in my own practice and also recommend to my students. This is the book.

Nurturing Massage for Pregnancy is so much more than a guide to massaging pregnant women. It perfectly balances theory and practice. Leslie helps us understand the delicate interplay of physical changes, emotional concerns, and cultural influences experienced by expectant and new mothers. She skillfully weaves case studies, ancient and modern traditions, and self care tips for the mothers and helpful hints for the mothers' partners.

It is amazing to me that, given the growing popularity of massage and specifically pregnancy massage, a book like this hasn't come along sooner. Like Goldilocks tasting the porridge, I have read all the pregnancy massage books that have come before. One book had almost no anatomy and physiology; another had some theory, but little actual massage technique; a third book focused mainly on pregnancy complications and contraindications and was way too scary. This book is just right.

I am excited that Leslie's book is so well researched. It contains everything massage practitioners and students need to work knowledgeably and safely. It is seasoned with just the right amount of medical information—an inevitable part of most North American women's pregnancies and births. We need facts to educate women and sometimes other healthcare providers about the safety and effectiveness of the work we do. This evidence-based approach is essential because there is so much misinformation circulating about the perceived dangers of massage during the perinatal period.

I am astonished that one of the most common ways for people to find my own website is to type "pregnancy massage dangers" into a search engine. These massage-danger myths prevent some mothers from seeking the healing benefits of massage. Likewise, some massage therapists are afraid to massage pregnant women.

Research shows that women who receive massage during their pregnancies, and especially during labor, are better able to provide loving touch to their infants. Infants need touch—and lots of it—to survive and develop normally, both physically and emotionally.

Through our loving professional touch we can help mothers form an essential bond with their infants. In this way, our work has the potential to change the world. In a time when many people are touch-deprived and disaffected, we massage therapists can help break cycles of alienation and violence with each new life. This fabulous book shows us how. Thank you, Leslie.

Carol Gray, Midwife, LMT

$\mathcal{F}$inally, a comprehensive book on nurturing massage for pregnancy, birth, and postpartum written by an experienced massage therapist/nurse. Leslie's extensive background in both massage and perinatal nursing is evident in each page of this book. The book covers not only massage techniques and their rationale in pregnancy, but Leslie has had the foresight to also cover the important physiological and emotional changes during pregnancy as well as massage for the stages of labor. When massage therapists, nurses, midwives, and doulas are touching a client, they are also touching the mother's emotions and state of mind. Massage helps facilitate healthful pregnancy, birth, and postpartum and provides an avenue of relaxation and touch that is very much needed in our lives.

Pregnancy massage shares many of the goals of regular massage but is tailored specifically to the needs of pregnant women and their changing bodies. Leslie brings her vast knowledge and technical expertise and has expertly covered the whole perinatal massage cycle. The information in this book serves as an excellent guide to perinatal massage for all who are assisting women in pregnancy, birth, and postpartum. With the high and climbing cesarean rate here in the United States, the section in the book on healing from a cesarean section will be put to good use.

Readers also will find helpful the quick reference list of contraindications (Appendix A). In this very valuable textbook, Leslie has included information for massage students and practitioners, but *Nurturing Massage for Pregnancy* can also be used as an addition to doula trainings, continuing education for perinatal nurses, and an extension to the work of postpartum doulas and lactation consultants.

Paulina G. (Polly) Perez, BSN, FACCE,
LCCE, CD
Author of *Special Women: The Role of the Professional Labor Assistant* and *The Nurturing Touch at Birth: A Labor Support Handbook*,
Cutting Edge Press
Johnson, Vermont

Nurturing Massage for Pregnancy: A Practical Guide to Bodywork for the Perinatal Cycle is a textbook for massage students and certified massage therapists who treat clients who are pregnant or laboring, or who have recently given birth. The book focuses on general soft-tissue and Swedish massage and assumes the reader is already familiar with those techniques as well as the basics of anatomy, physiology, and kinesiology. The book also integrates some myofascial release and trigger point techniques, as well as occasional complementary bodywork methodologies, such as the use of breath and visualizations, acupressure, aromatherapy, and hydrotherapy.

While educating the massage therapist in anatomical, physiological, pathological, and emotional realities of the perinatal cycle, the text integrates information that highlights birthing as a transformative event in a woman's life, thereby preparing the massage therapist for meeting her or his childbearing clients with a holistic understanding of their changing lives. To support this perspective, *Nurturing Massage for Pregnancy* incorporates into the text traditional and indigenous global birth wisdom gleaned from anthropological research and midwifery knowledge.

To address the concerns of many practitioners with regard to working with pregnant clients, contraindications and precautions are examined thoroughly, along with a review of basic obstetrical practices and conditions that a massage therapist might encounter if working with women throughout a pregnancy and birth. The book dispels common myths about the dangers of particular bodywork, such as massage or reflexology to the ankles, and highlights the areas where a practitioner *does* need to use caution, such as in regard to the increased risk for blood clots and varicose veins.

ORGANIZATION AND STRUCTURE

The book is divided into three parts: Pregnancy, Birth, and Postpartum. Each part includes chapters that prepare the massage therapist for meeting client needs, including physiology relevant to that phase of the perinatal cycle and how that physiology affects the bodywork practice. Each part also includes precautions and contraindications pertinent to that phase, general massage techniques appropriate to that phase, and common conditions or complaints with specific bodywork techniques to address them.

Part I: Pregnancy (Chapters 1–7) begins by describing the ways in which pregnancy massage is unique. It discusses the benefits it can have for both mother and baby and research that supports these benefits. Issues and concerns that prevent women from receiving pregnancy massage are explored along with ways the massage therapist may help to mitigate some of these issues. Part I also introduces images of the global honoring of pregnancy and birth.

The growth of an embryo and fetus after conception is reviewed and the experiences of a pregnant woman during each month or trimester are described, along with bodywork concerns specific to those times. Medical conditions during pregnancy that could necessitate precautions or contraindications in bodywork are explained and a sample medical release form is included, along with clarification of when its use is most highly recommended. Proper positioning and draping for each trimester are described, along with tips to help the therapist address particular issues of a pregnant client, such as appropriate positioning if she complains of heartburn or nausea. Cause, treatment, and specific bodywork techniques for some common complaints the practitioner is likely to encounter are then described in detail, with drawings and photographs to help facilitate understanding of the techniques.

Part II: Birth (Chapters 8–10) describes the basic physiology of labor and birth, a mother's experience through various stages of labor, and tips for addressing her care during each stage of labor. Contraindications and precautions with regard to labor are addressed. One chapter focuses on bodywork techniques to help relieve particular conditions and complications during birth. Readers are reminded in this chapter that their role in birth is to support a woman with touch, not to interfere with the role of family members, a midwife, or a doctor.

Part III: Postpartum (Chapters 11–13) focuses on the areas of the body that may become particularly stressed after many hours of labor, followed by months of nursing and carrying a growing baby. Common complaints, such as "nursing neck" and engorged breasts, as well as recovery care for the abdomen and womb are addressed with helpful bodywork techniques. Massage for the woman who experienced a cesarean delivery is discussed in the final chapter of this section.

PEDAGOGICAL FEATURES

Features to aid practitioners are integrated throughout the text, along with topics of special interest.

- *Self-Care Tips for the Mother* are practices a client can learn to relieve some of her discomforts. These include stretches and general health activities.
- *Massage Therapist Tips* are highlighted bits of wisdom that can help the massage therapist address or understand certain conditions. For instance, one tip describes how to create a nurturing space for pregnant clients, while another looks at why some clients may have sinus congestion and how to add to their comfort by having a fan available in the massage office.
- *Complementary Modalities* provides information about bodywork modalities which massage therapists may wish to investigate further, when treatments besides massage are especially effective for a particular condition.
- *Traditional Birth Practices* highlights methods of touching used by people of various cultures around the world when caring for pregnant, laboring, and postpartum women.
- *How the Partner Can Help* provides ideas that the massage therapist can teach to partners or birth supporters to give them confidence in offering nurturing touch during pregnancy or labor.
- *Case Studies* help address some concerns a practitioner may have, by sharing stories of therapist encounters with pregnant, laboring, or postpartum clients. Some of these studies describe how a therapist might approach a common condition of pregnancy. Others address a potentially difficult situation, such as a case of a pregnant client's bag of waters breaking while receiving a massage, and a home-birthing woman finding that touch increased her ability to relax during labor so that her cervix dilated more readily and she avoided going to the hospital.
- *Dispelling Myths* is a feature that dispels common erroneous beliefs about bodywork and pregnancy.

- *Common complaints* during pregnancy and birth are presented alphabetically for the practitioner's ease of use (Chapters 6 and 10).
- *Contraindications and Precautions* are identified by a special icon throughout the text.
- *Resources for the Practitioner* are provided in Appendix B, which includes contact information of perinatal organizations and prenatal and infant massage organizations.
- *Key terms* are boldfaced in the narrative and are defined in a glossary at the end of the book.
- *Illustrations and photographs* provide useful visuals of how to implement particular bodywork techniques, and offer inspiration about pregnancy and birth.

ADDITIONAL RESOURCES

Nurturing Massage for Pregnancy includes additional resources for both instructors and students that are available on the book's companion website at thePoint.lww.com/Stager. This website features the following:

- Answers to the end-of-chapter review questions
- A four-color image bank of all the illustrations and photos that appear in the book
- Video clips, narrated by the author, of techniques and concepts indicated in the book by this icon:
- Syllabi for 4-, 6-, and 8-hour classes, 1- or 2-weekend classes, and a 3-month class

SCOPE OF PRACTICE

Each state has different laws governing the practice of massage therapy. I am unaware of any that prohibit or regulate massage during pregnancy; however, it is the responsibility of practitioners to learn and practice by the laws of their state of licensure. Here are some general reminders when practicing massage for women in the perinatal cycle:

- Breast massage can be very beneficial at various stages of the perinatal cycle, however, breast massage is prohibited in some states. Know your states guidelines.
- In all states it is outside scope of a massage therapist's practice to recommend medications, orally-ingested herbs, or medical treatments for any client, including pregnant, laboring, or postpartum women.

- While certain behaviors are known to be dangerous for pregnant and breastfeeding women or a fetus, it is outside the massage therapist's scope of practice to instruct a woman to stop these behaviors, such as smoking or drinking alcohol. Your job is to nurture the client with your touch, not with your advice about topics outside of the realm of massage. If you feel a woman's choices may be putting her pregnancy or unborn child at risk, or that your own opinions are affecting your work with a client, you may decide to get a medical release from her care provider or decide it is not in your or her best interest to continue being her massage therapist during this time.
- It is the practitioner's responsibility to be familiar with the contraindications and precautions for working with the variety of conditions that can arise during pregnancy, birth, and postpartum, to know when to refer a client, and when to request the signing of a medical release form.
- There are many bodywork methodologies that are appropriate for various conditions in the perinatal cycle. This book focuses on general soft tissue bodywork, along with some simple hydrotherapies, visualization, breathing, and facilitated stretches. For interest, it mentions the use of acupressure, aromatherapy, and reflexology for some conditions where they are especially helpful or particularly common to use, but expects that the massage therapist will practice these only after receiving specific training.
- During labor and birth, the massage therapist may be in the role of providing comfort care, but unless the therapist is trained as a birth professional, it is not her or his responsibility to determine or suggest what choices are appropriate with regard to the progress of the labor. You may suggest position changes if your advice is requested by the mother or support team which may promote the benefits of particular touch, or may provide easier access for massage and touch.

A NOTE TO PRACTITIONERS

This book shares essential knowledge and practical skills that a massage therapist needs to provide safe, competent, and nurturing bodywork to women during one of the most psychically influential and physiologically challenging times of their lives. The organization of the book according to the three perinatal phases—pregnancy, birth, and postpartum—is intended to help the therapist working with clients during each phase. Observing the appropriate precautions, practitioners can feel confident that their work will never harm a pregnant, laboring, or postpartum client or a woman's in utero child.

There are many beneficial and complementary bodywork methodologies that can be integrated into perinatal work. I encourage students and practitioners to go beyond what is offered in this book and explore many modalities to support their work with pregnancy and birth. It is my hope that *Nurturing Massage for Pregnancy* will help to cultivate knowledge of, skill with, and respect for the perinatal cycle in all who choose to work with clients during this time of their lives.

—Leslie Stager RN, LMT

ACKNOWLEDGMENTS

Writing this book has been a long adventure in persistence and patience. I relied on numerous supporters without whom this could not have manifested into its finished form. I gratefully acknowledge the following people for their invaluable contributions to this work.

First and foremost, I must thank Linda Francis, my managing editor at Lippincott Williams & Wilkins, who was always quietly kind and encouraging through my bouts of doubt and frustration, and who stuck with me through these years of effort.

Thanks to David Payne, development editor, for agreeing that photos would be the most appropriate art-form in the book and who was thorough in his suggestions and revisions.

Those who edited the first draft of the book gave me specific, detailed suggestions that significantly improved the quality of the content.

Rick Giase, photographer extraordinaire, brought a calm focus to the photo-shoot that helped us all relax during the limited time we had, and gave us beautiful images.

I want to express my gratitude to all the models—pregnant and nonpregnant alike—who so generously and patiently allowed themselves to be photographed for this book. They are: Amy Baggett, Laura Brooks, Clint Chandler, Crystal Dougherty, Tai Quesada Dougherty, Kelli Dunn, Tess Gallegos, Jessica Garcia, Rob Killam, Jaimee Lind, Ken Mueller, Hiromi Nakada-Johnson, Pam Peppard, Mark Perez, and Victoria J. Robertson.

Many thanks to those who read and reread various drafts of various chapters, offered important clarifications of information, and gave continuous encouragement for the project, including Asha Stager, Terri Nash, Carol Gray, and Sue Firman. Thanks also to Carol Gray for her fearless determination to promote massage for the perinatal cycle as safe, and for supporting this project by editing, reviewing, and writing a Foreword.

Much appreciation to Karen Searls and Shoba Satya, for their hours of time invested in helping with acupressure information, although it was ultimately not included.

My gratitude extends to the Oregon School of Massage for giving me the opportunity to teach multitudes of students over the past 16 years, helping me hone my skills and motivating me to research the topic in depth. And to all my students, for sharing and growing their enthusiasm, asking questions, and spreading the benefits of touch.

REVIEWERS

Linda A. Boucher, MAMFT, BSN, RN, LMT
Branford Hall Career Institute
Windsor, Connecticut

Gary Bruce, NCTMB, LMT
Massage Therapy Institute
St Augustine, Florida

Diane Charmley, RN, LMT
Seattle, Washington

Carol Gray, Midwife, LMT
Portland, Oregon

Suzanne P. Reese, BA, NCTMB, HHP, RYT
Compassionate Child
Ramona, California

CONTENTS

Preface   *vii*

PART I
PREGNANCY   1

1   Massage During Pregnancy: A Unique
    Opportunity   3
2   Physiological and Emotional Changes
    During Pregnancy   13
3   Postural and Muscular Adaptations
    Related to Pregnancy   31
4   Precautions and Contraindications for Bodywork
    During Pregnancy   49
5   General Massage for Pregnancy   82
6   Common Complaints During Pregnancy   107
7   Bodywork in Preparation for Birth   132

PART II
BIRTH   141

8   Supporting Women During Labor and Birth   143
9   Massage for the Stages of Labor   152
10 Common Complaints During Labor   181

PART III
THE POSTPARTUM PERIOD   195

11 Reincorporation: The Postpartum Period   197
12 Bodywork for the Postpartum Client   208
13 Massage After Birth-Related Surgery   235

APPENDIX A: REFERENCE LIST
OF CONTRAINDICATIONS   Online
APPENDIX B: RESOURCES FOR THE PRACTITIONER   Online
GLOSSARY   245
INDEX   249

PREGNANCY

Touch is a primordial communication that is before words; it is in fact a language beyond words. The art of skillful touch brings depth to the experience of pregnancy, integrating the changes a woman undergoes while communicating nurturing, safety, and comfort.

TERRI NASH, MS, CPM

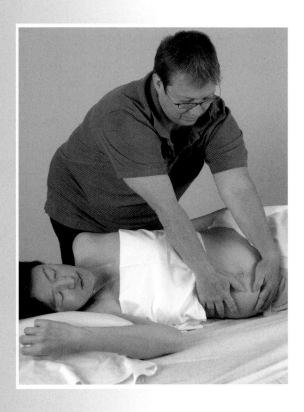

CHAPTER 1

MASSAGE DURING PREGNANCY: A UNIQUE OPPORTUNITY

LEARNING OBJECTIVES

After reading this chapter, you should be able to:

- Understand the unique aspects of working with pregnant, laboring, and postpartum women.
- Describe an overview of the worldwide prevalence of touch traditions during pregnancy and birth.
- List and explain the benefits of touch during the child-bearing cycle.
- Describe the multiple levels on which touch during pregnancy affects a woman and her baby's life.
- Discuss the myths and facts about the dangers of touch during pregnancy.

*M*assage therapists who work with women during their perinatal cycle have an exciting and unique opportunity to share in what is often the most life-changing and important experience of a woman's life—the process of creating, nurturing, and birthing life. Massaging pregnant women can be extraordinarily different from working with other clients. For instance, over the span of 9 months, a massage therapist observes and feels under her or his hands the subtle and dramatic changes that are occurring in a pregnant mother's body: changes in shape, composition, hormonal flow, fat and weight distribution, and posture. The therapist will see the normally nonpregnant client grow into a woman who is carrying 30 pounds or more of extra weight, mostly on the anterior side of her body, and some of it kicking visibly through her growing belly.

Additionally, in the course of her pregnancy, a woman often experiences important changes emotionally, energetically, and spiritually. The massage therapist who sees her regularly may witness the client's fluctuating sense of identity and her ultimate transformation into her new role as mother.

When working with pregnant, laboring, and postpartum women, massage therapists practice specific positioning to guarantee the safety of both the mother and baby. More pillows, supports, and cushioning as well as creativity will be needed to ensure comfort for each individual on your table. The use of sidelying and semi-reclining positions is a necessity, as well as learning to be mobile with your massage when a woman is in labor. Massage therapists who work often with pregnant women develop skills and versatility that will improve their ability to serve and meet the needs of a varied population.

Most amazingly, a massage therapist working with a pregnant woman has an opportunity to affect two people at once, while touching the skin of only one person. Each time a pregnant woman is massaged, the baby in utero, as well as the mother, is affected energetically and physically.

Massage therapists working frequently with pregnant clients also have an indirect and beneficial role in the birth passage of both mother and infant. With encouragement from the massage therapist, the client learns skills for relaxing when touched. When nurturing touch and emotional support is then offered during labor, the woman may find that she can more readily cultivate relaxation in this new situation,[1,2] reducing pain[3] and her risks of medical interventions and premature birth,[4,5,6] and increasing her potential for a more satisfying birth experience. Additionally, the sessions of nurturing massage that the therapist has offered the mother during pregnancy or labor will give her first-hand experience in the therapeutic benefits of touch. Because of this, she may find that she naturally increases the frequency and duration of the nurturing touch and massage that she offers to her newborn.[7,8]

After the birth, the massage therapist might have the opportunity to meet the baby whom she saw moving inside the mother's belly and whom she had actually massaged through the maternal abdomen. Some women may choose to bring their infant with them to a massage session, and so the therapist will find herself or himself continuing to use sidelying position to support the mother who wishes to hold or nurse her infant during the massage. As she or he massages, the therapist will notice that physical adjustments in the postpartum client's body are continuing to occur for months after birth. Massage can assist the new mother's recovery from the musculoskeletal strains and hormonal stresses of pregnancy and birth and can continue to be an important aspect of a new mother's life. When trained in infant massage, the therapist may be asked to share with the parents ways of offering nurturing touch to their new baby.

The massage therapist has a unique role in the life of a childbearing woman who relies on the therapist for help with relief of discomforts and for enhancing the sensory experience of her pregnant body. Pregnancy, birth, and mothering are impressive events in a woman's life, and the memories of the massage therapist who supported her through those phases may remain imprinted in her mind for a lifetime.

The purpose of this chapter is to introduce you, the massage therapist, to the unique aspects of massage for pregnant women and to lay a theoretical foundation on which later chapters are built. Later chapters will cover the specifics of working with laboring and postpartum women. Covered below are a few traditions of touch for pregnancy that have been a foundation of perinatal care around the world, and some key benefits and issues to consider when offering massage to pregnant women.

TRADITIONS OF TOUCH FOR PREGNANCY

For centuries, midwives, doulas, and families have known well the benefits of supporting women through pregnancy, birth, and postpartum and have

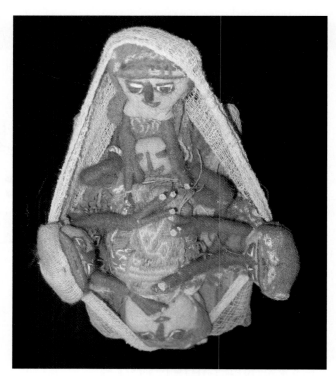

FIGURE 1.1   Ancient Peruvian doll imagery displaying women's hands-on support of the birthing woman.
Used with permission from Aaron Rubinstein.

nurtured them with the healing tools of hands, words, water, and warm herbal oils (Figure 1.1).

Massage accompanies childbirth nearly everywhere in the traditional world (except, of course, where the mother births alone).[9] According to Navajo tradition, the midwife was known as the "one who holds," referring to how she would often hold the pregnant woman from behind and massage her belly throughout labor while the woman birthed the infant.[10] In Indonesia, the term for "midwife" literally means, "someone who knows how to massage."[11]

In Guatemala and Belize, the midwife or *comadrona* teaches young women to care for their wombs with herbs and uterine self-massage prior to pregnancy (class notes from Rosita Arvigo's Mayan Abdominal Massage Professional Training, Massachusetts, 2000) then supports them throughout their pregnancy and in labor by massaging their backs, bellies, and legs.

In India and Bangladesh, a woman is often supported throughout her childbearing year with massage and touch from experienced women elders or the traditional midwife or "dai." In labor, according to ancient Ayurvedic prescription, a pregnant woman might be massaged by these elder women, who rub scented oils into her back, legs, arms, breasts, and belly to assure good baby positioning and a healthy, comfortable birthing. For weeks after birth, the mother and baby both are massaged daily to aide in their recovery from the birth experience.[12-14]

While actual massage practices vary worldwide, touch has commonly been used during the perinatal cycle for similar reasons: as a means to reposition the baby during pregnancy, to ease pregnancy discomforts and labor pain, to assist the progress of labor, to stimulate release of the placenta and prevent post-delivery hemorrhage, to speed postpartum recovery, and to encourage lactation and ease engorgement discomfort.

Furthermore, it is important to note the tradition of respect that surrounds pregnancy and birth in many cultures and to continue that tradition in our approach to clients. As we learn to support women with touch and revive the practice of honoring women for their creative ability, we can remember others worldwide who still actively revere and honor women who have the capability of birthing. This is evidenced by people in Assam, India, where their ancient temple honors the "yoni" or vagina of the Goddess Khamakya (Figure 1.2). Once a year at this temple, the goddess is said to be menstruating and the stream that flows deep inside the temple turns red. People stand in line for days to be able to kneel by this stream and collect the red healing water — the menstrual blood of Khamakya. Men and women from around the country stop work and come to the temple to honor this symbol of her fertility. Women often run out of the temple, moved by their contact with the Great Mother goddess, crying, and calling out, "Ma, Ma, Ma"[16] (J. Thompson, Anthropology Professor, personal communication, 2002).

"Ma, Ma, Ma". . . it is a universal sound that has called for mother for thousands of years. It is a word that is embedded in our language in the words: *Mama, Mammal, Mammary*—words related to mothering. It is a sound that often emanates naturally from a newborn's voice when calling for mother.

The specific word that we know as "mama"—mother—exists in numerous languages: Russian, Mayan, Quechuan, Swahili, Albanian, Hungarian, Indonesian, Swahili, Turkish, Hawaiian, Arizona Hopi, Chickasaw, Chinook, Creek, and Koasati. Many other languages have words related to motherhood that sound similar (Table 1.1).

The cycle of pregnancy, birth, and becoming a mother, and a woman's role as creator and bearer of life, is revered and acknowledged with elaborate ceremonies by many. Women are respected, feared, and recognized as the source of all creation, or as "vessels of spiritual fire."[15] In some cultures, simply to touch the pregnant woman brings one closer to what is considered a divine energy. People have recognized that it is no small matter that women bleed on a monthly cycle and do not die, that women bleed in a way that is related to creative energy rather than to wounding, to birthing rather than dying. It is no small matter either to have two people making use of one external body or to have women nourish life with milk produced in her breasts. An Orthodox Jewish woman described that in her tradition, a woman in her menses is revered for reflecting the creative power of the Divine: the power to bring another human being into life. Thus, she is treated deferentially by men, especially during this time in her monthly cycle (Y. Ableman, Chabad House, personal communication, 2002).

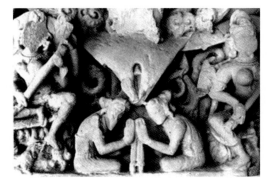

FIGURE 1.2   Reverence for the Yoni.
A twelfth-century Indian stone sculpture at Sixty-Four Temple. From Mookerjee A. Kali, the Feminine Force. Rochester, VT: Destiny Books, 1988. Courtesy of Thames and Hudson Ltd.

Table 1.1	Words for "Mother" Around the World
Language	**Word(s)**
Afrikaans	Ma, Moeder
Armenian	Mayrig
Czech	Matka, Matinka
Danish	Mor
Hopi (Arizona)	Maama
Hungarian	Mama
Mayan	Mamah
Old English	Modor
Polish	Matka
Quechuan	Mama
Slovak	Mamika, Mamka
Spanish	Madre
Swahili	Mama
Vietnamese	Me, Me de
Zulu	Umame

Traditional Birth Practices:

Japanese Pregnancy Massage

*M*ore than 120 years ago, Dr. George Engelmann described the methods of a Japanese healer caring for pregnant women after their fifth month of pregnancy: the healer "manipulates the abdomen of the patient, who clings about his neck, pressing his shoulders against her breasts; and pressing his knees between hers, so that she is firmly supported. Then he practices a lateral massage with his hands, beginning at the seventh cervical vertebra, and rubbing downward and forward, rubbing also the [buttocks] and hips with the palm of his hands, repeating the movement from sixty to seventy times every morning after the fifth month."[16]

As a massage therapist supporting and touching a woman through the journey of pregnancy, you might remember her as a powerful creator and consider yourself to be the "touch midwife," not as one who helps deliver babies, but in the Old English meaning of the word as one who is simply "with woman," holding, massaging, and supporting her with a particular type of nurturance on her birthing journey. In this role as a somatic supporter, you can help women find comfort in and get "in touch" with their physical, emotional, and spiritual selves during pregnancy, birth, and postpartum to help them feel comfortable, safe, and empowered by their choices.

Though touch has long been used as a significant healing tool for women in their childbearing years, its use diminished in industrialized cultures during the intensification of allopathic obstetrical practices and growth of medical technologies. Now it is being revived again and hailed as an important supplemental support during pregnancy and birth at hospitals, birthing centers, and at the home. Recent research, discussed below, has helped to promote touch as a useful and powerful tool for the perinatal cycle by drawing attention to its benefits.

BENEFITS OF TOUCH DURING PREGNANCY

We know that touch has significant effects on our lives; it is critical to our survival and the survival and health of all mammals.[17-23] Touch is a form of communication, a language that has the potential both to support and nourish, as well as to hurt. Children in some orphanages in the late 1800s had a mortality rate of 100%, attributed in large part to a lack of touch.[17] For a childbearing woman, touch holds increased significance because skin stimulation, such as massage, may support the pituitary's mobilization of "mothering" hormones that influence breast development, enhance the critical function of the placenta, help the body stay pregnant and prepare for birth and mothering, and stimulate mother-infant nurturing.[24,25]

Tiffany Field, PhD, a leading researcher at the Touch Research Institute in Miami, has studied the impact of touch in premature infants and, more recently, the effects of touch and doula support for women in labor. These studies have shown that women who are touched compassionately in pregnancy and labor end up touching their children more regularly, effectively, and sensitively.[7,8] In one of Field's studies, women were given a 20-minute back massage, five times a week during their pregnancy. These women described less anxiety, had fewer stress hormones in their blood, and experienced increased deep sleep, improved moods, and fewer painful back and leg complaints. Ultimately, the result was a decrease in premature delivery and obstetrical complications.[26]

Chronic stress, a condition many people experience in developed nations, contributes to numerous health problems, including some conditions that often plague a woman in pregnancy, such as altered regulation of blood sugar levels, decreased immunity, and increased occurrences of hypertension, insomnia, depression, and pain. When a pregnant woman lives with chronic stress, her baby in utero is also affected by the constant flow of stress hormones circulating in the maternal blood stream. X-rays of hands reveal specific markings and lines on the bones of children whose mothers underwent significant emotional stress during their pregnancy.[27] Some studies indicate that there may be an increase in attention-deficit/hyperactivity disorder in children who experienced intrauterine stress.[28]

While it may be difficult to eliminate excessive stress from one's life, therapeutic massage, especially combined with breathing and visualization, can help to decrease its intensity and reduce the potential for the above conditions. Furthermore, the massage therapist must remember that every massage affects not only the fetus, physiologically and emotionally, but also the mother and how she will later relate to her child. The following list outlines the benefits of massage during pregnancy:

- Improved Physiological Function: Massage improves venous blood flow and oxygen perfusion[29] while assisting removal of cellular waste by increasing lymphatic flow.[30-32] In pregnancy this helps decrease nonpathological edema, reduce blood pressure,[33,34] and relieve headaches.[35-37] With this improved circulation, especially through the large vessels of the inguinal region, the occurrence of edema and muscle spasms related to poor circulation can be reduced.

- Musculoskeletal Pain Reduction: Massage helps decrease strain on joints and muscles that are impacted by the extra weight gain of pregnancy, reducing muscle tension and back pain.[38,39]

- Improved Posture: Bodywork sessions are an opportunity to teach posture correction, relieving related musculoskeletal complaints such as low back pain, headaches, neck and shoulder pain, foot discomfort, and sciatica.[40]

- Enhanced Lactation and Increased Prolactin Production: Nurturing touch stimulates prolactin production, enhancing a mother's "nesting" instincts and abilities to nurture her infant.[24,25]

- Improved Emotional Wellbeing: Studies indicate that massage can decrease stress hormones, reduce depression and anxiety, and increase serotonin production, increasing one's sense of well-being.[5,26,41,42] All these benefits will also improve outcomes for the baby in-utero.[28,43]

- Increased Immunity and Decreased Intra-Uterine Stress: Touch enhances the immune system function by reducing stress.[44,45] Reduced maternal stress means a decrease in the possible detrimental effects of intrauterine stress on the baby.[28,43]

- Perineal Ease: Massage of the perineal area, before and during labor can help facilitate stretching of the tissues during birth.[46-48] Due to the intimate nature of this massage and limitation of scope of practice for massage, this massage technique is usually explained to the mother and performed by her partner, midwife, or a trained physical therapist, rather than actually practiced by the massage therapist. However, passing on the information as a massage technique to a client can be helpful, if that is within your scope of practice. By developing familiarity with the stretching sensations in that area, it may be possible to reduce a woman's resistance or fear when the sensations occur during birth, thereby reducing her risk of episiotomy and speeding tissue healing in postpartum. Many women have heard of this technique, and appreciate accurate information about how to do it.

- Improved Relaxation Skills and Self-Connection: Massage enhances a woman's body-awareness by bringing her attention to areas of muscular tension that can relax with bodywork and focused breath. Massage provides an opportunity for a woman to practice this relaxation and breath awareness in preparation for the birth process. Associating touch with relaxation *before* birth facilitates natural relaxation with touch *during* birth.[1,49]

- Increased Energy: Massage can reduce or relieve some of the common complaints of pregnancy including fatigue, stress, and insomnia — concerns that sap a woman's energy.[26,39,50-52]

- Increased Ability to Nurture Others: Massage provides an experience of nurturing, healing touch, which increases a woman's ability to touch her infant similarly. (This is particularly important for women with a history of sexual, physical, or emotional abuse.) As the mother experiences nurturing touch in pregnancy, she is reinforced with skills to touch her infant with nurturance; this in turn enables the infant to develop a positive experience of touch and caring and enter the world with more security, unlike infants who are not touched, who become withdrawn and aggressive, with more tendencies toward antisocial behaviors.[53-57]

Clearly, the massage therapist can provide an important service during a woman's pregnancy. Still, there are fears and issues that sometimes prevent pregnant women from taking advantage of the benefits of massage therapy. These are discussed below.

ISSUES WITH TOUCH DURING PREGNANCY

Considering the well-documented importance of touch, it ought to be a natural, common element in a woman's experience of pregnancy, birth, and postpartum. However, for a variety of social, medical, and legal issues, touch is often limited and restrained instead. Let us look at some of the situations and concerns that may decrease a woman's chances of getting touched during her pregnancy and how the massage therapist might take these issues into consideration.

Body Image

For some women, body image can become a source of concern that prevents them from seeking out massage. A healthy woman will typically gain at least 28 pounds during a normal pregnancy, some of which is naturally deposited in the thighs and buttocks. Without this extra weight, the baby would not thrive, the mother would not be able to adequately nourish her fetus, and the mother's body would not withstand the stresses of pregnancy. However, some women feel ashamed, unattractive, and nonsexual due to their weight gain and stop visiting their massage therapist at this time to avoid being seen with their added weight. They sometimes will avoid touch from their intimate partners as well.

In other cases, the woman's partner may avoid intimacy due to the changes in the woman's body. Although the woman may revel in her growing size and have a new sense of confidence related to her fertility and creative energy, her partner may become distanced or be subconsciously intimidated by the changes in the woman's body. As a result, their intimacy may diminish and familiar touching may become less frequent between them.

Be aware of the potential for a possible shift in a pregnant woman's relationship with her massage therapist or with her partner as a result of changes in her body. She may have emotional releases during a massage related to the stress in her changing intimate relationship or due to her changing self-image. Take note that in many cultures, a pregnant woman was and still is acknowledged as a Goddess—one who creates and brings forth life, like the great Earth Mother herself. Images of large, strong, and solid women in their fullness and sublime feminine nature have been created by ancient cultures that honored them for this ability. If your client expresses concerns about her body image, you might offer positive reminders that the extra weight in pregnancy indicates health, strength, and the ability to nurture her young as well as reinforcement of the growing "goddess" image.

Fear of Miscarriage

Another major concern of expectant mothers and their partners is the fear that touch—by themselves or others—could lead to a miscarriage. This becomes especially important after a woman feels the baby moving inside her belly for the first time, announcing the reality of its existence. At this time, the mother and possibly her mate may become more excited and simultaneously more overprotective and nervous. The partner may view the mother as fragile and the whole pregnancy unstable and believe that if she is touched the "wrong" way or in the "wrong" place, the mother or fetus could be harmed. If either the woman or partner entertains these fears, they may lose much familiar touch between them simply because of the distance that respect or ignorance can sometimes breed.

Receiving massage from a knowledgeable therapist can help to ease some of these concerns as the

woman feels how confidently she is touched, while being reassured that nurturing massage will in no way be harmful to her pregnancy or baby. As the massage therapist learns appropriate and safe ways to touch pregnant women throughout the childbearing cycle, she or he can educate women and partners about safe and nurturing touch during pregnancy that can help them improve their connection with one another.

Violation of Personal Boundaries

To create the most supportive atmosphere for the pregnant client and to avoid common actions or comments which may be disturbing to her, it is helpful to understand how the client's normal personal boundaries may be inadvertently violated during her pregnancy. Physical changes are rapid in pregnancy, and many women soon feel unfamiliar with their bodies and their bellies, which protrude into the world, bumping into things and sometimes getting in the way. As much as a pregnant woman may feel a stranger to the new sensations and image of her body, strangers themselves may be totally drawn to her in ways she has never experienced before. She finds that people commonly walk up to her, eye her belly with delight, and exclaim, "Oh, how wonderful, how far along are you?!" as they reach out and lay a hand on her bulging abdomen. This can be a frequent occurrence! The mother's belly has suddenly become public property, where strangers practice no restraint and normal boundaries and privacy have diminished. What would be inconceivable to do to a nonpregnant woman, suddenly becomes commonplace in pregnancy, causing some women to feel an aversion to touch, even from a massage therapist or others, apart from her family.

Along with this, many friends and strangers feel the need to relate their own birth stories to pregnant women, often telling stories of difficulty; of dismal, prolonged labors; or of terrible outcomes. A pregnant woman is like a sponge for energetic interchanges; the normal boundaries that may protect us from another person's issues are not as solid during pregnancy. Any negative birth stories that are told to a pregnant woman are likely to sink in immediately to her psyche and have an influence on how she approaches her own coming labor.

Create a sanctuary for the client who may feel overwhelmed in this way by offering a healing space where she can invite nurturing touch rather than ward off that which seems invasive. Avoid your own impulses to reach out and touch her belly immediately as she enters your office, looking much more pregnant than she was 2 weeks or 1 month before! Instead, greet her as an honored guest and client and welcome her into your sanctuary. Avoid offering your own advice and stories about birth, but instead help her to envision the beautiful, easeful type of labor that she would most like to have.

Body Memories

Many women have been subjected to sexual, physical, and emotional abuse and live with the memories and experiences impressed in the cells of their body. For some women, as their body uncontrollably and undeniably changes during pregnancy and birth, emotional responses attached to difficult life experiences may be invoked. Sometimes this may occur during a massage; somato-emotional responses are not uncommon to experience during attentive bodywork. Rising emotions can sometimes overwhelm and take both client and therapist by surprise, and if the therapist is untrained in supporting a client during these types of experiences, the client may feel unsafe to return. Some women may find that when already uncomfortable with their loss of control over their body during pregnancy, massage during their pregnancy may seem too frightening and uncomfortable to consider. The therapist can only offer support and safety to the degree that she or he is experienced, trained, and comfortable; but understanding that difficult emotions are often triggered by pregnancy, labor, and mothering may encourage her or him to get further training in the field of somato-emotional release work.

Education for the Massage Therapists

A lack of knowledge among massage therapists about how to massage during pregnancy can be another issue that pregnant women encounter. Many women have found that *during* pregnancy their regular massage therapist suddenly becomes unwilling to see them, as she or he is uncertain how to address the needs of a pregnant client. Many therapists who have not been trained are concerned about doing something "wrong" or creating a problem for which they would be legally liable. While causing problems is unlikely, this concern is valid and there certainly are contraindications for massage during pregnancy and times when certain types of touch are inappropriate. Bodyworkers should be aware of these issues. (See Chapter 4 for details on precautions and contraindications.) Acquiring the appropriate skills and knowledge to address pregnant clients will ease women's and therapists concerns.

Education for the Doctors

Massage therapists are not the only ones who need to become better educated about massage during pregnancy. Even though pregnancy massage is becoming much more commonplace, more education is still needed within the medical system to help touch become fully integrated. Many obstetrical physicians have hesitated when first approached about referring their pregnant clients for massage therapy. Massage can be a wonderful adjunctive tool to help women cope with the common discomforts of pregnancy; it is a loss when women are not told that it is safe and possibly an excellent choice for them to explore during pregnancy. However, these same doctors, after witnessing the results of clients who received massage and were then pain-free and much happier with their growing bodies, have come to accept that massage can indeed have a highly beneficial impact on a woman's experience of pregnancy. To help expand the use of massage throughout pregnancy, massage therapists may choose to offer in-services and educational packets about the benefits of pregnancy massage to doctors and midwives who may not yet have recognized these benefits.

Education for the Mothers

Finally, the mother's own lack of knowledge about the safety and benefits of massage during pregnancy can be an obstacle. It is helpful for you to have a span of knowledge about the perinatal cycle to work confidently and reassuringly, especially when working with women who have concerns regarding the safety of massage. By educating yourself about potential risks and contraindications related to specific types of bodywork modalities and understanding appropriate ways of doing massage, positioning, and touching the belly, you will be able to extinguish concerns and educate your client about practices that are safe and worry-free. Many women become voracious readers during pregnancy, researching everything they can get their hands on regarding conception, childbirth, and mothering. They learn that there may be various dangers on the pregnancy path; yet without detailed information, they may begin to grow anxious and uncertain about what is really safe or unsafe for this unborn child. For some, massage might seem too rife with potential for injury. Some women have experienced more than one miscarriage, and massage might, in their mind, seem risky for stimulating another. Many women have heard that certain acupressure points are dangerous or that massage to the ankles is contraindicated during pregnancy. Some may feel more comfortable avoiding massage or will need to know they have found a well-trained, knowledgeable therapist if they decide to see one at all. If you are chosen as her knowledgeable therapist, you will be able to alleviate her fears, rather than compounding your own and hers based on your uncertainty about safe practices.

DISPELLING MYTHS:

The Dangers of Pregnancy Massage

It is not difficult to learn about the dangers of pregnancy massage. Anyone who would like to be convinced of its dangers merely needs to use the topic words—Dangerous pregnancy massage—in an online Internet search engine and then review some of the massage and pregnancy sites that emerge. Some of the dangers reported include the following: massage should be avoided in the first trimester due to the risk of miscarriage from toxic overload after massage; first trimester massage is too much stimulation for the mother; massage to the feet, lower legs, and abdomen could cause miscarriage; abdominal massage should be avoided due to the potential for causing serious problems; abdominal massage should be avoided because babies don't like it and start kicking; massage to the low back is contraindicated during pregnancy, with no reasons given.

A newly pregnant woman or an untrained massage therapist might read this information and believe that it is just too frightening to receive or give massage during pregnancy. However, these bits of advice are not substantiated with research or documented reports of problems. We can examine and dismantle each of these fears.

The first trimester is indeed a time of great changes on many levels; all the more reason for receiving nurturing touch to help a mother integrate the changes that are occurring. There is no research that indicates that massage has caused toxic overload in a pregnant person and thereby caused miscarriage. Therapists are aware that massage can stimulate circulation and help flush metabolic waste into the circulatory system. Acknowledging this effect, many therapists are trained to work less intensely on people who have never had a massage before, encourage clients to drink water after a massage, inform the client that mild soreness for a day after massage could occur, and recommend the client rest briefly before recommencing her day again after a massage. Pregnant women are no different in this regard. Women should always be encouraged to drink water after a massage. Massage in the first trimester should generally not be exceptionally deep and stimulating if it is the first massage a woman has ever received or if she is experiencing nausea at times. Massage should not be avoided due to nausea, however, as many studies indicate massage can help to *reduce* nausea.[58-60] Usually, massage during the first trimester can help decrease anxiety and help a woman relax, have focused time to process the fact that she is pregnant, and offer her a wonderful way to enter into her new pregnancy.

Miscarriage is extremely common during the first trimester, yet it occurs whether women are massaged or not. Massage has never been clearly implicated legally or scientifically as a cause of miscarriage. In the majority of cases, miscarriage occurs because the fetus is nonviable. Touch to the abdomen, unless it is intentionally harmful, does not hurt the baby or the mother. The uterus during the first trimester is low in the pelvis and is not palpable without deep abdominal pressure, which is generally contraindicated for massage therapists during pregnancy. Instead, nurturing touch to the abdomen can be extremely relaxing for the mother, and most women feel that the baby is responding in a positive manner if she or he wakes up and starts moving during a belly rub.

Massage to the legs, feet, and belly during the first trimester *does not* cause miscarriage. There are acupressure points in the lower legs and feet that are contraindicated for acupressure or acupuncture, but general massage to the acupressure points areas will not stimulate them similarly.

With increased education regarding massage during the perinatal cycle, the fears and myths about its dangers can be reduced. Therapists can learn with accuracy when caution or contraindications are truly called for, and help dispel myths and assuage unwarranted fears. Armed with knowledge and gifted with the ability to offer nurturing caring touch, the massage therapist can help more pregnant women reduce anxieties and discomforts, and increase their chances for a pleasurable experience of their pregnancy.

CHAPTER SUMMARY

Throughout the world, touch has been used to improve and enhance women's experiences of their pregnancies and births. Ongoing research has helped to support the claims of the many psychological and physiological benefits of massage in general and specifically during the perinatal cycle. The massage therapist, trained in the benefits, contraindications, concerns, and techniques of perinatal massage, can continue this important tradition of touch. By honoring the natural wisdom of women's bodies, respecting the issues that can develop around pregnancy in our industrialized world, and minimizing fears with education, reassurance and competence, the therapist can provide the optimum individualized care for each pregnant, laboring, and postpartum woman.

CHAPTER REVIEW QUESTIONS

1. Name four elements of bodywork with pregnant clients that are different from working with non-pregnant clients.
2. What are some of the social issues that might prevent a woman from getting massage during pregnancy?
3. Name two reasons how touch has been used in traditional cultures to benefit a pregnant, laboring, and postpartum woman.
4. Discuss ways that you might consider childbearing as a significant rite of passage.
5. Discuss four benefits of touch for a woman during pregnancy.
6. What are the potential impacts of maternal stress on a woman or fetus during pregnancy?
7. What are some of the myths about touch during pregnancy and why are they myths?
8. Discuss concerns, issues, or stereotypical prohibitions to touch during pregnancy and how these can be mediated by a massage therapist. Examine any fears or beliefs you, or those in your community, have had about pregnancy massage.
9. Describe what effects, if any, massage may have with regards to the risks of miscarriage.

REFERENCES

1. Dick-Read G. Childbirth Without Fear. 5th Ed. New York: Harper & Row, 1984.
2. Klaus MH, Kennell JH, Klaus PH. Mothering the Mother. Reading, MA: Addison-Wesley; 1993.
3. Field T, Hernandez-Reif M, Taylor S, et al. Labor pain is reduced by massage therapy. J Psychosom Obstet Gynaecol 1997;18:286–291.
4. Hidarnia A, Montgomery KS, Bastani F, et al. Does relaxation education in anxious primigravid Iranian women influence adverse pregnancy outcomes?: a randomized controlled trial. J Perinat Neonatal Nurs 2006;20(2):138–146.
5. Field T, Diego MA, Hernandez-Reif M. Massage therapy effects on depressed pregnant women. J Psychosom Obstet Gynaecol 2004;25(2):115–122.
6. Janke J. The Effect of relaxation therapy on preterm labor outcomes. J Obstet Gynecol Neonatal Nurs 1999; 28(3):255.
7. Rubin R. Maternal touch. Nurs Outlook 1963;11:828–831.
8. Hofmeyer FJ, Nikodem VC, Wolman WL. Companionship to modify the clinical birth environment: effects on progress and perceptions of labour and breast feeding. Br J Obstet Gynaecol 1991;98:756–764.
9. Goldsmith J. Childbirth Wisdom From the World's Oldest Societies. Brookline, MA: East West Health Books; 1990:39.
10. Lockett C. Midwives and childbirth among the Navajo. Plateau 1939;12:15–17.
11. Kanagaratnam T. Coconut belly rubs: traditional midwifery care in Malaysia and Indonesia. International Midwife 1995;3:9.
12. Chawla J. Rites of Passage. Life Positive: Your Complete Guide to Holistic Living [serial online]. Available at: http://www.lifepositive.com/spirit/death/deathrites.asp. Accessed March 2007.
13. Chawla J. The dai's way to child birth: a unique project explores the indigenous knowledge of traditional midwives. InfoChange News & Features. [online resource base]. Available at: http://www.infochangeindia.org/WomenIstory.jsp?recordno = 81&section_idv = 1 No date given. Accessed March 20, 2007.
14. Reddy K, Egenes L, Mullins M. For a Blissful Baby: Healthy and Happy Pregnancy With Maharishi Vedic Medicine. Schenectady, NY: Samhita Productions, 1999.
15. Baker JP, Baker F, Slayton T. Conscious Conception: Elemental Journey Through the Labyrinth of Sexuality. Monroe, UT: Freestone Publishing; 1986: 222.
16. Englemann GJ. *Labor* Among Primitive Peoples. St. Louis: J. H. Chambers, 1884.
17. Bakwin H: Emotional deprivation in infants. J Pediatr 1949;35:512–521.
18. Schaefer M, Hatcher RP, Barglow PD. Prematurity and infant stimulation: a review of research. Child Psychiatry Hum Dev 1980;10(4):199–212.
19. Ruegamer WR, Berstein L, Benjamin JD. Growth, food, utilization, and thyroid activity in the albino rat as a function of extra handling. Science 1954;120(3109): 184–185.
20. Field T. Touch. Cambridge, MA: MIT Press; 1993.
21. Seay BM, Hansen EW, Harlow HE. Mother-infant separation in monkeys. J Child Psychol Psychiatry 1962;3:123–132.
22. Bowlby J. Attachment. New York: Basic Books, 1969.
23. Suomi SJ. The role of touch in rhesus monkey social development. In: Coldwell C. eds. The Many Facets of Touch. Johnson & Johnson Baby Products; 1996: 41–56.
24. Roth LL, Rosenblatt JS. Mammary glands of pregnant rats: development stimulated by licking. Science 1996; 264:1403–1404.
25. Serafim AP, Felicio LF. Reproductive experience influences grooming behavior during pregnancy in rats. Braz J Med Biol Res 2002;35(3):391–394.
26. Field T, Hernandez-Reif M, Hart S, et al. Pregnant women benefit from massage therapy. J Psychosom Obstet Gynaecol 1998;20:31–38.
27. Montagu A. Touch: the human significance of skin. New York: Harper Collins; 1986.
28. Linnet KM, Dalsgaard S, Obel C, et al. Maternal Lifestyle factors in pregnancy risk of attention deficit hyperactivity disorder and associated behaviors: review of the current evidence. Am J Psychiatry 2003;160(6):1028–1040.
29. Arkko PJ, Parkainen AJ, Kari-Koskinen O. Effects of whole-body massage on serum protein, electrolyte and

hormone concentrations, enzyme activities and hematological parameters. Int J Sports Med 1983;4:265–267.

30. Schweiz R. Manual lymph drainage as therapy of edema in the head and neck area. Med Prax 2003;92(7):271–274.

31. Zanolla R, Monzeglio C, Balzarini A, et al. Evaluation of the results of three different methods of post-mastectomy lymphedema treatment. J Surg Oncology 1984;26:210–213.

32. Premkumar K. Edema and lymphedema are they different? Implications for bodyworkers. Massage & Bodywork Dec/Jan 2005. Available online at: http://www.massageandbodywork.com/Articles/DecJan2005/edema.html. Accessed March 21, 2007.

33. Fakouri C, Jones P. Relaxation Rx: slow stroke back rub. J Gerontol Nurs 1987;12(2):32–35.

34. Hernandez-Reif M, Field T, Krasnegor J, et al. High blood pressure and associated symptoms were reduced by massage therapy. J Bodywork and Movement Therapies 2000;4:31–38.

35. Hernandez-Reif M, Field T, Dieter J, et al. Migraine headaches were reduced by massage therapy. Int J Neurosci 1998;96:1–11.

36. Quinn C, Chandler C, Moraska A. Massage therapy and frequency of chronic tension headaches. Am J Public Health 2002;92(10):1657–1661.

37. Goffaux-Dogniez C, Vanfraechem-Raway R, Verbanck P. Appraisal of treatment of the trigger points associated with relaxation to treat chronic headache in the adult. Relationship with anxiety and stress adaptation strategies. Encephale 2003;29(5):377–390.

38. Cherkin DC, Eisenberg D, Sherman KJ, et al. Randomized trial comparing traditional Chinese medical acupuncture, therapeutic massage, and self-care education for chronic low back pain. Arch Intern Med 2001;161(8):1081–1088.

39. Hernandez-Reif M, Field T, Diego M, Fraser M. Lower back pain and sleep disturbance are reduced following massage therapy. J Bodywork and Movement Therapies July 2006.

40. Moore K, Dumas GA, Reid JG. Postural changes associated with pregnancy and their relationship with low-back pain. Clin Biomech 1990;5:169–174.

41. Field T, Morrow C, Valdon SI, et al. Massage reduces anxiety in child and adolescent psychiatric patients. J Am Acad Child Adolesc Psychiatry 1992;31:125–131.

42. Ironson G, Field T, Kumar A, et al. Relaxation through massage is associated with decreased distress and increased serotonin levels. Presented at the 39th Annual Meeting of the Academy of Psychosomatic Medicine, San Diego, California. Oct 29–Nov 1, 1992.

43. Field T, Diego M, Hernandez-Reif M, et al. Pregnancy anxiety and comorbid depression and anger: effects on the fetus and neonate. Depress Anxiety 2003;17(3):140–151.

44. Ironson G, Field T, Scafid F, et al. Massage therapy is associated with enhancement of the immune system's cytotoxic capacity. Int J Neurosci 1996;84:205–218.

45. Diego MA, Field T, Hernandez-Reif, et al. HIV adolescents show improved immune function following massage therapy. Int J Neurosci 2001;106(1–2):35–45.

46. Renfrew M, Hannah W, Albers L, et al. Practices that minimize trauma to the genital tract in childbirth: a systematic review of the literature. Birth 1988;25(3):143.

47. Eason E, Labrecque M, Wells G, et al. Preventing perineal trauma during childbirth: a systemic review. Obstet Gynecol 2000;95(3):464–471.

48. Labrecque M, Marcoux S, Pinault JJ, et al. Prevention of perineal trauma by perineal massage during pregnancy: a pilot study. Birth 1994;21(1):20–25.

49. Kitzinger S. The Complete Book of Pregnancy and Childbirth. New York: Alfred A. Knopf; 2003.

50. Hernandez-Reif M, Field T, Largie S, et al. Parkinson's disease symptoms are differentially affected by massage therapy versus progressive muscle relaxation: A pilot study. J Bodywork and Movement Therapies 2002;6:177–182.

51. Sunshine W, Field T, Schanberg S, et al. Fibromyalgia benefits from massage therapy and transcutaneous electrical stimulation. J Clin Rheumatol 1996;2:18–22.

52. Field T, Sunshine W, Hernandez-Reif M, Quintino O, et al. Chronic fatigue syndrome: massage therapy effects on depression and somatic symptoms in chronic fatigue syndrome. J Chronic Fatigue Syndr 1997;3:43–51.

53. Gambill L. Can more touching lead to less violence in our society? It probably can if developmental neuropsychologist James W. Prescott's Pleasure Violence Reciprocity Theory is correct. The Human Touch Jan/Feb 1985.

54. Weller A, Feldman R. Emotion regulation and touch in infants: the role of cholecystokinin and opioids. Peptides 2003;24(5):779–788.

55. Diego MA, Field T, Hernandez-Reif M. Aggressive adolescents benefit from massage therapy. Adolescence 2002;37(147):597–607.

56. Harlow HE. The heterosexual affectional system in monkeys. Am Psychol 1962;17:1–9.

57. Goy RW, Wallen K, Goldfoot DA. Social factors affecting the development of mounting behavior in male rhesus monkeys. In: Montagna W and Sadler W, eds. Reproductive Behavior. New York: Plenum Press; 1974.

58. Grealish L, Lomasney A, Whiteman B. Foot massage. A nursing intervention to modify the distressing symptoms of pain and nausea in patients hospitalized with cancer. Cancer Nurs 2000; 23;237-243.

59. Billhult A, Bergbom I, Stener-Victorin E. Massage relieves nausea in women with breast cancer who are undergoing chemotherapy. J Altern Complement Med 2007;13(1):53–58.

60. Ahles TA, Tope DM, Pinkson B. Massage therapy for patients undergoing autologous bone marrow transplantation. J Pain Symptom Manage 1999;18(3):157–163.

PHYSIOLOGICAL AND EMOTIONAL CHANGES DURING PREGNANCY

LEARNING OBJECTIVES

After reading this chapter, you should be able to:

- Describe basic embryonic and fetal development
- Describe the maternal physiological and emotional changes that occur during each trimester of pregnancy.
- Name the primary influential hormones of pregnancy and their effects on the mother's body.
- Discuss relevant bodywork considerations related to the changes of pregnancy.
- Describe specific physiological changes to the organ systems that are unique to pregnancy.
- Explain the rationale for common bodywork and massage precautions during pregnancy.

As a massage therapist, you may see a pregnant client from the conception of her baby all the way through her birth and postpartum period. Understanding the physiological and common emotional changes occurring during this time will influence your work and help you better support her, as with each visit she will be a different woman, with a different balance of hormones, different energy of the baby within her, and different needs for bodywork. In this chapter we will review the process of conception and fetal development through the trimesters, hormonal changes and the maternal experiences of these changes, and general considerations for bodywork appropriate to each trimester. We will also consider how the pregnant client's various organ systems adapt during pregnancy.

CONCEPTION

Each pregnant client has had the experience of hosting a microscopic and energetic dance between hormones, sperm, and an egg. Each month hormones are released from a woman's pituitary gland with the special duty of helping one egg to mature in the woman's ovary. Simultaneously, the ovary sends estrogen to prepare the womb to receive the egg, just as a garden is fertilized to prepare for planting so that the seed will be well-nourished. Once the egg is fully matured, it emerges from the ovary and is urged into the waving tentacle arms of the fallopian tube fimbriae. The egg (the largest cell in the human body) is caught by these arms and propelled down the fallopian tubes. Microscopically viewed, the fallopian tube can be seen repeatedly undulating as it gradually squeezes the egg toward the womb. Meanwhile, millions of sperm (30 times smaller than the egg, and the smallest cells in the male body) which have been ejaculated—or, often these days, artificially inseminated—into the vagina or uterus are swimming toward the fallopian tubes, drawn by chemical attractants released by the egg. Of these millions of sperm, only about 2000 will survive long enough to get close to the traveling egg, and when they do, they begin to wiggle against her protective cell wall. Eventually, one sperm passes through the cell wall of the egg. The egg then secretes an impassable film around its walls, preventing other sperm from entering. Sometimes, two eggs are released during ovulation and make their way through the fallopian tubes. If each becomes fertilized, fraternal twins develop.

The sperm and egg—now a zygote—fuse their chromosomes and begin to divide repetitively for the next 3 to 7 days. On occasion, the zygote will split in two, and identical twins will develop. During this period, the zygote is being propelled through the fallopian tube to the uterus, dividing continuously until it is a clustered ball of cells called a blastocyst.

Meanwhile, the corpus luteum, a mass left in the ovary after the egg departed, produces hormones that continue to prepare the uterus for eventual implantation of the egg. The corpus luteum is a primary source of hormones for about 12 weeks, until the placenta is formed and fully functioning.

When the blastocyst enters the womb, it searches for the most desirable area of the uterine lining in which to implant itself, normally in the upper regions of the uterus. There it burrows into the endometrium and is nourished; the earliest development of a new life begins. A placenta begins to form from the trophoblastic cells on the outside of the blastocyst. This placenta will eventually take over the role of the corpus luteum, producing progesterone and estrogen and helping to nurture a healthy fetus.

All this has taken place in the span of 7 to 10 days *since ovulation*. Ovulation is assumed to be approximately 14 days after the last menstrual period, although that is merely an average. When calculating the length of a 40-week pregnancy, measurement usually begins from the last day of the woman's menstrual period, *not from ovulation and conception, even if the woman knows exactly when she conceived*; therefore, when we discuss a fetus at 3 weeks of *development*, the woman's dates of pregnancy may actually be measured at 5 weeks' *gestation*.

FETAL DEVELOPMENT AND MATERNAL SENSATIONS

What is a woman experiencing during this development of new life in her body? Pregnancy is divided into 3 time periods, each about 13 weeks long, called **trimesters**. We will now look at each trimester in more detail.

Traditional Birth Practices: Mysteries of Creation

Not all people believe our scientific stories describing the making of life as a journey of a microscopic egg and a sperm. Some tribal South Africans believe that conception occurs if a woman lies down in the rain, allowing the seeds inside her body to be germinated, just like those in the land.

A Nepalese way of understanding the creation of life is that the souls of those who have died in the past 40 days visit with couples who are making love, slipping into the woman's body during intercourse. It is the "buttermilk," or semen, that creates the baby's bones and the mother's menstrual blood that forms the baby's body.[1]

In Malaysia, it is believed that the fetal spirit is conceived in the father's brain and heart, where it learns first of the world through the father's perspective. The spirit then enters its mother in the father's semen during intercourse.[2]

The Trobriand Islanders of New Guinea, whose culture is entwined with the sea, believe that the souls of babies float in seaweed and attach themselves to women as they swim in the ocean. This soul, carried on a surge of the mother's blood rising to meet it, enters her womb and is nourished by the mother's menstrual blood.[2,3]

First Trimester: Weeks 1 to 13

The most critical development and growth for an embryo and fetus occurs in the first trimester and begins immediately on implantation of the blastocyst in the landscape of a woman's body. All of the mother's vital energies shift at once to support and nurture the growing embryo with increased blood, oxygen, and nutrients. The organs, brain, spine, and the fetal nervous system all begin to form early on. This early time period in the first trimester is developmentally critical, and a woman's well-being should be protected carefully (Figure 2.1). It is during the first trimester that a mother is urged to avoid extended immersion in hot water, drinking alcohol, and partaking in other activities that might disrupt healthy formation of this nervous system. The first trimester is also critical in that it is the most common time for **miscarriage** (delivery of the fetus before 20 weeks' gestation) to occur. Of women who know they are pregnant, 15% to 25% experience miscarriage, while the rate is speculated to be as great as 60% to 70% when including in the statistics of the women who had not yet realized that they were pregnant before they miscarried.[4,5] *Eighty percent of these miscarriages occur within the first trimester.*[5] Some important bodywork restrictions, covered in detail in Chapter 4, are related to this risk of miscarriage in the first trimester.

While a tiny life is developing deep in a mother's womb, this newly pregnant woman may have a variety of experiences. Some women soar through the first trimester feeling strong and healthier than ever. Others experience fatigue, indigestion, nausea, and vomiting. For many, it is a time of great joy and excitement, while for some it may be a time of ambivalence, irritability, or anxiety, especially if the pregnancy is unplanned, unwanted, or particularly challenging. A massage therapist will want to know if her or his pregnant client is in the first trimester, respecting the client's possible vulnerability due to any of the above issues and while offering nurturing and supportive touch to this mother who is incubating new life. Massage can be extremely helpful at this time, as a woman comes to terms with the physical, emotional, and possibly spiritual changes and prepares to transition into a new role and identity.

See Table 2.1 to review embryonic development, maternal experiences, and bodywork considerations in the first 3 months of pregnancy.

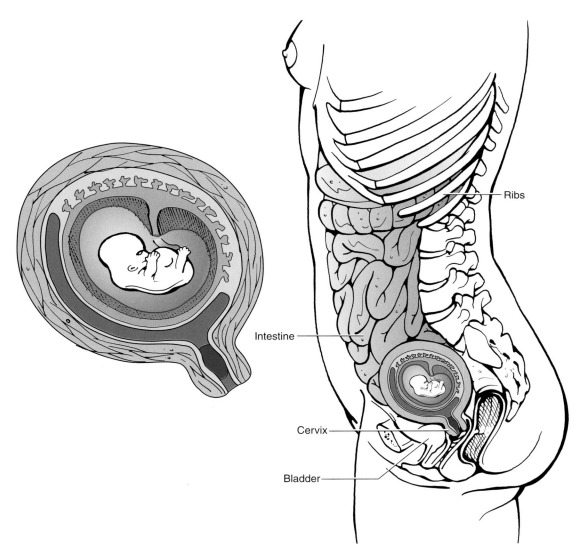

FIGURE 2.1   First trimester, second month.
The fetus is approximately 2 cm long and the nervous system is forming. The mother may be experiencing nausea, breast tenderness, and more frequent urination.

Table 2.1   First Trimester: Embryonic and Fetal Development, Maternal Experience, and Bodywork Considerations

Embryonic and Fetal Development	Possible Maternal Experience	Bodywork Considerations
First month of pregnancy **Overall:** • Lungs, brain, digestive tract, neural tube develop—the rudimentary nervous system. **1st week:** • Fertilized egg divides. • Corpus luteum produces progesterone and estrogen to prepare uterine lining. • Day 7–10, egg implants itself in uterine lining. **2nd week:** • Distinction of amniotic sac and yolk sac begins. • Pre-placenta cells produce human chorionic gonadotropin (HCG) and estrogen 10 days after fertilization. • HCG encourages the corpus luteum in the ovaries to produce high levels of estrogen and progesterone. **3rd–4th week:** • Embryo is the size of rice grain or smaller. • Embryo is attached to uterus. • Placental circulation is established. • Definitions of tiny head with rudimentary eyes, ears, nose, and tail with yolk sac. • Heart has begun a rhythmic beat.	• Many know instantly they are pregnant. • A woman may feel shifting, swirling energy in her core. • Food cravings are common. • Increased urination occurs. • Breast soreness develops. • Hormonal mood swings are common. • Some choose not to share with others about their pregnancy until after the first trimester when it is more secure. • Anxiety about miscarriage may be present.	• Avoid deep abdominal work. • Avoid scented oils that may trigger nausea. • If nausea present, may need to position in semi-reclining. • Study acupressure points that alleviate nausea. • Place pillow under ribs or position side-lying if breasts are sore in prone positioning. • Avoid deep, intensive work on sacral area, which can be stimulating to uterus. • Do thorough health intake especially assessing history of miscarriage or previous high-risk pregnancies. • Avoid electric heating pads on massage table in first trimester due to unknown effects of electromagnetic radiation on developing fetus. • Avoid contraindicated accupressure points.
Second Month of Pregnancy **Overall:** • Facial features, gonads, and brain development are foremost. **5th week:** • Rudimentary brain and spine form. • Embryo floats in oceanic amniotic fluid, attached to uterine wall and pre-placenta by tiny veins and arteries that will become umbilical cord. **6th week:** • Embryo is size of large raisin. • Clearly defined head with basic eyes, ears, and brain. • Brain grows rapidly. • Tiny buds of arms and legs appear. • Two-chambered, beating heart. • Defined bloodstream. • Digestive organs developing.	• There may be a growing excitement. • She may not have told others about pregnancy. • Breast soreness and size increase. • Nipples become more prominent. • Nausea or "morning sickness" may occur. • Urination frequency increases. • General fatigue occurs. • Increased vaginal discharge develops. • May only now become aware of pregnancy with missed menstrual cycle. • Anxiety about miscarriage may be present.	• Same as first month. • Avoid vigorous stimulating massage in the first trimester. • Check for diastasis recti if she has had previous pregnancies, and teach abdominal strengthening techniques.

Table 2.1	(Continued)	
Embryonic and Fetal Development	**Possible Maternal Experience**	**Bodywork Considerations**

7th week:
- More facial details: nostrils, lips, tongue, and teeth buds.
- Spine and brain mostly formed.
- Spine straightens.
- Legs grow.
- Heart develops two more chambers.

8th week:
- By 8—10 weeks, embryo is called a "fetus," from Latin meaning "young one" or "offspring."
- Fetus is 2 cm long.
- Ear becomes more fully defined.
- Functioning 4-chambered heart pumps blood through vasculature.

Third Month of Pregnancy

Embryonic and Fetal Development	Possible Maternal Experience	Bodywork Considerations
• Fetus grows from size of small quarter to about 3 inches long, weighing about 1 ounce. • Eyes develop with eyelids covering but not yet opened. • Skin is translucent. • Elbows and knees develop. • Hands and legs start to move. • Fingers and toes webbed but developing with fingernails. • Genitalia become defined. • Fetal heart beats 160 180 beats per minute.	• Feeling more settled in security of pregnancy. • Constipation may begin. • Headaches may develop. • Dizziness may occur. • Anxiety about miscarriage may be present. • Mood swings are common. • Fatigue is common.	• Same as first two months. • Address chronic postural issues before advanced and problematic in pregnancy. • Suggest client empty bladder before massage.

Second Trimester: Weeks 14 to 27

Rapid changes continue in the second trimester, and by its end, the pregnancy will be much more obvious with an enlarged belly and fetal movements felt by the mother. By the time a woman reaches the second trimester, the majority of concerns for miscarriage are alleviated (though all risk is not gone).

At the beginning of the second trimester, the fetus is still only 6 to 9 inches long and the placenta—which has taken 3 months to form—is now ready to replace the corpus luteum in estrogen and progesterone production. The placenta also takes on the role of the still-developing fetal lungs, stomach, intestines, and kidneys by filtering blood and waste. Through her own circulatory system, a woman processes her baby's cellular wastes, yet the baby's blood does not ever actually make contact with its mother's; their circulatory systems are separated by the placental membrane, and thus they may have different blood types.

Fetal skeletal muscles become more functional. Maternal blood nourishes the baby. With every breath a mother takes, oxygen travels through the placenta and the umbilical cord, oxygenating the baby's blood. Encouraging full belly breathing during bodywork sessions helps "feed" the baby while the mother is relaxing and enjoying the benefits of increased oxygen to her cells.

A woman may grow especially excited around 5 months of pregnancy, as she feels the baby's tiny flutters or movements, called **quickening**. According to some theories, quickening indicates the baby's first consciousness of its physical form.[6] The signs of life inside are undeniable. The mother will feel and begin to look more pregnant this trimester and may have more energy than earlier. Her breasts grow larger, and hormonal changes cause new discomforts that she

*F*atigue is a normal experience in the early stages of pregnancy. Many women fight fatigue, trying to keep up with the normal demands of their daily lives. They may complain about their exhaustion to their massage therapist. Gently remind your client that she is harboring and growing a human being in her body—no small task.

Every body system and every cell in her body is adjusting itself in some way to support fetal development. It is no wonder that she is tired. In most creation stories, it is only a supernatural being who can do this, and usually even he or she had to rest after creating the world!

may be coping with, such as nasal congestion, nosebleeds, mild swelling in the legs, leg cramps, the appearance of varicose veins, and an increase in vaginal discharge. The massage therapist can be assured that these are common and generally normal experiences for some women during this time.

Now the uterus is the size of a cantaloupe, and the woman's center of gravity is shifting backward to accommodate the forward-growing weight. Without postural adjustments, she may begin to experience cramping of the legs and feet, low backache from increased lumbar lordosis, and overstretching of her abdominal muscles (Figure 2.2).

Your client will probably feel less nauseous and have less urgent needs for urination since the baby is higher and putting less pressure on the bladder. Energetically, a woman's sleep may be filled with more vivid dreams as her connection deepens with the kicking and pulsing life inside. Many women may now come to terms with any previous ambivalence and rest more comfortably in the reality of their emerging role as mother, with fewer mood swings. For those whose history precludes a happy resolve with this pregnancy, the ambivalence or resentments may continue or increase. This may be especially true for women with a history of abuse or with financial, emotional, or medical challenges associated with the pregnancy.

Table 2.2 reviews embryonic development, maternal experiences, and bodywork considerations in the second trimester of pregnancy.

Third Trimester: Weeks 28 to 40

The third trimester is the time of the most perceptible fetal growth as a woman's belly continues to grow large and fetal movements become palpable and noticeable by observers. By the early part of the third trimester, the average baby weighs about 2 to 3 pounds and has at least a 50% survival rate outside the womb. The lungs are not fully developed yet, and this

will be a serious liability if the baby is born too early. The vital organs have been formed, and the baby is developing reserves of energy and thermoregulation abilities for outside the womb by growing "baby fat."

Some women feel better than ever now, and onlookers may comment on the woman's proverbial "rosy glow" of pregnancy. But it is not uncommon for the mother to have one or more complaints that interrupt her potential enjoyment of feeling the now-frequent baby movements. The top of the uterus is near her xiphoid process, and the baby may be pushing up into her diaphragm, causing her shortness of breath. She may have back pain, pelvic heaviness, ankle edema, and uterine ligament spasms. Her organs are compressed in the abdomen, and she may experience constipation, heartburn, indigestion, and leg cramps.

The mother may have an increase in hair and nail growth, sweating, and skin allergies, and the development of stretch marks, also called **striae gravidarum**. The etiology of stretch marks is still uncertain,[7] but there seems to be a genetic component that increases the effects of the rapid stretching of the abdominal skin and underlying collagen and elastin. Many women ask if massage can help with these marks. Moisturizer or oils can help nourish the skin, but there is very little research that indicates it will prevent these marks from developing, and none that proves a way to reduce them once they have developed. [8] Accepting their presence, some women choose to appreciate these lines as the permanent story of their child written on their body.

After 36 weeks, the baby drops down into the pelvis and maternal breathing difficulties are relieved—this drop is called **lightening** (Figure 2.3). She now has more pressure on her bladder and may need to urinate more frequently. Your client may be more anemic, as blood composition changes, increasing chances of her feeling dizzy or fatigued. She may be restless at night, awakening frequently to urinate, to process dreams or nightmares, or to try to find a

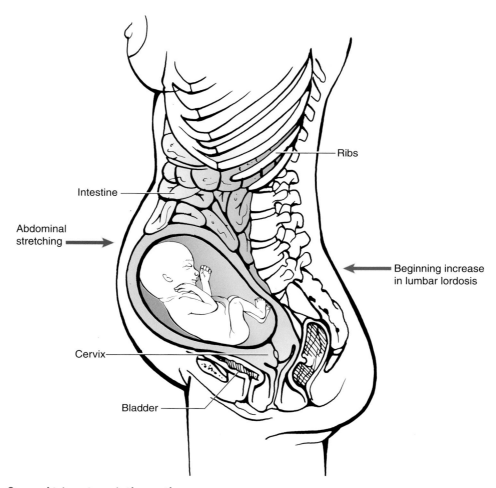

FIGURE 2.2   **Second trimester, sixth month.**
The fetus may be in any position. Her movements are felt regularly by the mother. Signs of pregnancy are quite obvious now, with changing posture and a visibly protruding belly.

comfortable position. Her joints begin to feel "wobbly," as the hormone **relaxin** loosens the pelvic joints in preparation for birth. She may be having irregular "practice contractions," called **Braxton-Hicks contractions**, as the uterus prepares for labor. These are mild and irregular contractions or uterine tightenings, and do not cause changes to the cervix, but are thought to help the uterus and pelvis prepare for labor. This uterine tightening is not to be mistaken for **preterm labor contractions**, which are contractions that occur before 37 weeks, are generally more consistent than Braxton-Hicks, and can cause cervical changes or delivery of a baby before fetal development is fully completed.

 CAUTION: Your client should always be directed to her prenatal care provider if she is having contractions that have not been positively identified as Braxton-Hicks.

Reading about all these symptoms at once may make pregnancy sound like a horrendous experience. Yet, many women do not experience any discomforts, and others find these symptoms are mild or perhaps only one of them is experienced. Rarely, for those who are happy about being pregnant, do these symptoms override the overall sense of enjoyment of the pregnant experience during this trimester, until the very end of pregnancy, when many women feel tired of carrying the extra weight and are ready for labor to begin. Offering comfortable positioning and relaxation massage during this time will help ease some complaints. Considering all the potential problems associated with pregnancy, we can appreciate why it was listed as the twelfth most stressful event in a woman's life on the Social Readjustment Rating Scale—one of the first life event stress-measuring scales. On the more contemporary "Peri Life Events Scale," the birth of a first child rates as the sixth most stressful life event while pregnancy ranks 32 out of

Table 2.2	Second Trimester of Fetal Development and Maternal Experience	
Embryonic and Fetal Development	**Possible Maternal Experience**	**Bodywork Considerations**
Fourth Month of Pregnancy • Fetus is 6−9 inches long, 5−6 ounces. • Body is completely formed, muscles contract. • There is an active sucking reflex. • Fine hair exists all over body called lanugo. • Tooth buds grow. • Eyes are large, eyelids still closed. • Lungs and organs are still developing. • Amniotic fluid is swallowed, producing meconium (the first feces) in intestines. • Fetus moves, kicks, making its presence known. **Fifth Month of Pregnancy** • Fetus is 8−12 inches long, weighing about 1 to 1.5 pounds. • Placenta and umbilical cord are fully functioning. • Fingerprints form. • Fetus startles when stimulated with loud sound. **Sixth Month of Pregnancy** • Fetus is fully formed, 14 inches long and 1.5−2.5 pounds. • Eyes are open and have rapid movements. • Fetus sucks thumb, makes frequent gross body movements, cries, and practices breathing movements in water. • Brain is still developing. • Lungs are very immature, but baby may live, with assistance, if born at this time.	• There may be increased excitement as feeling baby movements and belly showing more. • Breast size increases and breasts may leak colostrum. • There may be darkening of linea alba, nipples, face. • Increasing forgetfulness may occur. • Body and self-image changes. • Energy and libido may increase. • There may be a sense of well-being or possibly an increase in anxiety. • There is increased vaginal discharge. • Increase in dreams or nightmares may occur. • There may be nasal congestion, nosebleeds, headaches related to vascular changes. • There is often less pressure on bladder with baby higher in abdomen. • Anemia-induced fatigue may occur. • There is an increase in lumbar lordosis/backache. • Varicosities and hemorrhoids may appear. • Mild edema of ankles and wrists may occur. • Carpal tunnel syndrome may occur. • There is stress to upper spine and pectoralis due to growing belly and breasts. • Uterine round ligament spasms may occur. • Stretch marks may develop. • Leg cramps can be common at night.	• Practice varicose vein and thrombosis precautions. • Avoid contraindicated acupressure points. • Avoid strong scents that may stimulate nausea. • Begin sidelying positioning. Generally avoid supine and prone positioning. • Encourage postural awareness. • Teach abdominal, perineal, and back strengthening exercises. • Belly rubs in late second trimester help mother connect with baby.

102 events. Still, plenty of women experience pregnancy as the most nourishing time of their lives and are reluctant to let go of that experience when labor begins.

Table 2.3 reviews embryonic development and maternal experiences in the third trimester.

Past the Due Date

Even though the baby may not be technically "overdue," the passing of the expected due date, which was determined early in the pregnancy and based on the last menstrual period, may leave a woman feeling nervous, frustrated, or impatient as the baby grows larger and more confined. For many, this may be a great time for extra brisk activities or deeply relaxing full-body labor-preparation massages. Despite people's attachments to the due date, few births actually occur on that day, and it is not unusual to go up to 2 weeks past the due date. You might remind your client that forces beyond our understanding are at work that can delay or speed a labor. When the time is optimum for the baby, labor will commence.

Table 2.4 reviews embryonic development and maternal experiences when past the due date.

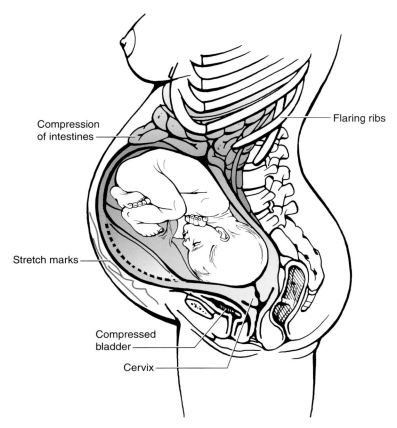

Compression of intestines

Flaring ribs

Stretch marks

Compressed bladder

Cervix

FIGURE 2.3 Third trimester, ninth month.
After lightening, the baby has dropped into the mother's pelvis, compressing her bladder but making maternal breathing easier. The baby will now be in vertex, or head-down, position 98% of the time.

HORMONAL CHANGES DURING PREGNANCY

We have looked at cellular, embryonic, and fetal development and maternal experiences of these changes. Now let us consider more specifically the effects of maternal hormonal changes and relevant bodywork concerns.

As soon as conception occurs, hormones begin to flood a woman's body. Progesterone, estrogen, relaxin, and prolactin are a few of the hormones that help prepare her body for nurturing new life. To supply the pregnant woman with extra hormones, some of the endocrine glands actually increase in size during the pregnancy, including the pancreas, thyroid gland, and the pituitary gland, which increases in size by 30% to 50%.[9,10]

Progesterone

"I hate being pregnant these days! I'm always constipated, I have hemorrhoids and a bladder infection, and my feet keep swelling." These complaints are not uncommon in the last months of pregnancy, and **progesterone** is the prime culprit behind them. The massage therapist will likely encounter some of the effects of progesterone during pregnancy massage.

The corpus luteum produces progesterone for the first 2 to 3 months of embryonic development. When the placenta is formed and fully functioning, it takes over production of this hormone. Progesterone helps prepare the uterus for the implanting of the egg by thickening the uterine lining and increasing the lining's secretory and nourishing qualities. Progesterone also aids breast development and relaxes the smooth muscle of the body, including the uterus, thereby preventing preterm labor contractions. This relaxation of the smooth muscle is vital for preventing uterine contractility, but progesterone affects more than the uterus—the primary organs such as the intestines, vasculature, and bladder are all composed of smooth muscle and are therefore all affected by progesterone.

What happens when these smooth muscles relax? The common complaints of pregnancy develop. Constipation occurs as a result of decreased

Table 2.3	Third Trimester of Fetal Development and Maternal Experience	
Embryonic and Fetal Development	**Possible Maternal Experience**	**Bodywork Considerations**
Seventh Month of Pregnancy • Baby is 15 inches long, 2–3 pounds. • Vernix covers entire body. • Movements clearly visible through abdomen. • By 26 weeks, baby can recognize voices outside womb and respond with movement. **Eighth Month of Pregnancy** • Baby is about 16–18 inches long, 4–5 pounds. • Body fat and lung surfactant are still developing. • By 7th or 8th month, baby is head-down in vertex position. • One quart of amniotic fluid surrounds baby, made up of albumin, urea, fat, fructose, lecithin, bilirubin, white blood cells. **Ninth month of pregnancy** • Baby is about 20 inches long and 6–7.5 pounds, and gaining 1/2 pound/week. • Rapid brain cell development occurs. • Lanugo starts to disappear. • Inner ear forms. • Lungs mature. • Ideally, baby has dropped further into pelvis. • By 9 months, heart circulates 300 gallons of blood daily.	• There may be symphysis pubis separation; sacroiliac pain; sciatica. • Diastasis recti may develop. • Edema of extremities may develop. • There is often increased heartburn, constipation, hemorrhoids, varicose veins, indigestion. • There may be lower and upper backache, hip pain, pelvic ache, calf cramps, wobbly hips. • Uterine ligament pain may occur. • Carpal tunnel syndrome may occur. • There may be shortness of breath and sore ribs. • Baby typically drops in last weeks, easing shortness of breath, increasing urinary frequency. • Stretch marks may develop. • There may be increased dependence on others for help. • Baby movements are usually visible. • Breasts are sore and enlarged. • Braxton hicks "practice" contractions occur. • There may be insomnia or dreams about baby. • There may be bouts of general discomfort; sometimes frustration, irritability, impatience with process. • There is anticipation and excitement about pregnancy, birth process, and baby. • There is changing identity, especially if no longer working.	• Avoid contraindicated acupressure points until 38 weeks. • There should be no supine positioning for greater than 5 min. Use only if client is comfortable. • Do not use prone positioning. • Do not perform hip mobilizations with diastasis symphysis pubis. • Attend to hip pain, sciatica, low back pain. • Perform labor preparation massage. • Offer belly rubs in low-risk pregnancy. • Teach perineal massage methods. • Teach partner massage techniques for labor. • Use varicose vein and thrombosis precautions. • Provide postural awareness education. • Teach visualizations and breathing to help relax with current discomforts. • Massage all stressed muscle groups. • Perform frequent passive pelvic tilts, lengthening low back.

gastrointestinal motility and increased water reabsorption in the intestines. Swelling in the ankles and hands also increases due to the new permeability of the vascular system. Progesterone increases heartburn due to prolonged gastric emptying; bladder infections due to urinary stasis; and increased body temperature, perspiration, and varicose veins due to vasodilatation and distention of the veins.

The progesterone level rises steadily from the tenth day of conception until 36 weeks of pregnancy, at which point it begins to decline, bringing on the Braxton-Hicks contractions.

Following is an overview of progesterone effects:

• Carpal tunnel syndrome (due to increased edema involving peripheral nerves)
• Constipation
• Dyspnea (shortness of breath)
• Heartburn
• Epistaxis (nose bleeds)
• Edema from vasodilatation
• Nasal congestion
• Orthostatic hypotension
• Spider angioma, varicosities in legs or vagina, hemorrhoids (hereditary and due to increased pelvic pressure)
• Urinary tract infections

Following is an overview of bodywork considerations for progesterone effects:

• Use semi-reclining positioning for women with heartburn.
• Avoid prone position that increases nasal congestion.
• Ask client to sit up slowly and wait before standing after massage to avoid dizziness from orthostatic hypotension.

Table 2.4 Past the Due Date (After 40 Weeks)		
Fetal Experiences	**Possible Maternal Experience**	**Bodywork Considerations**
• Baby activities continue but less room to move. • Lanugo—downy fetal body hair—decreases, and vernix—the creamy skin protector—is absorbed • Lines of hands and feet become more defined. • Placenta gradually deteriorates, losing best ability to nourish baby. • Amniotic fluid production may begin to diminish.	• Impatience increases for labor to begin. • Tension may develop impeding natural commencement of labor. • Friends and family may call often, questioning whether she is in labor, increasing pressure and anxiety. • Irritability increases. • Crying episodes and anxiety may occur. • All discomforts are magnified. • Insomnia may occur.	• Perform massage to hips, thighs, low back. • Perform full body massage for relaxation. • Perform acupressure and labor stimulating massage. • Teach visualizations and breathing for releasing tension, other fears, and obstacles to birth. • Offer belly rubs in low-risk pregnancy. • Provide nurturing supportive space for possible emotional release. • Teach resistance techniques with hip adductors to help relaxation of pelvic area. • Encourage long walks, hikes, and distracting activities. • Encourage meditation, observation of breath and thoughts, reminding mother that baby knows best when it's time to be born.

- Massage intercostals and diaphragm area to help relieve shortness of breath.
- Practice varicose vein and thrombosis precautions.
- Beware of low backache that could be related to urinary tract infection.
- Keep office cooler than normal if client is warm due to progesterone-related vasodilation.

Estrogen

"My breasts are sore and I am still throwing up several times a day." These are common estrogen symptoms in the first trimester. **Estrogen** is a hormone normally produced by the ovaries and adrenal cortex, but during early pregnancy its principal source is the corpus luteum, until the placenta takes over production. Along with the hormone relaxin, estrogen helps soften connective tissue, contributing to musculoskeletal aches and pains.

Estrogen helps build tissues in smooth muscles, preparing the endometrium for taking care of the fertilized egg, embryo, and fetus. Estrogen also affects the mammary glands by increasing breast size, vascularity, and the number and size of milk-producing ducts and lobes.

Estrogen and adrenocorticoid hormones contribute to the arrival of "spider veins" or **spider angioma**—tiny thin blood vessels near the surface of the skin. They also contribute to the darkening of the skin on the nipple areola and the **linea alba**—a fibrous band down the center of the abdomen where the abdominal muscles join. As the linea alba line darkens during pregnancy, it becomes known as the **linea negra** (black line). The skin of the face may also darken with a so-called "pregnancy mask," known as **chloasma**. These changes will disappear after pregnancy.

Estrogen contributes to extra blood flow to the nasal mucosa, causing swelling, stuffiness, and sometimes bloody noses. Estrogen decreases production of hydrochloric acid and pepsin, thereby contributing to heartburn already increased by the effects of progesterone. In late pregnancy as progesterone decreases, the relative increase in estrogen allows uterine contractions to begin.

Following is an overview of estrogen effects:

- Enlargement of uterus and breasts and lactation preparation.
- Breast tenderness
- Palmar erythema (red palms)
- Softening of connective tissue; backache, flank pain, tenderness of symphysis pubis
- Decreased secretion of hydrochloric acid and pepsin causing nausea, indigestion, and heartburn
- Chloasma, linea negra, freckles, darkening of nipples
- Change in substernal angle from 68 to 103 degrees, expansion of intercostal spaces
- Increased blood, lymph, and nerve supply to uterus

Following is an overview of bodywork considerations for estrogen effects:

- Beware of possible nausea with horizontal positioning, passive range of motion, incense or scented oils.
- Beware of breast tenderness if positioning prone in first trimester.
- Exercise caution with hip mobilizations and potential for symphysis pubis pain.
- Massage in intercostal spaces to address spreading angle of ribs.

Relaxin

"I feel like I'm walking on water—-I'm so loose in my hips." The effects of the hormone relaxin are felt by every pregnant woman. Relaxin is produced by the ovaries beginning in the tenth week of pregnancy and increases 10-fold, peaking in the last weeks of pregnancy between 38 to 42 weeks of gestation. Its primary effect is to relax and loosen connective tissues and ligaments, including the cervix and the pelvic joints, to provide just the extra mobility needed for the baby's head to pass through the birth canal. Relaxation of the symphysis pubis and sacroiliac joints is considerable. The symphysis pubis may expand from its normal 0.5 mm to as much as 12 mm or more. A separation of 10 mm or greater is called a **diastasis symphysis pubis** and can cause severe pain in the pubic area. Relaxin can also cause hypermobility of the sacroiliac joint, causing anterior or posterior rotation of one or both ileum and sometimes causing sharp pain in the sacroiliac area and low back.

Just as relaxin *relaxes* the skeletal body, a woman's emotional-psychic body relaxes as well. Boundaries become less distinct between her and the world at large. She may feel like she is melding into a unity with an energy much greater than herself as she harbors within her body the processes of fetal development, which have a life of their own; the growing baby, who has her or his own personality; and the psychological and emotional shifts that occur through dreams, hormonal surges, and cellular changes. The therapist can help support the client during a relaxation massage through this sometimes overwhelming loss of distinct personal boundaries by encouraging slow, deep respirations and positive visualizations that the client has indicated help her feel supported and safe.

Following is an overview of relaxin effects:

- Increased joint mobility and instability of sacroiliac joint, sacral area, and hips
- Breast tenderness

- Increased skin elasticity
- Relaxation of the articulation between sacrum and coccyx allowing coccyx to move posteriorly at birth to increase pelvic outlet

Following is an overview of bodywork considerations for relaxin effects:

- Maintain awareness of hypermobility of joints if doing mobilizations and passive range of motion.
- Avoid passive movements or resistance on legs/hips with separated symphysis pubis.
- Be aware of possible anterior or posterior ileum rotations causing sacroiliac pain or sciatica.
- Be aware of client's relaxing boundaries psychically, physically, psychologically, emotionally; reinforce positive visualizations about self, pregnancy, birth.

Other Important Hormones in Pregnancy

You may hear mention of the following hormones as your pregnant clients share about their experiences. **Oxytocin** is released from the hypothalamus. It causes the uterus to rhythmically contract during labor and stimulates the milk "let down" or **milk ejection reflex**—the stimulation of contractions in the milk glands that squeeze breast milk toward the nipple during lactation. Its presence is also thought to support mothering behaviors and the feelings of "maternal love."[11]

Prolactin is a hormone released from the anterior pituitary gland. It stimulates milk production, reduces anxiety, and has such strong analgesic effects that it may be considered for use with opioid dependency treatment. [12,13]

ORGAN SYSTEM ADAPTATIONS DURING PREGNANCY

The changes in pregnancy are not limited to musculoskeletal and hormonal ones. All organ systems undergo changes, some of which can be quite dramatic. This section reviews specific changes in several systems along with relevant bodywork considerations.

Respiratory System

The massage therapist may notice some of the effects of pregnancy on the client's respiratory system by observing the rate and depth of her breathing or by the increase in trigger points as the intercostal spaces widen. It is normal for pregnant women to breathe faster than when not pregnant, and after the twenty-fourth week of gestation, they also begin to breathe in the chest more than in the abdomen. As the baby presses up against a mother's diaphragm, the ribcage will actually expand laterally by 50%. Intercostal spaces become wider, ribcage circumference increases to 2 to 3 inches, and the substernal angle widens to 103 degrees, all helping to increase her respiratory ability. As these changes occur, the intercostals may develop trigger points and tight areas in response to the flaring ribs and shift in breathing.

The entire respiratory tract is affected by the extra blood volume of pregnancy. The trachea, larynx, Eustachian tubes, and nasal passages all become congested with blood, and a woman's tone of voice may actually change because of this. See the Massage Therapist Tip regarding bodywork considerations related to maternal respiratory changes.

Gastrointestinal System

Many women will experience an increase in or new development of constipation from uterine pressure against the intestines and from progesterone slowing intestinal motility. Heartburn and burping with reflux will increase due to the delay in gastric emptying time and relaxation of the sphincter at the junction of the esophagus and stomach. Nausea and vomiting increase, probably due to hormonal changes, but also due to the slowed motility, increased reflux, and general laxity of the GI system. See the Massage Therapist Tip for bodywork considerations related to heartburn.

Cardiovascular System

A pregnant woman is carrying, processing for, and feeding two people. Her heart must work harder and needs more blood. Total blood volume increases by 30% to 40% during pregnancy (nearly 2 to 3 *pounds* of extra blood!), and by mid-way through her pregnancy, her heart will be beating more rapidly and pumping nearly twice as much blood with each beat as when not pregnant. (By 6 weeks postpartum, the blood volume will have returned to normal.) This increased volume causes heart murmurs and new heart sounds in many pregnant women. According to one source, 93% of women develop nonpathological heart murmurs during their pregnancy.[14]

The heart literally grows larger in pregnancy—the heart weight increases and the cardiac chambers increase in size to compensate for the increase in volume. As the heart enlarges, it moves up in the chest to make room for the baby, perhaps even lying horizontally or rotated to the left. With extra blood and a whole new circulation flowing between the mother and the baby, your client may feel warmer than usual and sweat more. Fluctuations in blood pressure are normal. It is not uncommon for pregnant women to experience **orthostatic hypotension**—a sudden drop in blood pressure due to reduced peripheral resistance and pooling of blood. This may occur after lying down for a period of time and then standing.

 CAUTION: Be aware that your client may feel sudden dizziness, nausea, blurred vision, headache, or fatigue when standing after a massage due to orthostatic hypotension. Instruct her to move slowly, and to sit for a moment before standing, allowing her body to adapt between position changes.

Your client also will have nearly twice as much **interstitial fluid** as a nonpregnant woman has, and some of this fluid may end up as edema in her ankles and hands. This interstitial fluid is made up of water and electrolytes and is similar to plasma, though with much fewer proteins.

The extra blood that the body produces during pregnancy is needed at birth to replace the blood and fluids that are lost during delivery, so that the mother does not go into hypovolemic shock. To help prevent serious blood loss, there is also an increase in the **fibrolytic activity** of the blood—the blood clots faster than normal. This is helpful in cases of hemorrhage, but it also means that *a woman has 5 to 6 times greater risk for developing dangerous blood clots during pregnancy.*[15-17] This risk is further increased because of decreased circulation in the iliac, femoral, and saphenous veins of the legs caused by increased pelvic pressure and relaxation of the vascular system (Figure 2.4). If a woman has a high-risk pregnancy and is limited to bedrest, the risk for clots rises even further.

Bodywork Considerations Related to the Cardiovascular System

Due to the increased blood volume and adaptations of the cardiovascular system during pregnancy, there are some special points to consider when performing bodywork:

- Always use care when your client sits up after a massage. Encourage her to sit for several moments before standing.
- Keep your massage office cooler than usual, or keep a fan blowing if your client desires, to compensate for her increased warmth.

MASSAGE THERAPIST TIP   Maternal Respiratory Changes

*S*hortness of breath or difficulty filling lungs to capacity are common complaints during late pregnancy due to the baby pressing up into the mother's diaphragm and ribs.

CAUTION: This is not related to more serious shortness of breath that may be manifested as wheezing, sweating, faintness, and increasing anxiety. Difficulties breathing of this nature need to be referred to a medical health care provider immediately.

Below are some ways to address respiratory complaints when performing bodywork:

- A fan blowing fresh air across client's face can provide comfort for stuffy sinuses.

- After the first trimester, avoid prone positioning, which increases nasal congestion and compresses ribs and abdomen.
- Massage the superior chest area, including the scalenes, pectoralis attachments, and intercostals superior to the breasts to assist respiration and reduce trigger points.
- Use stretches and strokes that lengthen, open, and expand the chest, countering the compressing forces of weight and gravity on the chest and increasing respiratory capacity.

- Follow the precautions for varicose veins and deep vein thrombosis indicated in Chapter 4.
- Be aware that your client may be encouraged to elevate her legs and rest several times a day on her left side to help improve circulation and reduce edema, circulatory-related leg cramps, and varicosities. (The left side is believed to be more efficient for blood circulation during pregnancy due to the slightly right-sided location of the inferior vena cava.)

CAUTION: With the excessive circulatory load in pregnancy, women who have a history of cardiac problems will be at increased risk in the third trimester when the cardiac load is greatest. Do a particularly thorough health intake interview for such women, and avoid performing excessively stimulating circulatory massage, especially in the third trimester.

MASSAGE THERAPIST TIP   Heartburn

*I*t is not uncommon for pregnant women to complain of heartburn during their pregnancy. This can become uncomfortable for women during a massage. Below are several considerations when addressing gastrointestinal complaints during bodywork:

- A client with heartburn may be more comfortable in the semi-reclining position, with her head above her stomach.
- Encourage your clients to avoid heavy meals and foods that she knows cause her heartburn before massage her sessions.

- Be aware that if your client has found relief from her heartburn by using prescribed antacids and she begins to experience heartburn and reflux during your massage, she may ask to stop the session for a moment to take her antacid. If this is the case, she may find that she is more comfortable during the rest of the massage. It is not in the massage therapist's scope of practice, however, to suggest that a client use antacids.

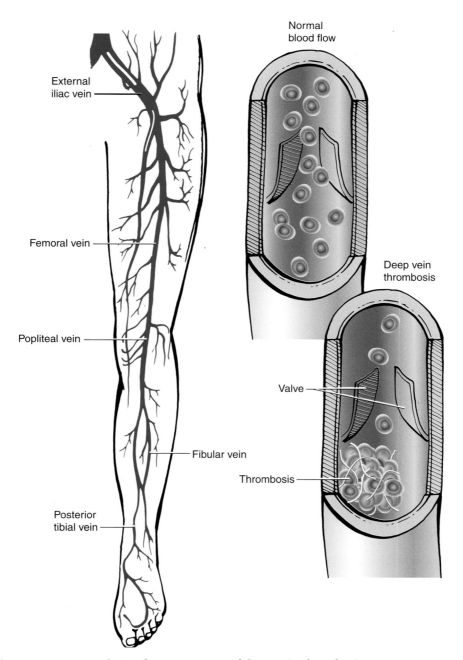

FIGURE 2.4   Most common vasculature for occurrence of deep vein thrombosis.

Great saphenous, femoral, and iliac veins of legs and groin. Clots are 5 to 6 times more likely to develop during pregnancy due to increased blood fibrinogen and decreased lower extremity circulation.

Excretory System: Kidneys, Bladder, and Skin

While the kidneys clear waste more efficiently during pregnancy, the risk of developing a urinary tract infection (UTI) increases significantly. Women with bladder infections have more risk for preterm contractions and kidney infections. Two physiological causes of UTIs are as follows:

1. Progesterone's effect of relaxing the entire urinary tract, including the ureters, causes urinary stasis in the bladder. As the bladder is emptied less completely or effectively, the risk for infection increases.

2. The angle at which the ureter enters the bladder shifts to perpendicular due to uterine pressure, resulting in a reflux of urine out of the bladder and back into the ureters.

With blood volume nearly doubled, there is an increase in blood flow through the kidneys. However, the blood flow and the rate of glomerular filtration (the kidneys' processing of fluids) actually *decrease* when a woman is standing or sitting since uterine pressure on the groin impedes the return flow of blood from the legs to the heart. When your client lies on her side, both kidney and cardiac functions and rates are increased and she produces more urine. This leads to the common frustrated comment, "It seems like I have to get up and use the bathroom every hour at night!" It also means that your client may need to use the restroom in the middle of a massage session.

 CAUTION: Sharp, unrelenting back pain or a dull aching in the low back could indicate a bladder or kidney infection. Do not assume that all back pain is necessarily musculoskeletal.

Bodywork Considerations Related to the Excretory System

The therapist must remember that the client's excretory system undergoes certain stresses during pregnancy. Remember the following tips in relation to this system when doing pregnancy bodywork:

- Offer your client water after each session. Massage will increase cellular waste release into the bloodstream. To help maintain blood volume and maximize waste processing, it is recommended that pregnant woman drink at least 4 quarts of water per day.
- Have the client empty her bladder before massage, and ask if she needs to use the restroom before changing position during a massage.

CHAPTER SUMMARY

Each trimester of pregnancy presents significant physical and emotional changes and challenges that your pregnant client must adapt to. Some of these physiological changes are tremendous, including enlargement of endocrine glands and cardiac chambers, increase in blood volume and shift in position

of the heart, and loosening of ligaments and expansion of the pelvic joints. Accompanying these changes are occasional discomforts, such as nasal congestion and orthostatic hypotension due to hormonal and cardiovascular adjustments, or feeling warmer than usual or having more urinary frequency. To accommodate some of these possible conditions, the massage therapist can offer simple modifications during a massage session to increase the pregnant client's comfort. A few practical and common ways to support your client are: having a fan available in a massage room if the client complains of stuffy sinuses or increased warmth, shifting her position to semi-reclining if she complains of heartburn, or offering the use of the restroom before shifting positions. In the following chapters, you will learn specific techniques of bodywork as well as contraindications during pregnancy so that your massage will be optimally oriented to the special needs of this population.

CHAPTER REVIEW QUESTIONS

1. Why might a mother experience an increase in urinary frequency and a decrease in shortness of breath sometime after 36 weeks' gestation?
2. Explain why some women may develop an increase in trigger points in their ribs during pregnancy.
3. What type of positioning might be most appropriate for a woman experiencing heartburn during pregnancy?
4. Describe four changes in the cardiovascular system during pregnancy and the risks and complaints that may develop because of these changes.
5. Name three office accommodations you might need to make specifically for your pregnant clients.
6. Explain why is it important to have your client sit for a moment on the edge of the table, before standing up to walk after a massage.
7. Compare the scientific view of conception and fetal development with some of the traditional views of conception and explore possible similarities in the beliefs. Consider whether a woman's spiritual view of her pregnancy would impact your work with her in how you approach her body and pregnant belly, or in the direction of your conversation.
8. What kinds of physical complaints might a mother have during the third trimester of pregnancy?
9. What effects caused by the hormone relaxin would be of concern to the bodyworker?

Case Study 2.1:
MAKING THE CLIENT COMFORTABLE

As was often necessary with her pregnant clients, Pearl made several accommodations during a massage to ensure that Tobin, who was 36 weeks pregnant, was comfortable and safe.

Tobin said that one of the things she was enjoying about being pregnant was that she was much warmer than normal for her. In bed at night she did not have cold feet anymore and did not need as many covers as usual. She said she often felt warm and was currently wearing a T-shirt, while Pearl needed a sweater when not doing massage. Tobin mentioned that the other new thing she was noticing was the development of a brown discoloration on her face which the doctor had said was not unusual and would go away. Pearl knew this was called chloasma and was a result of the extra estrogen in Tobin's system.

Tobin requested to have her feet uncovered during the massage and appreciated the fact that Pearl had aired out the room and decreased the temperature so that it was not stuffy. Tobin said that she at times felt congested nasally, and she liked to have air moving about her. The therapist offered to turn on the fan so that the air could blow lightly across the client's face, which she agreed to.

Pearl massaged Tobin in the left-sidelying position, and before repositioning on the right, asked if Tobin needed to use the restroom. Tobin said she needed to urinate frequently, and did need to do so now, as the baby was pushing down on her bladder often. Before Pearl could slow Tobin down, she had pushed herself up and gotten off the table. Suddenly Tobin leaned back against the table, saying she felt lightheaded. Pearl stood by her until she felt stable, a moment later. Pearl explained that it was not uncommon to experience orthostatic hypotension during pregnancy—a sudden drop in blood pressure when changing positions from lying or sitting to standing, and that she just needed to move more slowly when shifting from one position to another to give her body a chance to adapt. Tobin said that this happened to her now and then at home as well when she jumped out of bed or stood up from the couch too quickly.

Before getting off the table at the end of the massage, Pearl reminded Tobin to push herself up to a sitting position, and then to sit for a moment before standing up. She had no further episodes of lightheadedness. If she had continued to feel lightheaded, rather than being a momentary passing event, Pearl would have had Tobin lie down again on her side to improve blood flow to the head and avoid a fall, and then would have helped her to call her prenatal care provider if it seemed Tobin's symptoms were not going away.

10. Name three comfort measures a massage therapist might take for a client experiencing mild shortness of breath due to the pressure of the baby against her diaphragm.

REFERENCES

1. Dunham C. Mamatoto: A Celebration of Birth. New York: Penguin Books, 1991.
2. Vincent Priya J. Birth Traditions and Modern Pregnancy Care. Rockport, MA: Element Books, 1992.
3. Weiner AB. The Trobrianders of Papua New Guinea. New York: Holt, Rinehart, and Winston, 1988.
4. Feinberg RF. Pregnancy Loss: Approaches to evaluation and treatment. Obgyn.net http://www.obgyn.net/displayarticle.asp?page = /infertility/articles/feinberg_spotlight.
5. Puscheck E, Pradhan A. First trimester pregnancy loss. Emedicine from WebMD. June 25, 2006.
6. Brennan B. Hands of Light: a guide to healing through the human energy field. New York: Bantam Books, 1987: 62.
7. Chang AL, Agredano YZ, Kimball AB. Risk factors associated with Striae Gravidarum. J Am Acad Dermatol 2004;51(6):881–885.
8. Young GL, Jewell D. Creams for preventing stretch marks in pregnancy. Cochrane Database Syst Rev 1996;(1). Art. No.: CD000066, DOI:10.1002/14651858.CD000066.
9. Dundas K. Obstetrics: the physiological changes. Hospital Pharmacist June 2003;10.
10. Elster AD, Sanders TG, Vines FS, et al. Size and shape of the pituitary gland during pregnancy and post partum: measurement with MR imaging. Radiology 1991;181(2): 531–535.
11. Bartels A, Zeki S. The neural correlates of maternal and romantic love. Neuroimage 2004;21:1155–1166.
12. Ramaswamy S, Bapna JS. Effect of prolactin on tolerance and dependence to acute administration of morphine. Neuropharmacology 1987;26(2–3): 111–113.
13. Ramaswamy S, Viswanathan S, Bapna JS. Prolactin analgesia: tolerance and cross-tolerance with morphine. Eur J Pharmacol 1985;112(1):123-125.

14. Goldberg LM, Uhland H. Heart Murmurs in pregnancy: a phonocardiographic study of their development, progression and regression. Chest 1967;52:381–386.

15. Richter ON, Rath W. [Thromboembolic diseases in pregnancy.] [Article in German] Z Geburtshilfe Neonatol 2007; 211(1):1–7.

16. Broffman J. Clinical Vignette. Deep vein thrombosis and pregnancy. Los Angeles: UCLA Dept. of Medicine, 2007.

17. Adcock D. Pregnancy related risks associated with Thrombophilia: maternal and fetal issues. Clinical Hemostasis Review 2003 March;17(3):1–6.

CHAPTER 3

POSTURAL AND MUSCULAR ADAPTATIONS RELATED TO PREGNANCY

LEARNING OBJECTIVES

After reading this chapter, you should be able to:

- Describe the effects of weight gain, hormones, self-esteem, and pre-pregnancy muscle tone on posture.

- Describe postural and muscular stresses and adaptations during pregnancy and their relation to common complaints during pregnancy.

- How to assess posture and help a woman readjust her posture during pregnancy to decrease some of her strains and discomforts.

- Understand the need for teaching clients or partners tools for self-care as a way to address certain pregnancy discomforts.

- Describe symptoms of strained uterine ligaments and their similarity to other muscular complaints.

- Explain under what conditions a separation of the rectus muscle may occur during pregnancy, and describe the symptoms, assessment, and prevention or correction of a separation.

*I*n this chapter, we will examine the effects of weight gain, hormones, self-esteem, and pre-pregnancy muscle tone on posture and the changes that develop during pregnancy relative to these effects. We will look at how postural adaptations and muscular stresses can cause back and neck pain, psoas and uterine ligament spasms, headaches, and leg cramps. Next, we explore ways to improve a woman's experience of pregnancy

with postural assessment and adjustment, as well as with assessment of the rectus abdominus. You will learn about areas of the body that are especially stressed as well as teaching tools to share with your clients that can address muscular areas that need strengthening. By combining this knowledge with skilled bodywork, as discussed later in the book, along with client education, you will be able to effectively address specific pregnancy discomforts.

POSTURAL ASSESSMENTS AND CORRECTIONS DURING PREGNANCY

Within the 9-month gestational period, a woman normally gains between 20 to 35 pounds of extra weight. This weight is distributed among the placenta, baby, uterus, additional breast tissue, and extra fluids and blood (Box 3.1). While a mother may flourish with this extra blood flow, increased oxygen intake, hormonal boosts, and the energizing enjoyment of a secret world developing between herself and her growing child, her musculoskeletal structures are making adjustments to accommodate the extra load. As the muscles adjust, a woman's posture must shift as well, bringing with it new or unusual aches and pains.

These adjustments become more dramatic by the latter part of pregnancy, when a woman is gaining nearly 1 pound per week, most of it on the anterior side of her body. The muscles most affected by this

BOX 3.1 | Weight Gain in Pregnancy

In a normal 9-month pregnancy, the average weight gain of 20 to 35 pounds is made up of the following:

- 4 to 7 pounds of fat and muscle
- 2 to 5 pounds of cellular fluids
- 2 to 4 pounds of blood and plasma
- 2 to 4 pounds extra breast weight
- 6 to 9 pounds of baby
- 2 pounds of uterus
- 1.5 to 2 pounds of amniotic fluid
- 2 pounds of placenta

gain include those that support the weight of the abdomen anteriorly, posteriorly, laterally, and from below. These muscles include the abdominals, iliopsoas, paraspinals, spinal erectors, adductors, lateral hip rotators, and the pelvic floor group. The muscles supporting the increasing weight and size of the growing, and soon-to-be lactating breasts, are also affected, including the rhomboids, pectoralis, subscapularis, scalenes, and levator scapula.

In response to the extra weight and anterior expansion of the belly, a woman's posture must change. As the abdomen stretches, the spine naturally compensates by developing more curvature in the lumbar area. This can cause low back pain due to compression of the lumbar nerve roots and strain to the deep lumbar and paraspinal muscles. As the abdominals stretch, the connective tissues of the thorax, shoulders, and throat area are also affected, pulled caudally with gravity, and causing strain to the spine as it attempts to support an erect posture. Excessive lumbar

lordosis and consequent low back pain increase drastically as each muscular area supporting the pelvis responds to the rapid structural changes. As the pelvis tilts anteriorly, a typical stressful pregnancy posture might develop to compensate.

If a woman has weak musculature and pays little attention to her posture, she may develop a variety of discomforts or dysfunctions, including low back, shoulder, neck, and upper back pain, brachial plexus syndrome, leg cramps, diastasis recti, sacroiliac joint dysfunction, headaches, and shortness of breath. The client can often avoid these conditions by increasing postural awareness and correcting her posture as needed, along with receiving therapeutic massage and taking part in regular exercise to help diminish stresses as they occur. Box 3.2 outlines muscular influences on lumbar lordosis.

Contributing Factors to Poor Posture

The following factors have the strongest effects on posture during pregnancy.

Gravity

Gravity and the continual growth of the uterus and baby cause the forward and downward pull of the growing uterus, increasing lumbar lordosis and stressing the abdominals. Improved self-awareness about posture will help to avert the constant influences of gravity.

Hormones

Posture is also influenced by the effects of relaxin on connective tissue and ligamentous structures (see

BOX 3.2 | Muscular Relationships to Lumbar Lordosis

- A shortened psoas pulls on the anterior lumbar spine.
- The quadratus lumborum (QL) and erector spinae complex pull the sacrum and iliac crests up toward the thoracic spine.
- Shortening of the lumbar intervertebral muscles, such as the multifidi, decreases the spaces between the vertebrae, pulling them tighter and increasing lordosis.
- Rectus and transverse abdominus, in a constant stretch from the growing abdomen, become weaker, unable to fulfill their role of pulling the

pelvis posteriorly and supporting the abdominal contents and back.
- The gluteal muscles help stabilize the pelvis and extend and medially rotate the hip. If these are weak, lumbar lordosis and lateral hip rotation increases.
- The hip flexors iliacus, tensor fasciae latae, sartorius, rectus femoris, and quadriceps—shorten as the pelvis rolls forward toward them.
- The hamstrings are in constant stretch, weakening and decreasing their ability to stabilize the pelvis posteriorly at the ischial tuberosity.

Chapter 2). While ligaments are critical for helping humans to stand comfortably erect, during pregnancy, women cannot depend on their newly lax ligaments to adequately support them. Muscles take on a more prominent role in stabilizing joints and, unlike ligaments, become fatigued, possibly leading to strains and spasms. Elastic or cloth **abdominal support binders** that wrap around the belly and support its weight during the later stages of pregnancy may be effective in mediating some of these hormonal effects.[1] Figure 3.1 shows one example of an abdominal support available for pregnant women. See Appendix B, Resources for the Practitioner, for sources of maternity abdominal supports.

Muscle Tone

Poor muscle tone greatly affects a woman's ability to hold herself erect during pregnancy. Imagine trying to maintain your normal daily activities while carrying 28 pounds of solid weight on your belly with a thin,

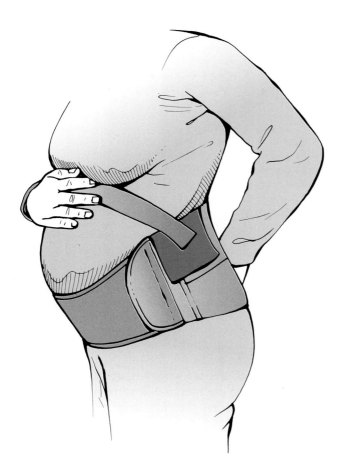

FIGURE 3.1   Maternity abdominal support.
These are often recommended for women with pendulous abdomens, or with complaints of sacroiliac, hip, and low back pain. There are numerous styles and sources for such supports.

stretchy fabric for support. The cloth would stretch in front, the weight would bear down, and the strain in your back would increase as your muscles attempted to hold the weight closer to the center of your body. As a massage therapist, you might encourage your client to strengthen the muscle groups that help to support this weight. These especially include the perineals, abdominals, psoas, hip extensors (gluteals), QL, lateral shoulder rotators (teres minor and infraspinatous), rhomboids, and spine extensors (erector spinae).

Muscle Tension

Pain-producing posture can develop when weak primary muscles cannot support the structural changes of pregnancy; when this occurs, secondary muscle groups become shortened and strained in their effort to compensate for the lack of support from others. Pelvic stabilizing muscles that may need strengthening include the gluteals, hamstrings, and perineal groups, transverse abdominus, perineals, and the hip adductors. The QL, psoas, and lateral hip rotators are notoriously tight and often are a source of discomfort in pregnancy. A woman may develop a kyphotic-type posture in the upper back as the medial or internal shoulder rotators tighten, pulled forward by the anterior weight of the breasts. Stretching and lengthening these tight muscles can help to improve postural balance.

Size and Position of the Baby

Some babies rest close to the mother's spine, whereas others lie forward, making the mother's belly pendulous, with all the weight extended out in front of her. If the baby is exceptionally big, or if she is carrying multiple babies, the mother's belly may become quite large, necessitating subtle or dramatic shifts in her posture to find balance.

Self-Esteem

Esteem can be a strong or minimal influence, but a woman with low self-esteem may carry her new weight less efficiently than a woman who feels healthy and empowered. Providing massage visits that foster positive self-esteem will help your client more easily incorporate suggestions for improved posture.

Assessing Posture

Look at the photographs in Figure 3.2, which depict healthy posture (A) and posture that will inevitably cause discomfort (B). It is not uncommon to see various elements of Posture B in pregnancy, most often

Healthy posture

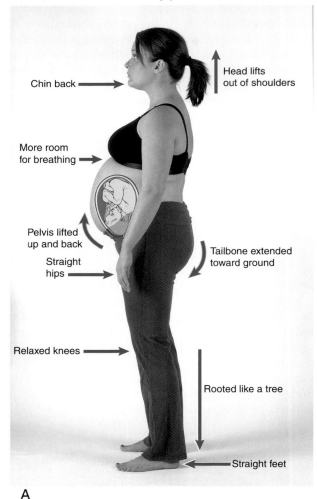

Chin back →

Head lifts
out of shoulders ↑

More room
for breathing →

Pelvis lifted
up and back

Straight
hips →

Tailbone extended
toward ground

Relaxed knees →

Rooted like a tree

Straight feet

A

**Posture causing
Structural strain**

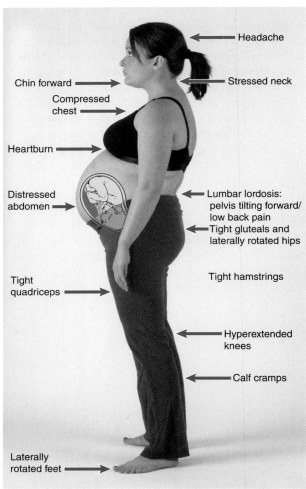

→ Headache

Chin forward →

→ Stressed neck

Compressed
chest →

Heartburn →

Distressed
abdomen →

← Lumbar lordosis:
pelvis tilting forward/
low back pain
← Tight gluteals and
laterally rotated hips

Tight hamstrings

Tight
quadriceps →

← Hyperextended
knees

← Calf cramps

Laterally
rotated feet →

B

FIGURE 3.2   Posture in pregnancy.
(A) Healthy posture and (B) posture causing structural strain. Note in (B) slumped shoulders, jutting chin, hyper-extended knees, laterally rotated hips and feet, and compressed chest. Her symptoms may include the following: shortness of breath, heartburn, headache, neck strain, low back pain, and calf cramps.

due to the influence of gravity and lack of awareness regarding one's posture.

Helping your client to readjust her posture can improve her experience of pregnancy. It is easy to remind your client at each visit of the importance of standing tall. Here are some suggestions for assessing your client's stance:

1. Observe your client walking or standing: ask her to walk around the room, or just observe her as she walks into your office. Are her feet turned out, in the "pregnancy waddle"? Her lateral hip rotators are likely very tight. Are her shoulders hunched forward, pulled by the weight of the breasts? Is her back arched? Is she holding her belly up with her hands? Is

her chin jutting forward in an effort to hold the head more erect? In what areas of the body do you think she will be feeling particularly stressed?

2. Try positioning yourself in her posture (or with the exaggerated Posture B in Figure 3.2) for 30 to 60 seconds, and note where you begin to feel discomfort. This will give you rapid evidence for where your client will be experiencing strain. Inevitably the hips, shoulders, neck, knees, and buttocks all begin to develop tension when the body is poorly positioned. In addition to the changes noted above, others occur. In response to extra lumbar lordosis, the knees hyperextend and lock,

compensating for the anterior pull of the belly and the posterior counter pull of the upper back. The psoas shortens and anteriorly tractions the lumbar spine. The tight erector spinae complex and QL pull up on the sacrum and iliac crests. The quadriceps and other hip flexors shorten, pulling down anteriorly on the pelvis. The minor stabilizing effect of the hamstrings and adductors decreases as they are stretched by the anterior pelvis. (Box 3.2).

Adjusting Posture

Keeping the pelvis in a neutral position and the low back lengthened requires conscious attention and exercise to maintain during pregnancy. Often, strengthening or stretching the muscles of support is necessary. The abdominal muscles must be strong enough to support the abdominal contents and keep the pelvis pulled up in front, and the psoas needs to be lengthened enough to prevent pulling down on the lumbar spine. Until this is achieved and can be maintained, help your client practice and develop the stance of solid, well-balanced posture in the following manner.

1. Show your client the illustration of optimal posture compared with that of stress-producing posture (Figure 3.2). Have her stand against a wall and flatten her low back against it. In this position, she can feel what it is like to have a straight back with her pelvis in posterior or neutral position.
2. Now have her stand away from the wall with her feet facing straight forward, hip-width apart. Ask her to relax her knees slightly out of a hyperextension and allow her sacrum and buttocks to drop slightly toward the ground. As she stands with feet apart and parallel, gently encourage her to envision her body naturally aligning itself.
3. Have her find a balance between her feet, by bringing her weight evenly between the heels and center of the sole of each foot.
4. Squeeze and hold the back of her heels, encouraging her to feel her feet grounded on the earth. Then run your hand from her sacrum up her spine to her head, suggesting that she imagine herself as a tree, rooted in the ground through her feet and reaching up to the sky through her spine, neck, and head. With this stroke up her body, ask her to inhale, as if she is bringing water up the tree trunk. Suggest that she loosen her knees, tuck her tailbone slightly to bring her pelvis more fully under her belly as support, lengthen her neck, drop her chin just slightly toward her

chest, and relax her jaw, face, and shoulders. If she can imagine her pelvis as a basket holding her growing infant, she may be able to feel how to position herself, imagining that if the basket is tipped too far forward, the baby will fall out.

5. Place your thumb and forefingers under her occiput, holding the occipital ridge and steadying her head with your other hand on her forehead. Ask her to take in a deep breath and lengthen her spine as you lift slightly, applying a gentle traction under her head toward the sky (Figure 3.3). In yoga, this is

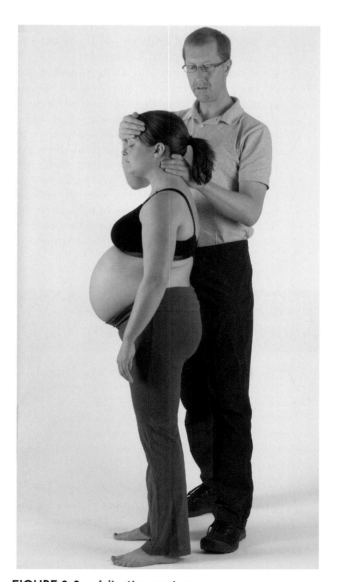

FIGURE 3.3   Adjusting posture

Lift from under the occiput, with another hand stabilizing on the forehead, encouraging the client to inhale deeply and allow her spine to lengthen.

similar to Mountain Pose, or Tadasana, which implies standing rooted and firm as a mountain and which brings clarity and fortitude to those who practice it.

6. Lift up from the occiput. Encourage her to lengthen her entire spine, rising from her hips and pelvis and again reminding her to lift toward the sky like a tree, or as if there were a cord extending from the earth up through her coccyx to the top of her head and pulling her upright. Encourage her shoulders to widen with a deep breath, allowing them to fall back as the chest expands and the breath flows into her chest and belly like an ocean tide. This practice will give her the sensate experience of length, strength, and ease. It will help her to realign herself, and to walk with this imagery impressed in her mind.

7. Continue holding and lifting under her occiput for several of her breaths as her spine extends from the sacrum to the neck. Allow her time to settle into this taller stance, noticing how that feels. She may be standing several inches taller than she was a moment ago. Of course, it is easy to be forgetful of one's posture and sink down again under the seductive lure of gravity! But with regular reminders of how to return to a tall and spacious posture, supported by massage that encourages opening and

How the Partner Can Help
Postural Support

The client may ask the massage therapist to share postural awareness and adjustment methods with the client's partner, so that he or she can assist her in cultivating more habitual awareness of her posture. You may choose to invite the client's partner or support team to a session where you can teach them your way of observing, assessing, and correcting imbalanced stances. People who are often in proximity to the client will have frequent opportunities to observe how and when the client begins to alter her stance in ways that may cause her discomfort later. The support person benefits from this awareness as well, as it is not only during pregnancy that postural awareness is essential. Establishing a practice of assessing one's own posture at regular intervals each day can help him or her avoid personal injuries in times of stress, as well as in daily life.

lengthening, a healthy posture can become a natural stance.

Sitting Posture

Problems develop for pregnant women who work long hours sitting at a desk, as the flow of blood from

MASSAGE THERAPIST TIP   A Postural Checklist

The massage therapist can help adjust posture by using touch to bring the client's attention to her feet and up her spine, then tractioning cephalically under the occiput. The incorporation of visualizations and breath will assist this work. You might consider using some of the verbal cues included in this checklist to help the woman embody postural change.

- Leg alignment: Turn the feet straight forward, hip width apart, and relax the knees slightly.
- Grounding: Imagine tree roots extending and sinking into the earth from the tailbone and soles of the feet.
- Lengthening: Envision lengthening, like a tall tree, extending through the top and back of the head with branches reaching to the sky. Lengthen in

the waist by allowing the upper torso to lift up from the hips.
- Breathing: Allow the breath to enter the chest like a rising ocean tide, deep and full, expanding the lower ribs and opening the sides and back of the thoracic cavity, then allowing the upper chest to fill with the final inflow of breath.
- Opening chest: Keep the shoulders broad, allowing them to fall naturally backward and relax downward.
- Lengthen the back of the neck: Lift the head up and away from the shoulders, feeling energy rise up from the earth-roots through the spine to the head, and envisioning the posture of one who feels strong, proud, or even regal.

the pelvis to the legs can be impeded. Positive posture can be practiced in the chair as well, remembering to lift the torso up out of the hips, and place the feet on a footrest so that the knees are at least at a 90-degree angle to the floor, and not dangling from the chair. This can help prevent the development of problems such as varicosities, pelvic congestion, hemorrhoids, edema, and leg cramps. Your client also may want to find a way to extend her legs frequently to relieve some of the congestion in her pelvic area.

MUSCULAR AREAS STRESSED BY PREGNANCY

As described earlier, specific muscle groups are particularly stressed during pregnancy. Minor muscular strains are not an uncommon experience during gestation. It may be useful to remind your client who is complaining of frequent muscular aches, that regular exercise can help decrease incidents of muscular discomfort, while having the additional benefits of cultivating a higher tolerance for pain during birth and generally improving birth outcomes.[2-5] Activities that are particularly beneficial during pregnancy for women beginning a new exercise regimen include low-impact or non–weight-bearing activities such as swimming, walking, biking, and yoga. Strengthening and stretching regularly also will help your client improve her posture.

Presented below are some of the most obvious muscles affected by pregnancy—including some at the core of postural support—and the consequences of the stress they endure: the uterus and its ligaments, perineals, abdominals, psoas, and QL. Most of these muscles can be addressed with massage during pregnancy, as well as with standard stretches and strengthening exercises.

Uterus

The uterine muscle undergoes perhaps the most dramatic adaptations to pregnancy, and its strained ligamentous support can sometimes cause a variety of discomforts. The uterus is a reproductive organ, but it is also the strongest muscle for its size in a woman's body. Before pregnancy, the uterus typically weighs about 2 ounces. By the end of a full-term pregnancy, the uterus alone, minus its contents, typically weighs about 2 pounds. It has increased its volume capacity by 1000 to 4000 times and is four to six times larger than it was before the pregnancy. The actual number of uterine muscle cells increases through the first trimester of pregnancy; then, the cells begin to enlarge and, eventually, in the second trimester, stretch until they are 10 times longer than their original size.

Uterine Ligaments

Six primary ligaments, along with the endopelvic fascia and other connective tissue, support and suspend the uterus. During pregnancy, any of these ligaments can spasm and refer pain to areas in the back, legs, or groin (Figure 3.4).

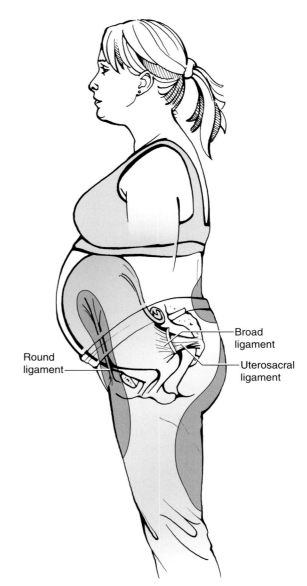

Round ligament

Broad ligament

Uterosacral ligament

FIGURE 3.4   Uterine ligaments and areas of referred pain.

The round ligament spasm will pull in the pelvic area and can cause pain in the lower pelvis, anterior leg, or most commonly, sharp pain in the groin. The broad ligament attaches in the wide area of the pelvis and causes discomfort in the low back and buttocks when in spasm. The uterosacral ligament attaches from the posterior uterus to the sacrum and, when pulled, causes pain in the sacrum, sciatic-like pain down the back of the leg, sacroiliac joint pain, and diffuse low back pain.

The two **round ligaments** are mostly a continuation of the uterine smooth muscle and originate on the anterior surface of the uterus below the fallopian tubes. They traverse the broad ligament to the lateral abdominal wall. There they pass through the inguinal canal to attach to the inner aspect of the labia majora of the vagina.

The two **uterosacral ligaments** arise from the posterior uterus and cervix, just inferior to the utero-cervical juncture. They attach to the periostium of the anterior mid-sacrum and near the sacroiliac joints.

The two **broad ligaments** spread out like a sheet from the lateral aspects of the uterus sinking into the fascia of the iliac fossa, the walls of the pelvic cavity, and into the connective tissue of the pelvic floor. Within the broad ligament are suspended the ovaries and round ligaments.

Bands of ligamentous tissue called the ligamentum transversalis colli, transverse cervical ligaments or **cardinal ligaments,** support the cervix and uterus. They arise from the lateral aspects of the cervix and traverse the broad ligament to insert into the anterior sacrum and lateral pelvic wall.

Referred Pain From Uterine Ligament Spasm

The uterine ligaments must stretch extensively during pregnancy, and it may be 6 months postdelivery before they, along with all the body's ligaments, return to their former nonpregnant state.[6,7] As they lengthen, these ligaments can spasm and cause discomfort that manifests as low back pain or pelvic discomfort. More severe ligament spasms may be misinterpreted as unrelated muscle spasm or as uterine contractions. Two of the most important actions a massage therapist can take to help prevent uterine ligament spasm are as follows:

1. Properly position a client on the massage table in a way that adequately supports the uterus.
2. Teach appropriate body mechanics for changing positions on the table, so that ligaments are not strained.

Uterine ligament spasms may be associated with the following types of discomfort (Figure 3.3):

- Round ligament spasm: Often experienced as pain in the lower pelvis, pain down the front of the leg, or sharp pain in the groin.
- Broad ligament spasm: Often experienced as discomfort in the low back and buttocks.
- Uterosacral ligament spasm: Experienced as pain in the sacrum, sciatic-like pain down the back of the leg, sacroiliac joint pain, or low back pain.

Bodywork Considerations Related to Uterine Ligaments

Below are some recommendations on how to alleviate pain from uterine ligament spasm in your clients:

- Educate your client to avoid sitting straight up from supine or lateral positions as instructed in Self Care Tip for the Mother: Preventing Abdominal and Uterine Ligament Strain (Figure 3.5).
- Support the client's growing belly with a small pillow or rolled towel when in the sidelying position to prevent strain on uterine ligaments (see "Positioning Techniques," Chapter 5).
- Suggest the use of an abdominal binder to help relieve backache caused by ligament pain (Figure 3.1).
- Teach your client to relieve round ligament pain by flexing the hip of the affected side and applying direct fingertip or palm pressure to the painful area near the groin.

Pelvic Floor

The **pelvic floor** or perineum refers to the muscles that hang like a hammock between the ischial tuberosity, the symphysis pubis, and the coccyx (Figure 3.6). These are generically and collectively known as the perineal muscles. The primary pelvic floor muscles include the group called the levator ani, the transverse perineal muscles, and the bulbospongiosus. They play a critical role in a woman's health, as they support the weight of the abdominal contents, including the organs and the baby-filled uterus. They also wrap like a figure eight around and control the three sphincters of the perineum: the urethra, the vagina, and the anus.

During birth, the perineal muscles must stretch and are sometimes cut or torn during delivery, weakening them. After this extreme stretching, or, as with any muscle, without exercise, the perineal muscles can lose their tone. Imagine a hammock, heavily loaded with weight, sagging toward the ground. The looser the hammock is woven and the heavier the load, the further it sags. Similarly, when the perineal muscles are untoned, the weight of the abdominal contents causes the muscles to sag. As many as one third to one half of all women in the United States experience problems caused by weak perineal muscles after age 55 and many of these pelvic floor dysfunctions develop after childbirth.[8,9] This includes symptoms of vague back and pelvic aches and heaviness, fatigue, vulvar varicosities and rectal hemorrhoids, urinary stress incontinence (urinating when coughing, sneezing, laughing, or straining) or

Self Care Tips FOR MOTHERS:

Preventing Abdominal and Uterine Ligament Strain

"Jackknifing" forward from a supine or sidelying position to a seated position causes strains and spasms to uterine ligaments and can contribute to diastasis of the rectus abdominus. Many women experience this discomfort, yet do not recognize this contributor to its occurrence.

Pregnant women on the massage table will need to reposition several times and possibly get up in the middle of session to use the restroom. It is particularly important for the mother to use care when moving from the lying to the sitting position. Whether on a massage table, in bed, or on a couch, she can use this method for sitting up without strain.

First remove any pillows between or under her legs. She should roll to her side first if she is not already lateral. Bending her legs, she will then use her arms to push her upper body up to a sitting position (Figure 3.5). Finally, she will swing her legs over the side of the table, keeping her knees together. This prevents straining of the abdominals when sitting up. She should always sit for a moment on the edge of the bed or couch for a moment before getting up, to avoid instability due to dizziness from postural hypotension.

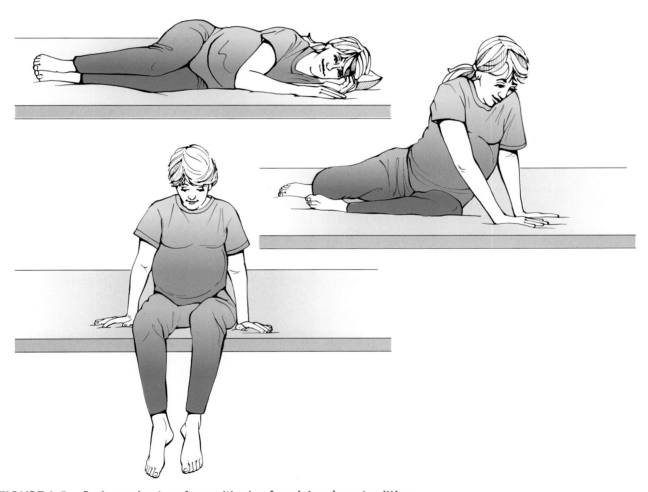

FIGURE 3.5   Body mechanics of repositioning from lying down to sitting.
To prevent strain to the abdominals and uterine ligaments, always remove the pillows first, then have the client roll to her side and push herself up using her arm and hand strength, rather than straining her abdominals. Have her sit on the edge of the table for several minutes if she feels dizzy.

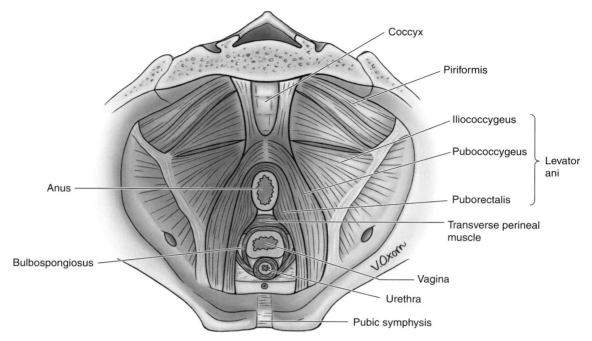

Coccyx

Piriformis

Iliococcygeus

Pubococcygeus

Levator
ani

Puborectalis

Transverse perineal
muscle

Anus

Bulbospongiosus

Vagina

Urethra

Pubic symphysis

FIGURE 3.6   Perineal musculature and pelvic bones.

The primary pelvic floor muscles include the group called the levator ani, the transverse perineal muscles, and the bulbospongiosus. These hang like a hammock between the ischial tuberosity, the symphysis pubis, and the coccyx. (From Moore KL and Agur A. Essential Clinical Anatomy, 2nd Ed. Philadelphia: Lippincott Williams & Wilkins, 2002.)

continual leakage of urine, and uterine or bladder **prolapse** (when the organ slips down toward or literally drops out of the vagina). **Kegel exercises** are an effective method for helping prevent these complaints by toning the muscles and improving circulation. There are many benefits to practicing Kegel exercises regularly, as described in Box 3.3.

Weak perineals are another possible cause of the common complaints during pregnancy of dull, aching low back and pelvic discomfort. As a bodyworker helping a woman cope with her physical changes during the perinatal cycle, passing on information about the benefits of Kegel exercises could be a great service to her. Awareness of the perineal support to the torso can be increased by combining client-activated perineal muscle contractions along with muscle-release techniques in the low back, hip rotators and adductors. The perineal contraction and release can enhance the effectiveness of the other muscular release.

BOX 3.3 | Benefits of Kegel Exercises

Kegel exercises improve the following:

- Circulation and health of the perineal area
- Bowel elimination
- Sexual pleasure and responsiveness
- Elasticity of perineal tissue
- Perineal strength for pushing during birth
- Familiarity with the perineal area, potentially easing associated psychological discomforts during childbirth

- Postpartum tone of vaginal muscles
- Perineal healing in postpartum

Kegel exercises reduce the following:

- Hemorrhoids and vulvar varicosities
- Occurrence of urinary incontinence
- Episiotomy or perineal tearing at birth
- Organ prolapse and low backaches associated with partial prolapsed

The following instructions can be offered to your client, but learn to do the exercises yourself first, so that you can describe them effectively. There are no contraindications to Kegel exercises; they are useful prenatally, in postpartum, and throughout a woman's life. Men can do Kegels as well.

General Instruction for Kegels

For more comfort, always be sure to empty the bladder before doing these exercises. To have the most beneficial effect, one must do the exercises several times a day. Dr. Kegel, who developed a successful perineal exercise routine in the 1940s, prescribed three 20-minute sessions per day, but even 10 minutes per day will strengthen the muscles as opposed to doing nothing at all. There is no need to stop all other activities to do these exercises once you are familiar with them; they can be practiced during work, at the movie, or driving a car, and no one else will ever know!

If you are uncertain how to do a Kegel exercise, try stopping the flow of urine mid-stream when voiding. These are the same muscles used for a Kegel. Use this as a way to identify the muscles to be toned, but do not practice with the urine flow regularly, especially with a full or irritated bladder, as the bladder can become aggravated by the practice.

Beginning Kegels

Once you know which muscles to use, begin with the following:

1. Sit in a chair with feet flat on the floor. Inhale.
2. On the exhalation slowly press the knees and inner thighs together, contracting the vaginal muscles at the same time. Hold until exhalation is completed or 6 seconds.
3. Relax with an inhalation and repeat the tightening and relaxing practice for 5 to 20 minutes.

Intermediate Kegels

When the beginning exercise is easy, start practicing Intermediate Kegels:

1. Sit or lie in comfortable position. Close your eyes. Allow your breath to fill your pelvic area and imagine there is a small elevator full of people in your pelvis that will rise from the bottom of your perineum up to your navel.
2. As you exhale, squeeze the perineal muscles, bringing the "elevator" slowly up toward the navel or to the highest level it can to go. Hold

there for at least 6 seconds and imagine all the people getting off! Breathe normally while holding the contraction.
3. Now, on another exhalation, slowly lower the elevator, one floor at a time, back to ground level.
4. Relax and repeat as many times as possible.
5. On some occasions, bring the "elevator" all the way to the "basement," pushing slightly downward and allowing the perineum to relax.

Abdominals

The abdominal muscles help maintain the position of the inner organs and uterus, stabilize the low back, and control the angle of pelvic tilt—all important jobs during pregnancy. They also assist with breathing and are activated with any trunk flexion, pulling, straining for bowel movement, coughing, laughing, and pushing a baby at delivery. They are lined and covered by connective tissue that joins together at the linea alba between the xyphoid process and the pubic symphysis.

Four layers of abdominal muscles cross the anterior torso, vertically, horizontally, and diagonally, and are often described as being like a corset, with the rectus abdominus as a front vertical panel, the transverse abdominus crossing horizontally and the external and internal obliques overlapping each other on the sides.

Diastasis Recti

By the end of pregnancy, the abdominal muscles have stretched considerably. If they are weak, the abdominals will not provide the necessary upward and interior support. As they stretch, the fascial linea alba where the rectus abdominus inserts, begins to thin and stretch as well, causing the abdominal muscles to spread apart from the linea alba. It is normal to have a slight separation during pregnancy: some diastasis develop in the second trimester while most occur in the third trimester or while pushing during labor. Statistically, most separations tend to occur at or above the umbilicus, but in personal practice, I have found most below the navel.

If the abdominals separate an inch, or 2 fingerwidths, the condition is known as a **diastasis recti** (Figure 3.7). With a 3- to 4-fingerwidths separation, low back pain increases as abdominal support decreases. A severe diastasis recti can impact a woman's pregnancy and birth and cause long-term back discomfort. Women who are more prone to a serious separation often have one or more conditions in which the abdominals become larger than normal.

MASSAGE THERAPIST TIP

More About Strengthening the Pelvic Floor

*B*elow are some tips on helping your client understand and perform Kegel exercises:

- There are many ways to do Kegels. They can be done rapidly or slowly. A client can invent her own methods of practice. Use imagery to enhance the client's ability to sense the muscles, such as visualizing wringing out a sponge and then relaxing like the soft petals of a flower bud as it opens.
- Advanced Kegel exercises include focusing on squeezing each separate sphincter muscle individually—the anal, vaginal, and urethral sphincters.
- Kegels are most effective when the muscles at the upper-third and middle-third of the vagina are developed. Encourage your client to think "high." She may place one hand over her pubic bone or at her navel and envision that she can tighten the vagina to that level.
- Remind your client that quality is better than quantity for improving muscle tone.

- Remind your client to practice relaxing her breath while doing these exercises. There can be a tendency to hold the breath or clench the jaw when tightening the perineum.
- To prevent general strain on the perineal muscles, encourage your client to brace her abdominal muscles and do a Kegel squeeze before and during coughing, straining, or lifting.
- Some women may have very weak perineal tone and may be unable to hold a Kegel contraction at all or only for a very short time. With a regular practice regimen, the improvement will be rapid and obvious.
- Some women have a greater need for learning to relax the perineum, as opposed to strengthening. If she finds this is the case, she can practice releasing and relaxing the perineum by visualizing a softening of the pelvic floor, and pushing outward slightly as she exhales.

Traditional Birth Practices:
Support for the Belly

*I*n many parts of Latin America and South America, women in traditional cultures wrap a cloth shawl around their abdomen during the second part of pregnancy. This cloth usually wraps beneath the abdomen several times and ties in the back. It acts as a support for the stretched abdominal muscles, holding the weight of the uterus and relieving stress to the low back. With this type of anterior support, as well as its constant pressure against the low back, postural issues may not develop as intensely as they could for a woman who has a large belly, weak abdominals, and no external support.

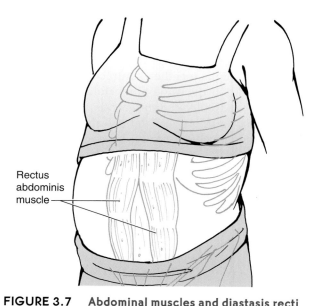

Rectus abdominis muscle

FIGURE 3.7   Abdominal muscles and diastasis recti
The abdominal muscles support the torso like a corset. With the stretching of the belly, the fascial linea alba thins and stretches, sometimes causing the rectus abdominus to separate in a diastasis recti.

Possible contributing factors to diastasis recti are listed in Box 3.4. Be aware of these risk factors as you work with your client, and teach her proper body mechanics for getting on and off your massage table to help avoid undue strain to the abdominals.

BOX 3.4 | Conditions Contributing to Diastasis Recti

Pregnancy Risks

- Large baby for the mother's size
- Multiple pregnancy (twins or more)
- Excessive amniotic fluid (polyhydramnios)
- Multiple births without sufficient recovery time between
- Pushing hard at birth with weak muscles
- Relaxin and estrogen softening and weakening connective tissue

General Risks

- Obesity
- General weakness due to lack of exercise
- Straining due to constipation
- Previous hernias or diastasis recti
- Improper body mechanics when repositioning from lying to sitting or standing

---

When Diastasis Occurs

Many women do not know when or if their abdominals have separated. There is often no obvious sensation or sign when it occurs; it may happen over a period of time, and it is not generally painful to the abdominal muscles. However, a woman with a diastasis of 3 or more fingerwidths will lack the anterior support for carrying the weight of the baby. Without the normal abdominal support, the posterior spinal muscles compensate and become strained and taut as they attempt to maintain a woman's posture without anterior assistance. The woman may complain of nagging low backache and may notice a strange bulging somewhere along her linea alba when her belly is flexed, as the abdominal contents are pushed through the opening. In extreme cases of diastasis recti, the bulge of the baby may be seen protruding through the opening quite distinctly.

Bodywork Considerations for Diastasis Recti

Below are some things to consider when adapting bodywork for women with diastasis recti:

- Ask your client whether she has experienced diastasis recti in pregnancy and/or postpartum, and if so, suggest that she consult with a physical therapist about preventative and corrective exercises, or read Elizabeth Noble's book, *Essential Exercises for the Childbearing Year,* which describes in detail methods of preventing and repairing diastasis recti. (See Appendix B, Resources of the Practitioner.) Many women find that prenatal Pilates and yoga classes, which focus on developing this core abdominal strength, can be helpful.
- Offer proper support for the pregnant belly in the second and third trimesters when positioning the client sidelying. (See Positioning, Chapter 5.)
- Teach the client proper body mechanics for rising from lying to sitting. (See "Massage Therapist Tip" below.)
- Suggest the use of an abdominal support binder in late pregnancy for women with especially large abdomens.

When to Assess for Diastasis Recti

Assessment for diastasis recti should be done when beginning work with a client *in the first trimester* who has had previous births (and therefore may have a diastasis already) and who you expect to see throughout pregnancy, or when you have a postpartum client. This will help you ascertain risk for and cause of some back discomforts, and establish the need for corrective exercises. An assessment can be done anytime there is reason to think a separation may have occurred. Remember that if this is a woman's second or more baby, she may begin this pregnancy with a separation which developed in a previous pregnancy and of which she may be unaware.

In the late second and through the third trimester, when the abdomen is large, corrective exercises could possibly aggravate or worsen her condition if she already has a significant separation. An *assessment* can be done however, if needed, if she has predisposing factors toward separation or she is complaining of chronic backache. If a diastasis is found, she can discuss with her prenatal care provider about the benefits of using an abdominal support girdle and about possible referral to a physical therapist who might be able to assist her in preventing further separation of the rectus during the final stages of her pregnancy.

Case Study 3.1:
EXTREME DIASTASIS OF THE RECTUS ABDOMINUS

Caitlin had been in labor for several hours and was now pushing when her massage therapist, Ann, came in the room to support her. This was Caitlin's fourth child. The other three were ages 5, 3, and 2. Caitlin's abdominal muscles had had little time to recover between births, and she had complained for months during this pregnancy about hip and back pain.

As Ann helped Caitlin lean forward to push with the coming contraction, she saw a large bulging shape in Caitlin's abdomen. As she pushed, a pointed, moving form slid and pressed out through the abdominal wall, looking, as Ann said later, like an alien emerging from Caitlin's belly. Caitlin had an enormous diastasis recti, and the baby's arms, elbows, legs, or feet kept pushing forward through the abdomen as the mother strained with pushing.

Caitlin said she had noticed the baby poking through now and then over the past months, but had not been instructed after the prior pregnancy in ways of correcting the separation. She had not realized that it was contributing to her back pain.

Several weeks after delivery, Caitlin came to see Ann for a massage. Ann subsequently assessed her abdominal diastasis and found a separation the size of 4 fingerwidths. Having watched how the baby pushed through the abdomen when Caitlin was holding her breath and pushing, Ann realized why it is important to do corrective exercises on an exhalation. The increased abdominal pressure with breath-holding forced the abdominal contents through the rectus separation. She showed Caitlin simple curl-up exercises and had Caitlin push her abdominals together with her hands when she did the curl-up. She also passed on contact information for a local physical therapist who could help her with more in-depth muscle strengthening to correct the separation.

It took Caitlin many months to begin to notice the gap in her abdominals getting smaller. It was difficult for her to find time to focus on corrective exercises, but she did her best to continue the abdominal strengthening and other exercises prescribed by her physical therapist. After 6 months, according to her report to Ann, she was feeling stronger and more stable in her hips and low back.

How to Assess

Essentially, to activate the abdominals to assess for a diastasis, the client must do an abdominal crunch. The following is the method for a client in her first trimester:

1. Have client lie supine with knees bent.
2. Place your fingers just below and above her navel in the center of abdomen.
3. Have the client exhale while slowly raising her head off ground. This will activate her abdominals. In the first trimester, if the abdominals do not tighten well enough to palpate, ask her to lift her shoulders off the ground along with her head (Figure 3.8).

 CAUTION: Ensure that the client exhales during the head lift muscle activation. Breath holding with exertion will increase intra-abdominal pressure and could increase the diastasis.

4. With her abdominals contracted, press lightly on the linea alba and slide your fingertips laterally until you reach the edge of the abdominals, which will feel rigid. If there is no gap, your fingers may not move at all before touching the muscular edge. If there is a gap, your fingertips may slide out to either side 1 or more inches. Measure in fingerwidths by extending your fingers together between the edges of the abdominal wall.

 CAUTION: If you feel the need to check in the late second or in the third trimester, the separation may be visually apparent as a bulge. Do not press your fingers into the abdomen, but instead observe for this bulge just above or below the navel.

A slight gap of 1 to 2 fingers is considered normal. Three fingers or more indicates the need for corrective exercises. Even without a gap, preventative exercises, such as abdominal crunches and those taught by a physical therapist, practiced in prenatal Pilates classes, or learned from Noble's book mentioned above, should be started in the first trimester and continued through the pregnancy. The good news about diastasis recti is that minor separations of less than 2 fingerwidths tend to correct themselves in postpartum even without specific exercise, and larger ones are generally correctible with exercise.

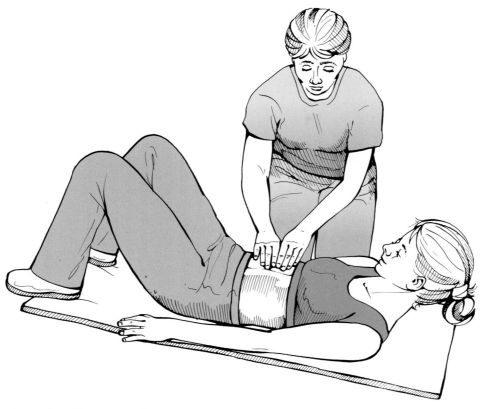

FIGURE 3.8   Assessing diastasis recti.

Have client lay supine and lift head while exhaling. Palpate above or below navel on linea alba for a gap between edges of rectus abdominus.

Psoas

The iliopsoas is a primary hip flexor that helps support the low back, the fetus, and the abdominal contents. It orients the tilt of the pelvis, helps hold the body upright, and stabilizes the spine and pelvis. In pregnancy, as the ligaments that normally stabilize the low back and pelvis are stretched and softened by relaxin and estrogen, they become less reliable and the psoas must work harder. When your client is standing, a tight psoas will pull down on the anterior lumbar vertebrae rather than flex the hip; this action will cause shortening of the lumbar spinal muscles and an increased anterior pelvic tilt (Figure 3.9).

A circular problem develops: when the psoas tightens, the anterior pelvic tilt increases; when the anterior pelvic tilt increases, the uterine weight shifts forward. With the weight fallen more forward, the abdominals stretch and lose tone, causing an even greater increase in pelvic rotation. In addition, if the psoas is tighter on one side than the other, pelvic alignment will shift, causing strain and discomfort on the entire side of the body that is trying to compensate for the imbalance. A tight or spasmed iliopsoas will

often be experienced as low back pain, sacroiliac pain, anterior thigh pain, sciatica sensations, and sometimes as pain in the iliacus area. It may also cause concomitant dysfunctional adaptations with the hips, knees, upper back, lower back, neck, feet, and ankles.

To address this issue, the psoas must be stretched and toned to release tension on the lumbar spine and to allow the pelvis to support the spine most efficiently (see the section "Low Back Pain" in Chapter 5). Postural education is also a very important tool to assist the psoas in supporting a properly balanced pelvis.

 CAUTION: The psoas should not be massaged with direct hand or finger pressure at any time during pregnancy. While the psoas can be accessed during the first trimester without touching the uterus, it is avoided, since deep abdominal massage is contraindicated during the first trimester due to the desire to avoid associations between bodywork and miscarriages that occur commonly in the first trimester. (This is discussed in more detail in Chapter 4.)

Case Study 3.2:
POSTURAL ASSESSMENT

Cindy saw her new pregnant client, Lynn, walking up the path to her office. Lynn was holding her back with one hand and appeared to be waddling slightly as she walked. She was 38 weeks pregnant in her fourth pregnancy, with three young children at home. Today was her first massage with Cindy. From her health intake form and through questions during the initial interview, Cindy learned that her client had been having generalized back pain for the past 4 weeks of her pregnancy, and had found little to relieve it. She said the pain was a general aching across her low back. She indicated the area by placing her hand just above her posterior ilium and along the QL. At times she felt twinges of pain down her left leg. She said she felt general tension in her neck and shoulders and was tired of being pregnant. Her doctor told her these were normal pains that she could expect from being pregnant. She otherwise had had no abnormal or high-risk conditions and no other discomforts, apart for some morning sickness in the first months. She stated that she was carrying an extra 25 pounds or so that she had gained during the last pregnancies and had not lost.

Cindy asked Lynn to stand in a relaxed posture for a moment so she could observe her stance. She noted that Lynn's hips, knees, and feet were laterally rotated. Lynn's tendency was to hold her low back with one hand, and arch her back to support the weight of her abdomen. Cindy also noted that Lynn's belly seemed larger than most clients' she had seen at this stage. She was aware that the size of the woman's belly at any particular stage of pregnancy was dependent on the size of the baby, the position the baby tended to favor, and the tone of the mother's abdominals. Lynn stated that this baby was bigger than her others, and that they expected it to be at least 8 or 9 pounds.

When asked about exercise, Lynn stated that she had never had an exercise routine. During the early part of this pregnancy, she had been so nauseous that she had stopped doing even the more basic activities that she had once participated in. She said she was busy enough as a mother of three and got exercise lifting and carrying the children.

Reassured that Lynn had presented her discomforts to her doctor and that no abnormalities had been found with Lynn's pregnancy, Cindy considered several factors that might be affecting Lynn's backache:

1. Mother of young children: Cindy knew this entailed frequent lifting, leaning over with the weight of a baby or child to put him or her in a car seat, and carrying children on one hip, shifting posture to the side to carry the child.
2. Fourth pregnancy: Cindy realized that the more pregnancies and deliveries a woman has had, the more risk she has for loss of abdominal tone, hypermobile ligaments, and diastasis recti.
3. Lack of exercise: Without regular strengthening exercise, Lynn was more at risk for developing stresses and strains during and after pregnancy.
4. Excess weight: With Lynn's extra weight gain on top of her pregnancy weight, she also increased her risk of diastasis recti and low back pain.
5. Poor posture: Lynn's poor posture, exacerbated by her weak muscle tone, also increased the strain on her muscles.
6. Large breasts: Lynn had large breasts, which influenced her posture as well, causing her to sink in her upper chest, resulting in upper back and neck pain.

Cindy helped Lynn notice how she was standing at the moment, and then suggested that she move her feet hip width apart, and turn her feet so they faced straight forward. Holding onto Lynn's heels, she encouraged her to sink her energy into the floor, feeling the soles of her feet grounded on the floor. Then she slid her hand up the back of Lynn's legs, sacrum, and spine to reach her cervical spine, where she pulled up under her occiput and encouraged Lynn to inhale deeply, expanding her ribs and chest. For several breaths, Cindy encouraged Lynn to imagine being 2 feet taller than she was, with that length rising up from her feet, all the way through her head. Lynn was shocked at how much more easily she could fill her lungs, and how much tension immediately left her low back. Postural awareness had not been something she had considered with regard to her pregnancy discomforts.

On the massage table, Cindy spent a moment assessing Lynn's abdominals in the supine position, asking her to exhale, and raise her head slowly. She immediately saw a bulging ridge in the middle of Lynn's abdomen and assumed she might have a diastasis of the rectus muscles. She explained what this was and all the factors that would contribute to this. Cindy suggested that Lynn have her doctor assess it further to confirm it, or have it reassessed after birth when she could begin strengthening exercise.

Cindy offered to work with Lynn on postural correction over the next weeks, and during postpartum, and showed her where to get information about corrective exercises.

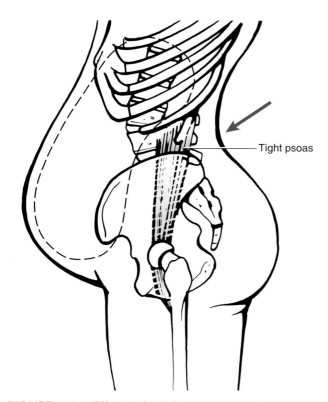

— Tight psoas

FIGURE 3.9   Effects of a tight psoas on posture.
When your client is standing, a tight psoas will pull down on the anterior lumbar vertebrae, rather than flexing the hip; this action will cause shortening of the lumbar spinal muscles and an increased anterior pelvic tilt.

Note: Despite the contraindication of abdominal massage during the first trimester, if useful and if agreeable to the client, gentle myofascial work just inside the iliac fossa without going deep into the abdomen, can be appropriate, even in the first trimester. Below are some bodywork considerations for the psoas.

- Encourage the client to explore comfortable ways of stretching the psoas herself, such as in the lunge position. (See Chapter 6)
- Assisted stretches while on the massage table will help alleviate problems associated with tight psoas.

Quadratus Lumborum

The QL is an important stabilizer of the low back that assists spinal extension when it bilaterally contracts, helps the trunk flex laterally, and fixes the twelfth rib during respiration. It extends from the posterior iliac crest to the lower border of the twelfth rib and attaches on the lumbar transverse processes. In pregnancy it becomes shortened due to anterior pelvic tilt and lumbar lordosis. Many women may experience

soreness, spasm, or general aching in the QL during pregnancy, yet many others are unaware of its tension and relation to their low back discomfort until it is touched with massage. Due to a mother's increased hip and waist size, it can be difficult, yet still important, to access this muscle during pregnancy and help it release with massage and stretches.

Below are some bodywork considerations for the QL:

- See the section "Low Back Pain" in Chapter 5 for specific ways of working with the QL.
- Passively stretch the QL while the client is in the sidelying position, by using a wedge or pillow under her waist, extending her waist on her upper side. (See Figure 6.2A.)
- Encourage the client to explore comfortable ways of stretching the QL herself. (See Chapter 6.)

CHAPTER SUMMARY

Primary musculature is stressed by pregnancy due to normal weight gain and necessary adjustments in posture to support the anterior weight of a growing baby. The psoas, QL, pelvic floor muscles and the abdominals are core muscles that support and stabilize the pelvis during pregnancy. Using the information in this chapter, you can help a client have a sensory understanding of appropriate posture for her stage of pregnancy. By reviewing her posture at each massage session or least once each trimester, along with suggesting resources for learning to stretch and strengthen primary muscles, you will give your client some tools that aid her search for comfort and stability. In this chapter you learned the importance of muscular strengthening and stretching, and of postural and abdominal assessments. In later chapters you will learn bodywork and particular ways to address these core stabilizing muscles.

CHAPTER REVIEW QUESTIONS

1. Name three muscle groups especially affected by the weight gain and postural changes of pregnancy.
2. Stand in an exaggerated strained pregnancy posture. Which areas of your body feel particularly stressed after just a few moments? Describe how to help a client make adjustments to this posture.
3. Name three factors that have particularly strong influence on pregnancy posture. What postural changes are common to develop during pregnancy?
4. Explain why the iliopsoas is an influential muscle in a pregnant woman's posture.

5. Explain why proper positioning on the table and body mechanics for getting on and off the table are particularly important during pregnancy.
6. Describe what kind of symptoms a woman with uterosacral ligament spasms might experience.
7. Name three benefits of perineal exercises.
8. If a client with three young children came to see you during her fourth pregnancy at 34 weeks, with a pendulous belly and complaining of low back pain, what condition might you suspect could possibly be contributing to her back pain? What would you suggest or how would you treat her?
9. Describe two ways of helping a woman with a large abdomen decrease her risk of straining uterine ligaments. Describe how a client should move from sidelying to sitting position to prevent uterine ligament strain.
10. After the late second trimester, corrective exercises for a diastasis recti are generally not recommended to be started. Explain why this is so and when they can be started.

REFERENCES

1. Carr CA. Use of a maternity support binder for relief of pregnancy-related back pain. J Obstet Gynecol Neonatal Nurs 2003;32 (4): 495–502.
2. Hall DC, Kaufmann DA. Effects of aerobic and strength conditioning on pregnancy outcomes. Am J Obstet Gynecol 1987;157(5):1199–1203.
3. Clapp JF 3rd. The course of labor after endurance exercise during pregnancy. Am J Obstet Gyneco. 1990;163(6 Pt 1):1799–1805.
4. Varrassi G, Bazzano C, Edwards WT. Effects of physical activity on maternal plasma beta-endorphin levels and perception of labor pain. Am J Obstet Gynecol 1989;160(3):707–712.
5. Bungum TJ, Peaslee DL, Jackson AW, et al. Exercise during pregnancy and type of delivery in nulliparae. J Obstet Gynecol Neonatal Nurs 2000;29(3): 258-64.
6. Polden M, Mantel J. Physiotherapy in Obstetrics and Gynaecology. London: Butterworth-Heinemann, 1990.
7. Schauberger CW, Rooney BL, Goldsmith L, et al. Peripheral joint laxity increases in pregnancy but does not correlate with serum relaxin levels. Am J Obstet Gyn 1996;174(2):667–671.
8. Health information. Pelvic floor disorders. National Institute of Child Health and Human Development. Last updated: 1/10/2007. Accessed at http://www.nichd.nih.gov/health/topics/Pelvic_Floor_Disorders.cfm.
9. Pelvic floor disorders. University of Southern California Center for Colorectal and Pelvic Floor Disorders. Last accessed 5-30-2007 online at: http://www.surgery.usc.edu/divisions/cr/pelvicfloordisorders.html.

CHAPTER 4

PRECAUTIONS AND CONTRAINDICATIONS FOR BODYWORK DURING PREGNANCY

LEARNING OBJECTIVES

After reading this chapter, you should be able to:

- Discern when the use of a medical release prior to massage is indicated and when to refer a client to her prenatal care provider based on symptoms that might indicate pregnancy-related problems.

- Describe the most common bodywork-technique precautions for pregnancy and be able to determine in which situations they would apply.

- Describe the difference between sedating and potentially stimulating type bodywork and the precautions or contraindications associated with each.

- Describe high-risk obstetric conditions and their relevant bodywork precautions.

- Develop health intake and medical release forms that address specific bodywork concerns related to pregnant clients.

- Identify specific acupressure points that are contraindicated for use during pregnancy.

- Ask discerning questions to help identify pain as possibly a concerning condition of pregnancy or as purely musculoskeletal.

- Understand the importance of a thorough health intake at an initial visit and update at each subsequent visit.

- Describe three potential consequences of improper client positioning during pregnancy massage.

- Name the three most important safety concerns for a therapist working with a pregnant woman.

*M*ost pregnant women in the United States will have a normal perinatal period without looming dangers to the safety and health of herself or her baby, and without need for medical interventions.[1,2] The majority of pregnant women who come for massage and bodywork sessions will also be healthy and will need few bodywork restrictions. However, while appreciating pregnancy as a normal physiological passage in many women's lives, all pregnancies do have associated risks, and some will become classified as "high risk." A bodyworker must be aware of precautions, contraindications, and various bodywork guidelines that are important to observe not only for the client with a normal pregnancy, but for those with minor or more serious risk factors. The massage therapist needs to be educated about what conditions are normal and what symptoms or conditions indicate that a client should be referred to her prenatal care provider (PCP) or perhaps to a more experienced pregnancy massage therapist. (See Box 4.1 for a list of these symptoms.)

This chapter begins by clarifying bodywork terminology that is used hereafter in the text, specifically what is meant by "Type I" and "Type II" touch. Then, information on health intake and assessment questions specifically relevant to working with pregnant clients is presented, including an explanation of obtaining a medical release. Next, we consider precautions that are needed for specific types of bodywork. General conditions considered by the American College of Obstetrics and Gynecology to increase risk during pregnancy, and which have a few particular

BOX 4.1 | Symptoms Requiring Referral to the Primary Care Provider

Refer a client to her primary care provider for the following symptoms:

- Abdominal Discomfort
  - Tender or painful abdomen or unexplained pain in abdomen
  - Right upper quadrant abdominal pain
- Leg pain
  - Pain or aching in the leg
  - Unidentified leg pain
  - Swelling, heat, tenderness in leg
- Uterine Cramping
  - Intermittent or regular uterine cramping before 36 weeks

- More than four preterm contractions an hour for 2 hours
- Malaise
  - Increasing malaise, dizziness, visual changes, right-sided upper abdominal pain, and/or nausea
- Bleeding or leaking fluid
  - Unexplained vaginal bleeding
  - Sudden gush or slow leak of liquid from vagina (amniotic fluid should be clear, but could also be greenish, or port wine color)
- Pain
  - Any unexplained pain or discomfort that is severe, sudden, nagging, or worrisome

---

considerations for bodywork, are then defined. The intention of these descriptions is to help the therapist understand *why* the situation is considered an obstetrical risk, and how massage can be adapted to the particular situation.

Finally, high-risk obstetrical complications that the prenatal massage therapist may encounter are explored.

PRIMARY CONSIDERATIONS FOR PREGNANCY MASSAGE

Most of the massage students' and therapists' fears about working with pregnant women are not actual dangers. The three most significant real concerns for a pregnancy massage therapist are listed as follows:

1. Proper positioning: Improper positioning of a client during pregnancy can be a danger for both mother and baby by interfering with uterine blood flow and resulting in maternal hypotension, nausea, syncope (fainting) and ultimately shock, along with consequent effects on a baby. Ligament strain, sacro-iliac pain and misalignment, leg cramps, and brachial plexus compression can all be aggravated by inadequate support and improper positioning on the massage table. Methods of positioning will be discussed in detail in Chapter 5.
2. Blood Clots: During pregnancy, the *risk* for developing a blood clot or *thrombus* is greatly

increased (see the section "Circulatory System" in Chapter 2). Because massage may have the capacity to stimulate circulation through the blood vessels and increase the risk for dislodging a clot, only gentle touch should be used on the legs of pregnant and postpartum clients, and at times, no touch at all. Massage is always contraindicated to legs with thrombophlebitis or deep vein thrombosis (DVT). Thankfully, despite the increased risk, the actual incidence of a clot becoming an embolism during pregnancy is low. This issue is discussed in greater depth later in this chapter.

3. High-Risk Pregnancies: Pregnancies that become categorized as high-risk hold the potential for serious complications to a mother and/or baby. In these situations, there are usually restrictions to the type or quality of bodywork given and a medical release is necessary before offering bodywork. When a mother has a high-risk condition, excessively stimulating or deep, full-body or abdominal massage could possibly increase risks in some situations. This is also discussed later in this chapter.

Consideration of these issues is of primary importance during each perinatal massage. Throughout this chapter, and throughout the book, these three topics are addressed where relevant, and recommendations for the massage therapist are provided. In addition to these areas of precaution, it is also important to remember that any standard massage contraindications and

Table 4.1 Review of Standard Massage Precautions for All Clients	
Local Contraindications	**Precautions for All Type I Bodywork (A medical release is required and possibly only Type II techniques may be permitted.)**
Acute skin injuries/burns	Cancer
Acute arthritis	Severe hypertension
Acute bursitis	Circulatory and cardiac conditions
Communicable skin conditions, irritation, or discharge	Convulsive disorder
Varicose veins	Type I diabetes
Vertebral disk problem	Infectious disease
	Pitting edema due to heart/kidney problems
	Kidney disease or kidney stones
	Thrombophlebitis or blood clot

precautions—such as avoidance of inflamed or infected skin—that are applicable to nonpregnant clients, still apply in pregnancy. The massage therapist is responsible to know these standard massage precautions (see Table 4.1 for a list of these precautions).

As you read this chapter, keep in mind that it is most important to understand *why* particular precautions and contraindications exist. With that knowledge, you can make skilled and sound decisions about what kind of bodywork is appropriate in each individual case.

Note: Many massage therapists will never encounter a pregnant client with a dangerous high-risk complication. Once trained, others will intentionally choose to offer massage to a higher-risk population. This chapter is meant to be a useful resource for all practitioners. Refer here for information regarding conditions of which you are uncertain about the appropriateness of bodywork. Rather than immediately refusing to work on a client who says she has a "risk" condition, turn to this chapter to see if you can determine if the condition actually poses a *bodywork* risk or not. By reading this chapter you may learn standard types of precautions that can then be applied to other situations not listed here. Keep in mind, however, that safety is always primary, so w*hen in doubt, give a shout: ask for advice from someone more knowledgeable to ensure safety!* Always obtain advanced training in perinatal massage before working with high-risk pregnancies.

CLARIFICATION OF BODYWORK TERMINOLOGY: TYPE I, TYPE II

There are numerous schools of bodywork and modalities of touch. For purposes of clarification and simplification, this book divides bodywork into two categories: stimulating touch and gentle or subtle energy touch. When listing contraindications to massage, it can be too limiting and ill-defined to simply state that "massage is contraindicated." When touch is gentle and nurturing, it can be used in nearly every situation. When it is vigorous or deep tissue, it will have some limitations. The differentiation between these two types of touch is made by referring to Type I and Type II styles of touch.

Type I: Stimulating

Type I massage and touch is generally more intensive and may be stimulating to the circulatory and/or musculoskeletal system, with a tendency to increase the release of cellular waste products. In this category are at least some of the techniques from the following modalities: vigorous Swedish, Rolfing, deep tissue, trigger point, sports massage, lomi lomi, and Shiatsu. This is not a comprehensive list. In the text, I may refer to this Type I work, as "deep," "stimulating," or "circulatory" bodywork. While Type I full-body Swedish massage may be contraindicated, this does not necessarily contraindicate all touch. Often, localized work on the extremities—hands, feet, neck, shoulders, head—or Type II full-body touch will still be appropriate.

Type II: Gentle

The second type of touch is physically gentle, nonforceful or nonintrusive, and does not stimulate the physical body in the same way as the above techniques. It is therefore appropriate in nearly every situation, even if Type I work is contraindicated. Type II techniques include, but are not limited to, the following: Swedish massage to the extremities or in localized areas, as well as light-touch, full-body Swedish massage, indirect myofascial release, gentle acupressure such as Jin Shin Jytsu, and subtle energy work such as Reiki, craniosacral therapy, or polarity therapy. I refer to these Type II bodywork modalities in the text as "gentle" or "energy-work." Except in the case of a communicable, contagious disease process, when contact with the infected person is contraindicated, *there is rarely a reason for Type II touch to be contraindicated.*

HEALTH INTAKE, ASSESSMENT QUESTIONS, AND MEDICAL RELEASE

Many massage practitioners use a standard health intake form with new clients. These forms generally do not address the specifics of pregnancy. Because a woman's pregnancy is constantly changing, with the possibility of developing risk conditions as the pregnancy progresses, it is important to have an intake form that addresses these special concerns of pregnancy. It is equally important to update your information *at each visit*, as a client may return with a new health condition that may indicate new precautions with bodywork. Obtaining and reviewing this information will not only give you perspective on the physical concerns your client may have, but can also enlighten you to emotional issues that she may be contending with and which may arise during bodywork sessions.

On review of the information received, you may, on rare occasions, need to cancel the session or resort to only Type II bodywork for the current session, asking her to return next time with a medical release indicating whether it is appropriate for her to have Type I bodywork. This will generally occur only if her symptoms have just recently developed and she has not yet been seen by her prenatal care provider. Some questions may be asked over the phone when an appointment is made to determine if a medical release seems appropriate prior to bodywork.

Figure 4.1 is an example of an acceptable health history intake form, which is devoted to pregnancy questions. The intake should include questions about how far along the client is in her pregnancy, what number pregnancy this is, and should identify potential risks or current complications. The form benefits the client as well as the therapist, as it indicates to her that you are aware of conditions of pregnancy. It also gives her a chance to review the health of her pregnancy relative to massage, and will bring to her mind the type of conditions that she should inform you of in the future, should her condition change. If the health intake is not done in writing, the therapist should at least ask the following questions:

1. *What number pregnancy is this? How many births has she had?*
   These are two different questions. A woman could have been pregnant five times but not have a child. She may have had miscarriages, abortions, or had a child die before or after birth. Her response to these questions will give you information to help evaluate risks during this pregnancy. If she has had three or more consecutive miscarriages, she will be considered higher risk for another miscarriage.[3] A woman who has had more than three full-term pregnancies, or has had two or more pregnancies following within a year of each other, will be more likely to experience varicose veins, diastasis recti, low back pain, and other back complaints. This information is useful to the massage therapist with regard to what type of bodywork precautions may be necessary, as well as to having an idea of the client's emotional state.

2. *How many weeks pregnant is she, which trimester is she in, or what is her due date?*
   Obtaining this information when an appointment is made will help you to determine ahead of time how to set up your massage table for her optimum comfort and safety and help you evaluate trimester-dependent precautions. It will also inform you if she is close to delivery time, which would allow you to use labor preparation techniques and prepare you for the possibility of her having early labor contractions during a session.

3. *Does she have a history of complications with this or other pregnancies?*
   Depending on what the previous complication or condition was, having formerly had a high-risk pregnancy may increase a woman's risk with this one, even if she is currently having no problems This would be particularly true with a history of preterm birth, placental abruption, or deep vein thrombosis, all of which have a risk of recurrence in a subsequent pregnancy.

4. *Is she currently having any high-risk conditions, complications, or physical concerns?*
   If she describes any conditions which indicate bodywork precautions, you will have to investigate further as to whether bodywork is appropriate at this visit, or whether you should obtain a medical release or have a discussion with her PCP before continuing.

CONFIDENTIAL HEALTH INTAKE FORM FOR PREGNANCY

Name _____   Date _____

Address _____

Phone _____

Emergency contact: Name _____   Phone _____

Prenatal Care Provider: Name _____   Phone _____

My due date is: _____

This is my _____ (1st, 2nd, etc) pregnancy and will be my _____ (1st, 2nd, etc) birth. I am _____ (number) weeks pregnant in my _____ (1st, 2nd, 3rd trimester).

In order to provide you with the best care possible during your pregnancy, it helps me to know of any complications or conditions that may require particular bodywork precautions. Please inform me, at each of our visits, of any changes in your pregnancy.

Please check ( ) current problems; mark with (+) if you have had one of these problems in the past.

_____ Sciatica   _____ Bladder infection*

_____ Nausea   _____ Uterine bleeding*

_____ Anemia   _____ Chronic hypertension*

_____ Edema/swelling   _____ Blood clot or phlebitis*

_____ Headaches   _____ High blood pressure*

_____ Low back pain   _____ Problems with placenta*

_____ Leg cramps   _____ Preterm labor*

_____ Insomnia   _____ Abdominal cramping*

_____ Carpal tunnel syndrome   _____ Preeclampsia*

_____ Skin disorders/athlete's foot   _____ More than 2 consecutive miscarriages*

_____ Separation of the symphysis pubis

_____ Diabetes (gestational or Type I)

_____ Separation of the abdominal muscles

_____ Any other problems in current or past pregnancy (provide details): _____

_____

I, _____, verify that I am experiencing a low risk / high risk (circle one) pregnancy according to my prenatal care provider. If I am currently having or develop complications (any conditions/symptoms listed above with *), I will discuss the condition with my massage therapist and wil have a medical release for bodywork signed by my prenatal care provider before continuing bodywork.

Signature _____

FIGURE 4.1   Health history intake form.

A health history should be obtained at the first prenatal massage visit, and updated at each subsequent visit.

5. *How is she feeling about this pregnancy?*
   This can be a casual question. It need not be direct, and may be assessed based on how she has expressed herself during the health intake. Do not assume that all women are enthusiastic about their pregnancy. Some are ambivalent about their situation and need time to adjust to this new reality. Some did

not plan to be or want to be pregnant. Other women have tried unsuccessfully for years to become pregnant or to maintain a pregnancy, and have finally resorted to vitro fertilization or other new technologies for becoming pregnant. Assess her relationship to her pregnancy to avoid making assumptions or an embarrassing faux pas with a casual comment. Your role as massage therapist is to offer a safe environment for her to receive nurturing touch and support for however she happens to be feeling at that point.

6. *Is she doing any exercise during her pregnancy?* This may give you an indication of her general health and orientation toward exercise and desire for referrals to others in your community should she have particular muscular aches that may benefit from prenatal yoga, swimming, or another exercise program recommended by her PCP. It will also give you a clue about her interest in self-care strengthening or stretching instruction.

Assessing Symptoms of Discomfort

Before beginning work with any client, it is important to collect the above health information that may affect your work. If a client presents at your office with a *new*

condition, or in the rare case of symptoms arising *during* a massage, a few discerning questions can help determine appropriate action and possibly identify whether symptoms indicate a problem of pregnancy. For instance, a symptom of mild abdominal pain could be a musculoskeletal concern, such as a tight or spasming psoas or uterine ligament, or could indicate a condition that needs medical attention, such as preterm contractions or urinary tract infection. Box 4.2 highlights common symptoms that may reflect both musculoskeletal and pregnancy-related conditions.

The client herself will often be aware of symptoms that should be assessed by her PCP, but the massage therapist should also be able to recognize a situation that requires bodywork precautions or is contraindicated for massage. As a massage therapist, you will never diagnose a condition of pregnancy, but do not hesitate to refer a client to her PCP for *any discomfort that has an unclear etiology, or which you or the client are concerned about.* If you encounter a concerning symptom, such as recent headaches and pitting edema (which will be explained later in the chapter) in the third trimester, first determine if the symptoms have been assessed recently by the client's PCP. If they have and it has been determined that the client is in no danger, your own worries can be alleviated. Avoid contemplating out loud all the possible ramifications of the symptoms. While at times they might indicate a

---

MASSAGE THERAPIST TIP
Addressing Client Health Information With Sensitivity

*P*regnant women in the United States have plenty of concerns on their minds. They are often consumed with thoughts about maintaining optimum fetal health, examining how their life will change with a new family member, or anxious about how they will fare through labor. Women come to their massage therapist to find renewal, relaxation, and recovery from their stresses and strains of daily life. It is the last place they expect to find more things to worry about or to feel judged for their choices. If, as a massage practitioner, you begin doing automatic assessment tests for deep vein thrombosis on every client, (as some students are taught to do), or requiring a medical release even when she has a low-risk pregnancy (as some spas require), or questioning every complaint with a fearful discussion of all the possible risks it could indicate, you could add to her stress, not relieve it. Simple, discerning questions, as discussed in this chapter, can indicate if a client should contact her PCP without overly increasing anxiety.

Care and respect in your responses is also needed when reviewing the personal information you receive during a health intake or while massaging your client. Everyone has personal opinions about sexuality, pregnancy, and birth choices. Common "hot" topics that may come up during a massage or intake process include abortion, in vitro fertilization, single parenting by choice, homosexual parenting, or birth control choices. Practice cultivating a safe environment by keeping your opinions to yourself, and letting your hands share their caring touch.

In accordance with creating a safe, nurturing space for your clients, remember that all your health-intake information and whatever your client discusses during her sessions is confidential and must remain within your office walls between the two of you. Letting your client know this ahead of time helps create that safe space.

BOX 4.2 | Common Symptoms That Could Indicate Problems of Pregnancy

Massage therapists may encounter pregnant clients asking for relief of the following symptoms. Some of these common complaints may indicate a more serious problem. Most musculoskeletal problems will get at least some relief from massage, whereas a medical problem will not improve with massage.

Mid to High Back Pain

1. Kidney stones or infection

2. Musculoskeletal

- Assess whether pain is sharp, shooting, or localized in kidney area, and unrelieved by massage.
- Kidney pain usually has more sudden onset.
- Musculoskeletal pain is likely relieved by massage.

Low Back Pain

1. Preterm labor.
2. Urinary Tract Infection (UTI)

3. Contractions

4. Musculoskeletal

- Musculoskeletal low back pain is common during pregnancy.
- Preterm labor may feel like backache, groin pressure, low abdominal ache, without sensation of contractions. May be irregular or constant.
- UTI symptoms include any or none of the following: low back pain, burning or frequent urination, low-grade fever, low abdominal pain. May be irregular or constant.
- Full-term contractions may be experienced in the low back, rather than abdomen.

Groin Pain and Pressure

1. Preterm labor

2. Urinary tract infection
3. Contractions

4. Separated symphysis pubis

5. Pulled round ligament

- Preterm labor may be experienced as groin pressure. May be irregular or constant.
- UTI may be experienced as low abdominal pain or pressure.
- Separated symphysis pubis is often painful with walking, and with abduction of hips. May feel tender to the touch in pubic area.
- Round ligament pain may feel like low abdominal or groin pain; often sharp and sudden like muscle cramp. May be relieved with flexion of hip.

Headache/Heartburn/ Edema/ Severe Persistent Back Pain/Nausea

1. Preeclampsia, gestational hypertension, HELLP syndrome
2. Normal aches and pains of pregnancy

- Headaches, heartburn, edema, back pain, and nausea are all common and nonpathological complaints during pregnancy, but above symptoms also can indicate preeclampsia.
- Client should see health provider if above symptoms have not been assessed and are experienced as a new group of symptoms, or if headache is unrelieved by Tylenol or massage, if client is seeing spots or visual changes, or has pitting edema.

Pain in Leg or Calf

1. Possible blood clot

2. Leg cramps common in pregnancy,

- Sharp pain or aching pain in calf or leg should be assessed for recent musculoskeletal injury or activity, new shoes, poor posture.
- Assess for redness, swelling, streaking, or inflammation in area indicating especially at night possible clot.
- Refer client to care provider for unexplained leg or calf pain.

problem, they can also be very normal conditions of pregnancy, with no concern for the mother's or the baby's safety.

If symptoms are new and the client is concerned enough about them to want to call her PCP, she should be immediately supported to do so. *Always listen to intuitive or "gut" feelings if they are urging caution.* Even if all other signs indicate there is not a problem, our intuitive mind often picks up on cues that we miss with our rational mind.

If the symptoms have not been assessed by the PCP, ask further appropriate, discerning questions that define the discomfort as specifically as possible, as discussed below. If you are uncertain about the condition, suggest that she call her PCP to verify if she should be seen right away, or if there are any restrictions for body-work in relation to this condition. By asking questions, the massage practitioner may avoid assuming that all sensations are dangerous and pregnancy-related, or that all sensations are musculoskeletally-based.

1. *Has this been assessed by her primary care provider recently? Has the discomfort increased since that visit?* If symptoms have increased and she was told to report changes, she should call her PCP before beginning body-work.

2. *Where exactly does she feel it?* To help clarify, have her point to the area of discomfort. Some describe a "belly ache" and point to the pubic bone, while others will point to the liver area. Knowing where it is located can help define it. Any sensations in the abdomen that are not easily identifiable, or sensations elsewhere that are not clearly musculoskeletal should be referred to the PCP for further assessment. Keep in mind that uterine sensations, such as contractions, may be felt in the legs, pelvis, and groin, as well as the abdomen.

3. *What is the quality of the discomfort?* Massage therapists generally learn to assess nerve, ligament, and muscular pain, such as sharp, shooting, and burning sensations that are often related to nerve pain or ligament spasm. Dullness and aching may be related to muscle soreness, uterine cramping, or possibly organ dysfunction of some sort.

4. *Is the sensation intermittent or is it constant? Does it refer elsewhere in the body?* Contractions are typically intermittent. Muscular spasms may be intermittent sharp pain that can radiate and may include a constant, localized aching. Constant unchanging or increasing pain in the abdomen may reflect developing problems with the uterus, placenta, or baby,

or a condition such as a urinary tract or kidney infection, and the client should call her PCP right away.

A note about contractions: Most women experience mild, intermittent tightening of the uterus in the latter part of pregnancy (or sooner for women who have had more than one birth). These have been commonly called Braxton-Hicks contractions, or "practice" contractions. They are irregular, nonrhythmic, sensations of the uterus that do not increase in amplitude and do not change the cervix. It is important not to ignore the potential for preterm labor by *assuming* that any mild uterine sensations are merely these types of normal tightenings. However, it is equally important not to be nervous each time a woman's uterus tightens. One contraction does not mean labor or preterm labor has begun. A general guideline is that if a woman is having *regular* or frequent tightenings of her uterus (more than four per hour for a period of 2 hours) her PCP should be called.

5. *Does repositioning or touch help relieve the pain? Does she know what relieves it and what makes it worse?* Generally musculoskeletal pain will increase with movement, and lessen with positional or postural changes that alleviate muscle tension or spasm. Massage will often help relieve muscular pain.

6. *Is it tender if palpated? Is it inflamed with redness, swelling, or heat?* Tenderness upon palpation might give more indication of muscular discomfort if you can touch a specific muscle where it hurts. Inflammation should be reported to the PCP.

A tender abdomen is not normal and the client should be referred immediately to her PCP if she feels pain on touching her abdomen. Sharp or aching pain in the leg, or unidentified leg pain, especially with redness, edema of the extremity, or localized swelling or heat associated with it, should also be referred to the PCP for evaluation of a possible blood clot.

Having the client describe the discomfort will give you some information to start with. You also might explore more about the discomfort in relation to her pregnancy. These questions would include the following:

1. *How long has she had the pain?* If it just started when she got on the table, perhaps she pulled a ligament or muscle while positioning herself. If she has had the discomfort for weeks,

she may have visited her PCP already and been given some idea of what is causing the discomfort. If her discomfort has increased since her last prenatal visit, she should call her PCP.

2. *When is her next appointment with her prenatal care provider?* If she has experienced the pain for days, but has not seen her provider recently, find out when her next visit is. She may want to call her PCP to determine if she needs to be seen sooner.

3. *What does she think is the cause of the discomfort? Has she experienced it before?* Many women will know or have a sense of what has caused the discomfort or it may feel familiar from a previous pregnancy.

4. *How far along in her pregnancy is she?* This should already have been discussed in your general intake process and be in your mind as you review her symptoms. Headache and nausea during the first trimester can be normal and would more likely be related to hormonal issues or dehydration, while in the third trimester, complications of pregnancy such as preeclampsia or HELLP syndrome might be considered. This will be discussed later in this chapter.

Medical Release

A written **medical release** is a form signed by your client's prenatal care provider which indicates approval, from an obstetrical viewpoint, for massage at this point during her pregnancy, and which can indicate restrictions or concerns applicable to massage. When working with women with a high-risk condition, obtaining a release may be valuable for several reasons:

- Clarification of limits and risks: While the client will normally have been told what types of restrictions her condition requires, a release from the PCP can clarify limitations, restrictions, or risks of which you must be aware of with bodywork. After obtaining this information you can decide whether you are comfortable working with a client with this condition. Your nurturing touch will never adversely affect the pregnancy, but if you have insecurities for any reason, your uncertain energy will be transmitted to the client through your tactile and verbal contact, and will not provide her with optimum comfort. The medical release may help to alleviate your worries.
- Liability: Some hope that a medical release form could reduce legal liabilities should a

lawsuit regarding the woman and baby's care arise. This is a concern that is especially pertinent in the litigious-prone United States, where 76% of obstetricians have reported to the American College of Obstetrics and Gynecology that they have been sued at least once, with an average of 2.6 times in their careers.[4]

- Building a referral base: Obtaining a medical release could help you to establish a relationship with the midwife or doctor by making the provider aware that the client is receiving or wants to receive massage. It will help you to become familiar with local medical providers and give you an opportunity to share with them the benefits of touch for pregnancy and ensure that you are included, at least peripherally, as part of a circle of support working to help a woman have the best pregnancy and birth experience possible. By sharing in this process, medical providers may also come to view you as a resource and may refer clients to you or allow you to display our business cards in their office.

Some practitioners choose to obtain a medical release before working with any pregnant client. This is due to perceptions of pregnancy as a dangerous condition, or concerns that the pregnant woman will not inform the therapist of relevant risk factors. If it is your policy to have a medical release for all your clients, then obtaining one for your pregnant clients would be consistent. However, *a release for massage is not necessary for clients with a normal, low-risk pregnancy,* unless the client (or therapist) would feel more at ease having a form signed by her PCP confirming in writing that massage is safe for her.

The most appropriate time to use a medical release form is if a new client presents to you with a high-risk condition or if a current client develops a condition of which you are uncertain about bodywork restrictions. See Box 4.3 for a list of conditions for which a medical release is most highly indicated and recommended. If you choose not to use a release, but have questions about a particular condition, do research, or call her PCP's office and ask what kinds of risks are associated with that condition. You will not be given information specific to your client, due to privacy issues, but you may be able to obtain general risk information or resources for obtaining more information about the type of condition she has.

You can develop your own release form that suits your practice and clientele. The form should include a list of contraindications, and/or of acceptable bodywork techniques that the PCP can check if pertinent to

BOX 4.3 | Conditions for Which to Obtain a Medical Release for Bodywork

- Hypertensive disorders including:
  - Preeclampsia
  - HELLP syndrome (Type II as well as Type I bodywork may be contraindicated, depending on the severity of the client's condition.)
  - Severe chronic hypertension
  - Moderate to severe gestational hypertension
- Placental dysfunctions including
  - Placenta previa
  - History of partial placenta abruption in this pregnancy
  - History of placenta abruption in former pregnancy
  - Symptoms of bleeding

- Miscarriage or premature labor or birth
  - Preterm labor in this pregnancy
  - History of more than one preterm birth
  - High risk for repeat miscarriage, such as three or more consecutive miscarriages prior to this pregnancy
- Polyhydramnios
- Blood clots: Thrombophlebitis, DVT, history of DVT or embolism
- Any client restricted to bed rest or modified activity
- Any client with a condition being managed in the hospital
- Any time the client requests to have a release from her doctor or midwife

---

this client. Your client can bring the form to her PCP, along with information or a brochure about the type of bodywork you do. Once the provider signs the form, the client brings or mails it back to you for review. Many times doctors or midwives do not know what concerns a massage practitioner could have, therefore it is still your responsibility to know prenatal bodywork contraindications and follow those guidelines, even if a doctor signs a form approving all massage with no restriction. For instance, if you know that a client has large varicose veins, has a history of clots, or is on bedrest and at higher risk for deep vein clots, you would still not massage her legs, despite the doctor's lack of written restriction. A sample medical release form is provided in Figure 4.2. The release may need to be updated or revised as the pregnancy progresses and the client's condition changes.

BODYWORK PRACTICES REQUIRING PRECAUTIONS IN PREGNANCY

Certain types of bodywork require special precautions when performed on pregnant clients. Below are some considerations to take into account when using specific methodologies, techniques, or tools with your client.

Abdominal Bodywork

Abdominal bodywork is contraindicated in a few situations. Because the majority of miscarriages occur during the first trimester,[3,5] avoid *deep* abdominal massage at this time. The primary reason for this

recommendation is to prevent any questioning or association of massage with miscarriage in your own mind and in the mind of the client, should this pregnancy result in miscarriage.

Note: Be aware that Type II, slow effleurage or energy techniques on the abdomen will not cause harm, and some advanced practitioners may still choose to use these techniques on the abdomen at this time, with the client's informed consent or request.

Along with first trimester contraindications, Type I abdominal massage is also contraindicated at any time during pregnancy that there are concerns or risks with the health of the uterus or placenta, as well as when the mother is having preterm labor risks, or if the baby is demonstrating signs of stress, as indicated by irregularities of the heartbeat. These are situations for which the client would be medically managed. You might see her in a hospital or at home with restricted activity or on bed rest. In this situation, it is highly recommended to obtain a release from your client's PCP that assures you and your client that gentle touch to the belly poses no risks to her condition.

Understanding *why* abdominal work is avoided can help you make the appropriate choices and communicate effectively with your client about touching her abdomen.

In the second trimester, once the pregnant belly has grown larger, abdominal bodywork can be offered if five other criteria are met first:

1. The client is not experiencing abdominal or pelvic pain, cramping, or bleeding.
2. The client is not considered at high risk for preterm labor.

RELEASE FOR THERAPEUTIC BODYWORK DURING PREGNANCY

Dear _____   Date_____

Your patient is interested in receiving therapeutic massage, which has numerous benefits, and few, if any risks during pregnancy.

The following describes the types of bodywork I may use, some of which may be contraindicated with certain types of conditions:

- **Nurturing therapeutic massage** uses long strokes, squeezing, kneading, and pressure on tight muscles, and is generally beneficial and appropriate for all pregnant clients.
- **Abdominal massage** can at times stimulate a few *Braxton-Hicks contractions* and is contraindicated with *placenta previa, risk of abruption, severe hypertension, or preterm labor.*
- **Deep tissue and circulatory stimulating work** can trigger a release of cellular waste into the circulatory system. Occasionally, some clients may experience mildly achy muscles for 24 hours after a session. This work may be contraindicated with clients who have a high risk of preterm labor or uterine irritability.
- **Deep leg massage** might stimulate circulation through the legs and may increase the risk of *dislodging a blood clot.* If your client is at high risk for blood clots and thrombophlebitis, leg massage, or possibly even full body circulatory massage, may be contraindicated depending on the severity of her risk and condition.
- **Range of Motion** and **Resisted Stretching** are not recommended when a client has an extreme *hypermobility of the joints.* As well, it is contraindicated to do hip mobilizations with *diastasis symphysis pubis.*

Please help me to work safely with your client by indicating what types of bodywork restrictions might be necessary.

This signed release confirms that I, _(Doctor or midwife name)_, verify that my pregnant patient, ___(patient name)__, would benefit from massage therapy during her pregnancy. I consider her pregnancy at this time to be *(circle one)*:

Low Risk   / Moderate Risk / High Risk

The following checked techniques ARE appropriate for my client at this time of her pregnancy:

_____ General relaxing massage (rare need for restrictions)
_____ Abdominal massage/belly rub (on occasion, mild Braxton-Hicks contractions may be stimulated)
_____ Stimulating or deep tissue massage (may stimulate blood circulation, causing the release of cellular waste products)
_____ Leg massage (not appropriate if client has problems with blood clots/phlebitis)
_____ Range of Motion, resisted stretching (not appropriate with extreme joint laxity and hypermobility)
_____ Client may only be positioned on left side
_____ Client is restricted to full bed rest and may not get out of bed onto massage table.
       (Session can be done with client on the bed)

Specific precautions and activity restrictions are as follows:
_____
_____

_____ Contact my office for clarification or review of these precautions for massage at the following number: _____.

Signature _____ Date _____

Printed Name_____

FIGURE 4.2   Sample medical release form.

Sample of the type of information you might ask on a medical release for pregnancy massage. Use this as an example, but create your own that applies to your own type of bodywork — acupressure, lomi lomi, cranial sacral, etc. — and its risks if different from those that appear here. Enclose with your release a brochure or fill in a description on your release that informs the PCP of the type of work you do.

MASSAGE THERAPIST TIP   Is a Medical Release Necessary?

*U*nless it is your policy to obtain a medical release for all clients, a release is generally not necessary for a low-risk normal pregnancy. Some women, however, who have concerns about what kind of activities are appropriate during their normal pregnancy, may feel safer if they bring a release to their prenatal health provider.

Once familiar with the providers in your area, you may find that some doctors and midwives state that massage is beneficial in all situations, as long as the pregnant woman wants massage, and nothing vigorous or stimulating to the abdomen is done. They may feel that when a massage therapist requires a medical release, it heightens fears for women who are likely already carrying various anxieties about the health of their pregnancy. If she did not need a medical release *before* she was pregnant, why should she need one now? Pregnancy is a normal, healthy condition of a woman's life, and generally is not dangerous.

For high-risk pregnancies, many bodywork practitioners determine that a medical release will help them offer the safest and most appropriate care to their clientele. Others will choose not to use medical release forms even for high-risk pregnant clients because they are familiar with local providers, are very knowledgeable about the conditions and contraindications of pregnancy, and are confident in their work with pregnant women. By using a medical release for a high-risk pregnancy, however, you assure and inform both the client and the PCP that you understand that this particular situation has more concerns than normal, that you will be observing any necessary special precautions, and that you are seeking the PCP's advice as to further precautions based on this woman's condition.

Considering the benefits of using a medical release, many practitioners will find its use logical and practical for high-risk pregnancies. In the context of this book, I will elucidate the times when a release is highly recommended.

---

3. You have asked permission first before touching the client's belly.
4. You always ask your client for feedback regarding your use of pressure and her comfort level.
5. You use firm (but not forceful) effleurage as opposed to very light touch on the pregnant abdomen, which can feel ticklish and uncomfortable, unless the client directs you otherwise.

Acupressure

The use of a few specific acupressure points is contraindicated during pregnancy. These points are based on the "forbidden" points of acu*puncture*. Not all of the prohibited acu*puncture* points are prohibited for acu*pressure*; however, many of the points are contraindicated for applying needles only, not for using finger pressure.

Since many massage therapists study a basic course of acupressure, or at least hear about acupressure points that are contraindicated in pregnancy, they are included here for reference and clarification. Be aware that contraindications for acupressure are sometimes misconstrued into contraindications for massage in general. These are different techniques that do not affect the body similarly; therefore, contraindicated acupressure points are *only* contraindicated for acupressure treatment. This is lucky for women, for if it were true that the regions of contraindicated acupuncture or acupressure points could not be massaged, then the shoulders, hands, abdomen, inner calves, and ankles would all have to be avoided for massage as well.

Generally, acupressure applied to points that specifically stimulate the uterus, ovaries, and downward flow of energy should be avoided or limited, as these points, used in combination with other practices, can be used to help initiate contractions when labor is imminent and desirable. This means that focused and sustained pressure and attention to these exact points, with the intention of inducing energy flow is contraindicated. It *does not* mean that you cannot touch that area of the body at all.

The two primary prohibited acupoints until 38 weeks' gestation are Spleen 6 (SP 6), located on the lower medial leg, and Large Intestine 4 (LI 4), located in the webbing between the thumb and first finger on each hand (Figure 4.3). These are two of the most effective points for helping to stimulate effective uterine contractions.[6-12]

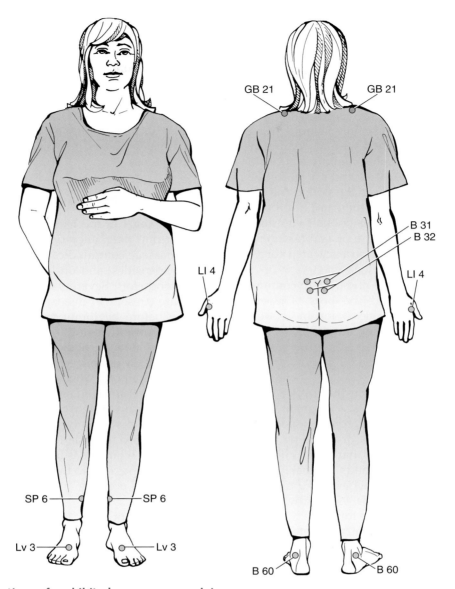

FIGURE 4.3   Locations of prohibited acupressure points.

Until the last 2 weeks of pregnancy, stimulation with acupressure of acupoints Large Intestine 4 (LI 4) and Spleen 6 (Sp 6) are contraindicated. Bladder 60 (B 60) and Liver 3 (Lv 3) are contraindicated by some sources, but others use those points during pregnancy. In the first trimester, use caution and avoid deep stimulation to Gall Bladder 21 (GB 21) and Bladder (B) 31, 32, in the sacral foramen.

Other points to consider (seen in Figure 4.3) are Gall Bladder 21 (GB 21), Bladder 31(B31), Bladder 32 (B32), and Bladder 60 (B 60): During the first trimester, some sources suggest using caution and avoiding deep stimulation to GB 21 on top of the shoulder.[6,13] Some sources also mention B 31 and B 32 in the sacral foramen, as potentially stimulating to the uterus when used in conjunction with other points.[6] B 60, lateral to the malleolus,[12] and Liver 3 on the dorsum of the foot are also sometimes contraindicated, mostly when used in combination with other points,[9] (D. Betts, Personal Communication, December 2006), though other sources do not mention them as contraindicated.[6,14,15]

One perinatal massage book warns against other points on the leg and feet, including Kidney 5, Bladder 61, Spleen 10, and Kidney 1;[16] but these points are not prohibited for finger pressure in most Traditional Chinese Medicine resources or prenatal acupressure books, nor by acupuncturists and acupressurists consulted for this text.

Be aware that there are not hard and fast rules, even within the practices of acupuncture and acupressure, about what points should definitely be avoided.[6,17,18] The most important rules to adhere to when doing acupressure with any client is to work gently with care and respect. The *method* of application of pressure, more than the acupressure point itself, is of primary importance. For instance, some contraindicated points can be used with special tonifying contact, whereas they would remain contraindicated when touched with a sedating type energy (K Ethier, L Ac, personal communication, May 20, 2007). Hence, we can list standard "forbidden" points, but there are times when the skilled and experienced practitioner may find their use appropriate. That is beyond the scope of this book. If you deepen your studies of a particular form of acupressure, you will learn which points are contraindicated for your type of practice.

See Figure 4.3 for location and a list of commonly prohibited points, and read the box, "Dispelling Myths: Massage of the Ankles," for more details about stimulating points around the ankles.

Aromatherapy

Many practitioners use scents in their office or add essential oils to their massage oils. A pregnant woman is likely to be more sensitive to aromas, especially in the first trimester when nausea or vomiting is common. Before using strong scents, have your client do a "sniff-test" to see if she responds agreeably to the odor. Avoid burning incense, which can permeate a room and be uncomfortable for some. Always have unscented oil or lotion available for use.

Many essential oils are contraindicated for use during pregnancy and postpartum. Until you have studied a full course in aromatherapy, it is advisable to assume all essential oils to be contraindicated in the *first trimester,* unless you have specific instruction for their use. In the second and third trimesters, some scents can be quite useful, while others are still contraindicated until labor begins. As a warning, the following essential oils have specific dilutions or restrictions for use in pregnancy, yet are commonly found in scented massage oils: lavender, rose, rosemary, geranium, chamomile. There are numerous useful aromatherapy resources written specifically about pregnancy. Refer to these if you plan to incorporate aromatherapy in your practice. See Suggested Readings in Appendix B for further information.

Breast Massage

Breast massage can be appropriate during a normal, low-risk pregnancy to help relieve aching of enlarging breasts; however, it is contraindicated in any high-risk pregnancy or preterm labor situation due to possible uterine-stimulating effects. Nipple stimulation promotes the release of the labor-inducing hormone, oxytocin, and is sometimes used by clients to help support or initiate labor. While the nipples are not touched during professional breast massage, there could be a minor risk of hormonal release due to generalized tactile stimulation of the breasts. Avoiding breast massage during a high-risk pregnancy eliminates this risk.

Massage to the Adductors and Inner Thigh

Varicose veins in the legs often emerge for the first time during pregnancy (Figure 4.5). Adhere to standard massage contraindications and avoid massaging over varicosities, and on legs with known phlebitis, and blood clots. Severe varicosities can indicate that clots are present in deeper veins. Obtain a medical release before beginning any bodywork for clients who are currently being treated for a blood clot.

Not all clots are obvious and symptomatic. Small ones often go unnoticed and eventually are broken down by the body. You will know when your client has a *symptomatic* clot, as she will be medically treated. Severe pain and swelling in the leg are likely to have come on suddenly, with an 80% to 90% chance that it occurred in her left leg or in the left iliofemoral vein.[19-21] If a woman has been medically managed for her clot, all massage to the legs will be contraindicated to avoid possibly dislodging the clot into the circulation.

You will not know if your client has a nonsymptomatic, but potentially dangerous clot, however; therefore, always practice safety. Because massage does have the capacity to release a clot with serious consequences,[22] a general recommendation during pregnancy and postpartum, is to use only gentle touch to the legs, especially in the hip adductor region. Discussions with several midwives, obstetrical doctors, and pregnancy massage specialists have indicated that the risk from nonsymptomatic clots is so low that there need not be this type of restriction on bodywork, however, a nonsymptomatic clot can still dislodge and become a pulmonary embolism. Therefore, some therapists choose to adhere to the following standard: throughout pregnancy and for at least 6 weeks postpartum, avoid tapotement, deep vibration, cross-fiber friction, petrissage, deep effleurage, and pressure in the hip adductor region of the leg between the knee and groin, and any work that involves tissue compression which can slow or block the blood flow momentarily, including firm acupressure. (This precaution could be for longer if she has not yet been released, for medical reasons,

DISPELLING MYTHS:

Massage of the Ankles

Many massage students learn: "Don't massage a pregnant woman's ankles." However, the idea that it is dangerous to massage a healthy pregnant client's feet or ankles is simply not true. The term "massage" is not specifically defined in that generic statement, but one would assume it refers to effleurage or other types of stroking or "Swedish" massage manipulations. There is no evidence that gentle stroking to the ankles is dangerous, and initiating effective uterine contractions during pregnancy is not that simple. As several obstetricians and midwives have stated in personal interviews, if labor could be started merely by massaging a woman's ankles, the use of medical interventions to induce labor would be stopped! *Effleurage to the feet and ankle area does not stimulate labor.*

The reasoning behind the prohibition of ankle massage during pregnancy has developed for two reasons. Under the medial and lateral malleolus are reflexology areas related to the uterus and ovaries (Figure 4.4). In a similar region are several acupressure points that can be used to support labor (Bladder 60 and Kidney 3). While reflexology and acupressure are different touch techniques from massage, some people still have had concerns that by massaging near these areas, they might stimulate miscarriage or preterm labor. I have found no documented evidence of this ever happening, and interviews with midwives, obstetricians, massage therapists, acupressurists, and reflexologists, have confirmed that there is no reason to avoid massaging the ankles.

Effleurage and general massage are very different techniques from reflexology. The uterus and ovary reflexology zones are very specific spots which massage does not stimulate in the same way. Additionally, reflexology itself, when applied to these spots, does not trigger miscarriage or contractions (D. Byers, Director of International Institute of Reflexology, personal communication, Dec 2006). According to Christopher Shirley, Director of the Pacific Institute of Reflexology, the beneficial results of reflexology to the ankles may actually help *reduce* the occurrence of miscarriage as it helps nurture a healthy maternal environment to support the developing fetus (C. Shirley, personal communication, January 2007).

As for stimulating acupressure points with massage, gentle effleurage in the ankle region with intention of relief of discomfort will not affect those acupoints in a negative way or induce contractions. To influence acupressure points, strong and continuous pressure, repeated over a period of hours or days, is necessary to have any hope of possibly stimulating a uterine contraction. Gentle *massage* can therefore be done without fear in the areas of points prohibited for acupressure.

Suzanne Yates, bodyworker, antenatal educator and author of *Shiatsu for Midwives*, states that she often gently massages around the ankles with light pressure as she connects with the mother's womb. "I have done this kind of work for 18 years now and not had any problems. Indeed I feel it is of benefit. In the first trimester it is calming and supporting the flow of the Jing, an important energy which nurtures the baby" (S. Yates, personal communication, December 2006).

The outcome is that a massage therapist can feel assured that gentle nurturing touch will not harm a pregnant client, and accidentally stimulating the acupressure points around the ankle with massage will not cause uterine contractions to suddenly begin.

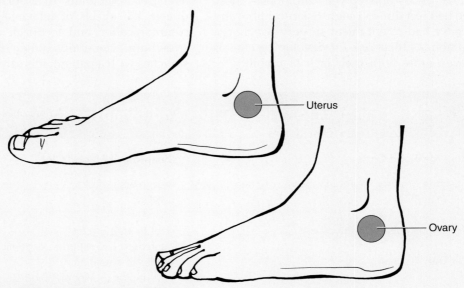

FIGURE 4.4   Reflexology zones of uterus and ovaries.
Small specific zones are stimulated with Reflexology to support and nourish the uterus and ovaries and do not stimulate contractions during pregnancy.

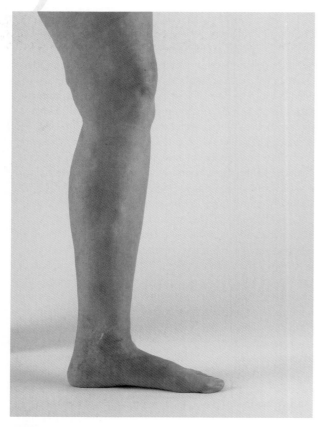

FIGURE 4.5   Varicose veins.
Varicose veins often develop during pregnancy and can be prominent and visibly bulging. Legs with numerous varicose veins have a slightly increased risk of developing DVT.

from her PCP's care.) This is especially true for women with a history of deep vein thrombosis, those on restricted bed rest due to a high-risk condition, and those who have had recent major surgery—such as a cesarean section, as their risk for developing clots is increased even more with their lack of mobility.[20,23]

See Box 4.4 and read more about blood clots in the next section.

Note: Direct pressure on the boney adductor attachments, which avoids compression of the blood vessels, can be used when there are no known clots.

Electromagnetic Fields: Electric Blankets and Heating Pads

There have been studies indicating negative effects from extended exposure to electromagnetic fields or EMF's[24-27]—the electrical force which surrounds electrical devices or wires. While the verdict is not final on the effects of EMF during pregnancy, electromagnetic radiation could theoretically have the capacity to affect the well-being of the fetus in subtle ways, including increasing risk for miscarriage.[25,28] Since there is no confirmed assurance of what level of EMF exposure is totally safe, it may be prudent to avoid the use of electric blankets and heating pads with pregnant clients. Instead, use moist, nonelectric warmth at 101°F or less if desiring the therapeutic benefits of heat on muscle tissue.

Passive Range of Motion

For women who have been experiencing nausea during pregnancy, the rocking or rotations of range of motion stretches, or Trager bodywork, could increase nausea, especially in the first trimester when morning sickness is more common. Avoid these techniques if a client has complaints of nausea.

Do not do hip mobilizations if there is a separation of the symphysis pubis (see Chapter 2). Avoid overstretching joints that are already hypermobile due to the effects of relaxin by maintaining active communication and feedback with the client when stretching. Generally, when facilitating isometric stretches with a patient, it is safer to suggest that your

---

BOX 4.4 | Risk Factors for Blood Clots and Symptoms

Risk Factors for Blood Clots	Symptoms of Blood Clot
Cesarean section or other recent hip, pelvic, or knee surgery	Pain in area of clot
Bedrest and immobility	Swelling
Leg injury	Redness
History of previous deep vein thrombosis	Heat in area of clot
Smoking	Decreased circulation to extremity
Age greater than 40 years	Tender to palpation
Obesity	No symptoms—Not all blood clots are symptomatic
Family history	

Case Study 4.1:
BLOOD CLOTS DURING PREGNANCY I

When Mary, a 25-year-old woman with her first pregnancy, came for her first massage, she marked on her health intake form that she had a blood clot. The massage therapist queried Mary further and learned that she had recently experienced pain, swelling, and heat in her left inner thigh and edema of her lower leg, and had been told she had a blood clot. She was placed on anticoagulants to prevent further clotting potential. Mary did not have a history of circulatory problems but had been told this was a condition that sometimes occurs in pregnancy. She did not express worry or concern over her condition but did state that she was having a lot of discomfort in her legs and hoped that the therapist could do deep work to her legs to help relieve it.

The therapist was alarmed at the request and at the client's apparent lack of knowledge about the risks involved with a blood clot, namely the potential for the clot to be dislodged with potentially life-threatening consequences. The therapist informed her client that she was unable to work on her legs at any time during the pregnancy because of this clot. She also told the client that until she had a medical release from the client's doctor approving Type I massage for the rest of her body, the therapist would only use Type II, non-pressure, energetic techniques during today's massage, along with deeper work to her shoulders, neck, arms.

The client stated that everything was fine, since she was on anti-coagulants and the doctor had not specified that she should avoid massage. She did not understand the therapist's concerns and was perturbed that she would not do deep work during the session. Mary did not reschedule a massage.

---

client position her muscle in the stretch, rather than you positioning for her.

Foot Massage and Reflexology

There are two considerations regarding foot massage during pregnancy. The first is that many pregnant women experience calf cramps. These are due to a variety of possible causes, such as overactivity, underactivity, changes in posture, and other influences. Plantar flexion of the foot during a foot massage, (pointing the toes), can stimulate calf cramps. Avoid

this action and ensure that the foot is well supported when the client is in the sidelying position to avoid drooping of the foot in a plantar-type flexion.

The second issue concerns safe touch when working with edema, a common development in the feet and hands during the latter part of pregnancy. Normal nonpitting edema, as well as sometimes **pitting edema** of the extremities can be normal. Pitting edema is evaluated by pressing a finger pad into the skin for 5 seconds and then lifting the finger up. If an indentation is formed by the finger pressure and remains for more than a brief moment, it is considered to be pitting. It can vary from mild to extreme (Figure 4.6).

Deep work on pitting edema can cause tissue damage, and so Type I deep techniques should be avoided. Only light touch, such as lymphatic and energy work should be used directly on pitting edema.

 CAUTION: Pitting edema can be normal, but it is also associated with pregnancy complications like preeclampsia, which will be discussed later in this chapter. If pitting edema has just developed since the last prenatal visit and has not been evaluated yet, the client should be instructed to call her PCP to determine if she needs to be seen sooner than planned.

Supine Positioning

Avoid supine positioning after about 22 weeks' gestation or any time a woman's pregnant belly is visibly obvious and she is uncomfortable lying supine for more than a few moments. When the client is supine, the weight of the baby and other uterine contents can press directly onto the large blood vessels (the aorta and inferior vena cava) along the mother's back (Figure 4.7). If it does, the blood flow will decrease, affecting both the mother and the baby. The baby's heart rate will decelerate, its oxygen saturation levels will drop,[29] and the mother may feel dizzy, nauseated, or generally uncomfortable or uneasy. If this should happen, the optimal treatment is to have her turn immediately onto her left side to relieve the pressure on the blood vessels and resume full blood flow. Encourage her to breathe deeply to increase oxygenation.

Despite this restriction of supine positioning, some women are comfortable lying supine. This is because of the baby's ever-changing position. If the baby is positioned such that its weight will not compress onto the mother's spine when supine, short periods of bodywork (3 to 7 minutes) may be allowable in this position. Sometimes this is convenient for

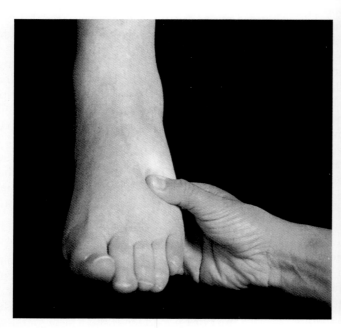
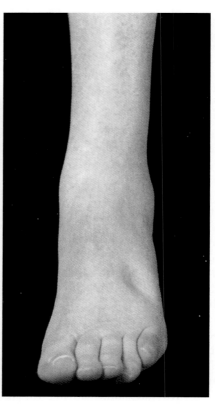

FIGURE 4.6   Pitting edema assessment.

Pitting edema can be normal in pregnancy, and can also be associated with preeclampsia. Assessment is done by pressing finger into swelling for 5 seconds, and looking for indentation after removing finger. Deep tissue work should not be done on pitting edema. (From Bickley LS and Szilagyi P. Bates' Guide to Physical Examination and History Taking. 8th Ed. Philadelphia: Lippincott Williams & Wilkins, 2003.)

a final neck traction or massage of the shoulders and face. Certain assisted stretches are also done with the client in the supine position. In either of these situations, it is imperative to maintain good verbal communication with the client about how she is feeling, and instruct her to roll over to her side if she feels the least bit uncomfortable.

 CAUTION: Any woman in the supine position who complains of nausea, dizziness, or uneasy feelings, however mild, should be repositioned immediately to her left side, which typically provides the most optimum blood perfusion to the baby and mother.[29-33]

As a general rule, when the position of baby is not definitive, always position your second or third trimester client in the sidelying or semi-reclining position for extended bodywork. An optional position is to place a foam wedge under the client's right hip; this tilts and displaces the weight of the uterus to the left,

preventing compression of the large blood vessels situated to the right of the spine.

Saunas and Hot Tubs

Practitioners who work in spas or other settings where saunas and hot tubs are available should take special care to ensure that temperatures are kept at a safe level for their clients. Hot tub water temperatures are best kept to 101°F or less, and immersions into heat kept to 5 to 10 minutes. Immersions in hotter water can be done as long as it is for less than 10 minutes, which avoids the risk of raising core body temperatures over 102°F.[34] Core body temperatures over 102.6°F *in the first trimester* may be associated with some neurological birth defects and may possibly increase risk of miscarriage, although study results are conflicting about this.[34-36] The issues of neural tube defects decline after the first trimester, since this primary development occurs very early in the fetal life.

Later in pregnancy, mothers tend to become dizzy or unable to tolerate heat for more than short periods

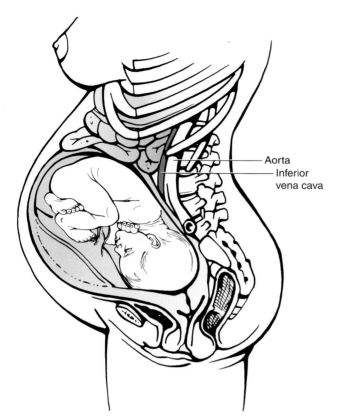

Aorta
Inferior
vena cava

Complementary Modalities:

Applications of Heat During Pregnancy

Most pregnant clients in their second and third trimesters will feel warmer than when they are not pregnant. This is due to hormonal effects and increased blood volume. While some may enjoy short immersions in hot water, your client in advanced pregnancy may not appreciate a heating pad or blanket on your massage table.

If she is experiencing muscle tension in a particular area, however, and you feel that the application of heat will enhance your work and the ability of her muscles to relax, use localized nonelectric warm packs. Hydroculator packs; heated flax seed bags; hot water bottles; or moist, hot towels, can be used to warm an area of tension. Avoid heat applications greater than 101°F for more than 10 minutes directly over the abdomen or low back where the heat may affect the developing fetus, particularly in the first trimester.

FIGURE 4.7   Supine positioning and pressure on inferior vena cava and aorta.
When the pregnant mother is positioned supine, risk exists for the weight of the gravid uterus to press onto the large blood vessels running along the spine. This compression will decrease oxygen flow to both the mother and child.

of time, thus self-regulating with regard to heat immersion. Interspersing short dips in hot water with immersion in cold can help prevent the development of hyperthermia.

HEALTH FACTORS THAT INCREASE RISK DURING PREGNANCY

Some pregnancies begin with or develop risk factors indicating minor or major concerns for the mother and/or the baby. These risks may lead to serious complications. Pre-existing risk factors include maternal age, obesity, history of repeat miscarriage, or asthma, while risks that can develop during pregnancy itself include conditions such as preterm labor and gestational hypertension. If the client has a condition that increases her risk for complications, massage restrictions are not always necessary unless

problems actually develop during the current pregnancy. Some of these conditions are discussed below, beginning with those that have a few extra bodywork considerations.

This is followed by a discussion of complications that can develop during pregnancy and that pose serious risk to the life and health of the mother and/or the infant. These conditions contraindicate Type I massage or require increased precautions for bodywork. Remember, however, as you read the following section that the majority of women you see will be having a normal, healthy pregnancy and can be supported fully with your nurturing touch.

Conditions Requiring Special Bodywork Precautions

The following conditions classify a woman's pregnancy as having some potential for problems. They are explained here to give you an understanding of why they are considered risks and to help inform you if you encounter or hear about the condition. Bodywork considerations are dependent on the history of the problem and the current level of severity, and they generally emphasize observance of precautions related to positioning, abdominal work, or use of Type I bodywork.

Traditional Birth Practices:
Keeping the Mother and Baby Safe

*C*ultural practices to keep both the mother and baby safe during pregnancy often include taboos against activities or foods that could cause baby to "stick" inside, bring on illness or weakness, cause problems to the placenta, or cause labor to not progress effectively. Traditional Yup'ik Eskimo practices from Western Alaska have included turning their pillows over prior to sleeping to encourage the baby to stay mobile, rather than stuck, inside the womb, and walking quickly through door ways to encourage a quick delivery. Women were sometimes instructed not to sleep on their backs to prevent baby from rising up in the womb, and to lean forward for several minutes each day to keep baby smaller and thus have an easy delivery. It was encouraged that eating only freshly made foods could help prevent fetal deformities, while no burnt food should be eaten, as this could cause the placenta to become stuck and not release after birth. Many practices around the world, including some of our own, involve maintaining positive thoughts and avoiding emotionally stressful situations, such as funerals.

Maternal Asthma

When a pregnant woman has severe asthma, her fetus is at risk due to the mother's use of medications and the decreased oxygen availability to the fetus during asthma attacks.

 BODYWORK PRECAUTIONS: Ask whether the client's asthma is affected by certain scents, and avoid the use of essential oils, scented oils, candles, and other scents that you or she suspects may trigger an attack.

Obesity

Obesity is defined as having greater than 20% of the expected weight for a woman's size and age. Beginning pregnancy with obesity increases the risks for gestational diabetes, a large baby, and hypertension.

 BODYWORK PRECAUTIONS: It is worthwhile to consider using the sidelying or semi-reclining position during the first trimester if it is more comfortable for your client. The supine and prone positions can increase breathing difficulties for extremely obese people. Semi-reclining position may be more comfortable than sidelying for some women as pregnancy progresses.

Tobacco/Drug/Alcohol Use

With any type of maternal addiction to drugs, alcohol, and tobacco, risks increase for fetal complications, lower fetal birth weight, preterm delivery, deep vein thrombosis, labor complications, placental abruption and previa, and miscarriage.

 BODYWORK PRECAUTIONS: For clientele for whom drug, tobacco, and alcohol use is common, the recommendation of a medical release is based on the severity of the client's drug use, the likelihood of her developing any of the above risks, your uncertainty of the client's veracity, or, if working in a clinic or environment with clientele for whom drug use is not uncommon, the clinic's standard protocol.

Chronic Hypertension

High blood pressure that develops before pregnancy and has been treated medically over a period of time, is considered to be chronic, as opposed to hypertension which develops during pregnancy and is called gestational hypertension. Chronic hypertension can lead to increased risks for preterm labor, placental abruption, and decreased fetal growth.[37-39]

 BODYWORK PRECAUTIONS: For a client with severe hypertension, a medical release is recommended to determine the level of risk your client's PCP considers her to be, and to determine if Type I full body techniques are appropriate. Abdominal massage is contraindicated with severe hypertension.

Thromboembolic Disorders

By the third trimester, many women have at least small, asymptomatic clots in their legs, most commonly in the deep vessels of the inner thighs in the area of the saphenous, iliac, and femoral veins. The development of blood clots that partially or totally block a leg vein is called **deep vein thrombosis (DVT)** (see Figure 4.8). It occurs, as its name implies, in the deep blood vessels of the legs, most commonly in the left iliofemoral vein. **Superficial thrombophlebitis**—a condition of venous inflammation in

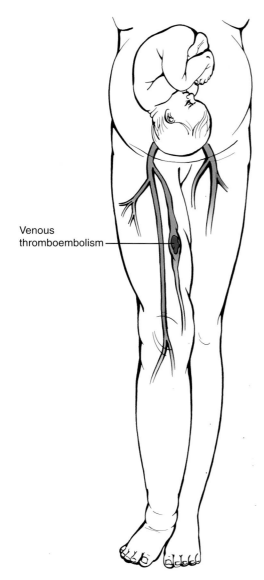

Venous thromboembolism

FIGURE 4.8   Deep vein thrombosis.
Risk for the development of clots increases during pregnancy due to impeded circulation to the legs and increased clotting factors in the blood, and during postpartum if postcesarean and having decreased mobility.

the superficial veins caused by a clot—occurs more often in the calf.[19]

The concern surrounding a blood clot is the possibility that it could become dislodged into the circulation, as an **embolus,** and become lodged in the lungs, causing difficulty breathing, chest pain, and possibly death. This is known as a **pulmonary embolism.** DVTs have a higher likelihood of causing a pulmonary embolism than superficial clots.[19]

During pregnancy, the risk of developing a clot increases by five or six times, as compared to

nonpregnant women.[19,40] The higher risk for clots occurs because of changes in the perinatal circulatory system, including expanded blood volume, increased clotting factors in the blood, and impeded blood flow to the extremities (see Chapter 3). Risk factors include smoking, being over age 35, being overweight, having had a previous DVT or embolism or having varicose veins, high blood pressure, preeclampsia, or being on bed rest or very inactive.[41]

DVT occurs in an average of one out of every 1000 to 1800 pregnancies[19,20,23,42,43] and can develop in any trimester of pregnancy. [20,21,44,45] During the postpartum period or after a cesarean section the occurrence of DVT may increase to about 1 in 700 women,[23] though the incidence of embolism is low. Out of 268,525 deliveries reviewed in one study, 165 women developed known clots in their veins, and 38 of those experienced a pulmonary embolism.[20]

> **BODYWORK PRECAUTIONS:** *Standard protocol is as follows:* If the client is complaining of leg pain that is unexplained by new activity or strain, or if you notice redness, swelling, and heat in an area of the leg, instruct her to call her PCP immediately for further assessment.

Follow standard clot precautions on the legs of all pregnant and postpartum clients.

Some perinatal massage sources recommend that a practitioner assess a client before each massage for signs of DVT.[16] The assessment recommended is the Homan's test, which involves abruptly dorsiflexing the client's foot and assumes that if the client feels sharp pain in the popliteal area or calf, the test is positive. However, the more accurate positive sign is a resistance of movement to the dorsiflexion action.[46]

I do not recommend this test for several reasons:

1. The use of the Homan's sign is generally no longer recommended as a diagnostic tool.[47,48] Ultrasound and venography along with visual assessments, such as localized swelling, heat, and redness are the primary diagnostic tools used by medical professionals.
2. The Homan's test has been demonstrated to be inaccurate, and is not useful for determining the presence of a clot.[49-51] Even when done correctly, its accuracy can be as low as 8%.[49] Whether the result is positive or negative, there is no assurance regarding the absence or presence of a clot.
3. Other physical issues can cause a positive result, including leg cramps, edema, cellulitis, and a change in shoes from high heels to low heels.[46]

A massage therapist who regularly tests for a positive Homan's sign can stimulate client anxiety about her safety. A pregnant woman has plenty of worries to occupy her mind. When she comes for a massage, she does not need to add to these by thinking about the remote chance that she may have a problematic blood clot. Instead, make it standard to practice gentle touch to the legs, and always visually assess for redness, pain, swelling, and inflammation, referring to the PCP if found.

Multiple Gestation (Twins or More)

While it can be exciting for the mother to be having more than one baby at a time, risks increase for the development of preterm labor. All other common complaints of pregnancy are further exacerbated due to the increased size and weight gain and hormonal influences (Figure 4.9).

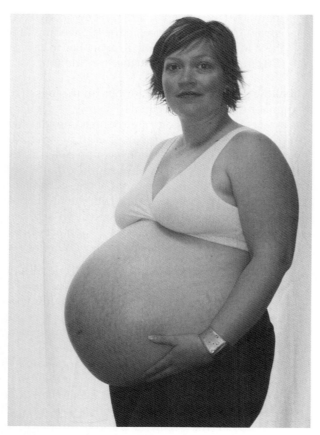

FIGURE 4.9   Large abdomen: mother of twins.
When a mother has a particularly large abdomen, as with multiple pregnancy, obesity, or extra large baby with smaller mother, extra care is needed to ensure adequate body mechanics instruction is given for getting on and off massage table and for repositioning. Extra abdominal support may be needed on the table as well.

 BODYWORK PRECAUTIONS: In the third trimester, if the abdomen is exceptionally large, extra care in teaching the client proper methods of sitting up from sidelying, as well as possibly using a foam wedge or rolled towel on the table to support under the belly is important. (See "Positioning" in Chapter 5.) The client with a large belly has an increased risk for diastasis recti, and for straining of the uterine ligaments. Help her to rest comfortably and well-supported on the table, and minimize her need for repositioning. Use only gentle abdominal massage for short durations to avoid stimulating contractions. Avoid excessively stimulating Type I work throughout the pregnancy until the last weeks. A medical release is recommended if premature labor has occurred with this pregnancy.

History of Repeat Miscarriage

Miscarriage is birth that occurs before 20 weeks' gestation. Miscarriage occurs in about 15% of pregnancies each year,[3,52] with the vast majority occurring in the first trimester before 12 to 13 weeks' gestation. According to the Centers for Disease Control and Prevention, of the 6.28 million pregnancies *reported* in the U.S. in 1999, miscarriage occurred in 1 million of those.[53] Since so many miscarriages happen too early to have even been reported as a pregnancy, we can conclude that there are many more than this that occur each year.[54]

The vast majority of miscarriages result from a healthy response to the early abnormal development of an embryo, but other known associations with miscarriage include maternal issues, such as problems with the cervix or uterus or conditions such as diabetes, infection, or virus. Miscarriage is also associated with increased *paternal* age[55,56] as well as maternal drug use, including tobacco.[57-59]

Women who have three consecutive miscarriages in the first trimester have a 35% chance of having another miscarriage.[60] Women with this experience will often have a significant level of anxiety during consequent pregnancies if the fear of losing the baby again overrides their ability to relax and enjoy the current pregnancy. Massage can be very helpful, by encouraging relaxation and self-care.

 BODYWORK PRECAUTIONS: If a client has had two or more consecutive miscarriages, avoid abdominal massage until 1 to 2 months past the date of the previous miscarriages, unless the client asks for belly massage and feels that this touch will help to allay anxieties. The contraindication is simply to avoid association between your touch and another miscarriage, should that unfortunately occur. With this in mind, if the client has a history of multiple miscarriages, has a high level of anxiety related to it, has had preterm contractions in this pregnancy, or is, for additional reasons, at higher risk for repeat miscarriage, avoid any stimulating touch, such as vigorous Type I bodywork that could alarm a client who already has concerns about receiving massage. A medical release is recommended for clients with three or more consecutive miscarriages to help ascertain risks and precautions.

Previous Premature Birth

A **premature birth** is one that occurs between gestational weeks 20 and 37. Each time a woman has a premature delivery, her risks increase for having another.

If her first and only pregnancy resulted in the delivery of a baby less than 3 pounds, her chances of it occurring in the next pregnancy are 50%.[60]

 BODYWORK PRECAUTIONS: practice caution with clients who have a history of a premature delivery in their last pregnancy and for those who have a current condition that was associated with the first preterm birth. Wait to offer abdominal massage until 1 to 2 months past the time of the previous premature labor, or until the mother's anxiety has diminished about preterm labor occurring again. Avoid Type I techniques until the mother has been told her risk for preterm labor in this pregnancy has decreased. A medical release is suggested prior to commencing work if she has had more than one pregnancy with issues of preterm birth or preterm labor, to help determine what level of risk she is at currently.

DISPELLING MYTHS:
Massage and Miscarriage

One of the greatest fears bodyworkers have about working with a pregnant woman is unintentionally doing something that could cause her to miscarry or experience preterm labor. Miscarriages occur in hundreds of thousands of pregnancies each year due to causes utterly unrelated to massage. The fears abound however, and if a miscarriage should occur after a massage, both client and therapist may harbor fears that the massage caused it to happen. This is a common misconception about prenatal massage. Other fears are also expressed about the potential dangers of prenatal massage. Here are some examples of erroneous beliefs collected from general public and from students in pregnancy massage classes:

"Massage releases toxins that poison and kill the baby, or cause a miscarriage."

"Overstimulation to the abdomen may shrink the uterus and negatively affect the baby, or even cause miscarriage."

"Avoid prenatal massages until the late second trimester. The massage moves fluid which the baby can feel is an attack, and it can cause miscarriage. Using the wrong pressure points with reflexology can also cause miscarriage."

"Don't press hard on the left side of the low back or sacrum, as that is where the baby attaches and you might hurt it."

None of the above statements are true. *Therapeutic massage does not cause miscarriage.* There are, however, two caveats to identify:

1. If one has a strong intention toward *causing* a miscarriage and does very deep, intensive, and invasive manipulations to the abdomen, especially in the first trimester, there is a possibility that problems could occur. Healing bodywork is not of that intensity, however, nor does it have nor should it have, that intention.

2. If someone is at high risk for miscarriage and is already on the verge of one, then circulatory and vigorous Type I full body massage or abdominal massage might possibly support and encourage the body to do what it was already beginning to do. This can actually be helpful during what is often a difficult experience for women and often their partners. While massage and bodywork can be supportive during a miscarriage that is already underway, nurturing touch will not cause a healthy pregnancy to miscarry. The general precaution during the first trimester, when most miscarriages occur, is to use respectful, gentle, and superficial touch to the belly or avoid the abdomen altogether. This way, if a miscarriage occurs soon after a massage, both the mother and massage therapist can avoid harboring any concerns that the massage was somehow the cause of this miscarriage. This is the primary reason for abdominal bodywork precautions in the first trimester of pregnancy—to simply avoid an association between bodywork and a potential miscarriage, for which any woman is initially at risk.

Note: If the client with a history of preterm labor in previous births has not been having preterm contractions with *this* pregnancy, gentle touch to the abdomen can be done for the client who requests it and feels it will help her cope better emotionally with her pregnancy.

Fetal Genetic Disorders, Intrauterine Growth Restriction, Oligohydramnios

Nowadays, with numerous blood tests, ultrasounds, amniocentesis, and chorionic villi sampling, women know a great deal about the health of their unborn baby. Knowing ahead that her baby may have abnormalities can cause increased emotional stress for the mother.

Intrauterine growth restriction means the fetus is small for its estimated gestational age, as indicated by measurements and ultrasound. This condition may indicate it has fetal anomalies or other problems.

In **oligohydramnios**, too little amniotic fluid is produced. It is associated with placental dysfunctions, fetal anomalies, or fetal death.

 BODYWORK PRECAUTIONS: Precautions are dependent on the history of the problem and the current level of severity. A woman may have increased fears or anxieties about her pregnancy. Abdominal massage may be contraindicated to avoid association of massage with potential problems with the baby. This contraindication will be based on the woman's anxiety level and her desire to receive or avoid abdominal massage. Some women may want gentle touch and energy work to the abdomen to ease anxiety and help them to deepen their connection with the baby. The massage itself will not affect the condition of the baby, but in some instances, a woman's uterus may be more irritable and contractile, increasing the risk for preterm labor or premature rupture of the membranes or amniotic sac and making abdominal massage, and sometimes Type I massage, a contraindication.

Fifth or Subsequent Pregnancy

With each pregnancy, a woman's musculoskeletal system is again stressed. Risks increase for diastasis recti, varicose veins, ineffective uterine contractions in labor, and postpartum hemorrhage.

 BODYWORK PRECAUTIONS: A woman in her fifth or subsequent pregnancy will tend to have more low back pain and need extra abdominal support. She should be encouraged to do abdominal strengthening from the start of her pregnancy (or sooner) and should be assessed for diastasis recti as a cause of low back pain. Abdominal support binders can be helpful as well. (See Appendix B, Resources for the Practitioner.)

Prolonged Infertility or Hormone Treatment

Any woman who has had difficulty becoming pregnant will have increased emotional concerns and anxiety over the health of her pregnancy. If she has taken fertility hormones, she is at a much higher risk for multiple conception and has increased risks in general.

 BODYWORK PRECAUTIONS: In this situation, a woman's need for comfort and reassurance will be high. Abdominal massage and vigorous Type I massage may be contraindicated throughout pregnancy until the last few weeks before delivery, depending on the history of attempted pregnancy or miscarriages and the client's anxiety level. Discuss her expectations of bodywork so your work can support her needs. A medical release may be recommended if the client has a history of repeat miscarriage or if she has a great deal of anxiety about this current pregnancy and would feel more relaxed having a medical release.

Gestational Diabetes

Gestational diabetes (GD) occurs in about 4% of all pregnancies.[62] It is different from the common Type I or Type II diabetes, as it only occurs during pregnancy, and is a condition that usually resolves after delivery. Excess maternal blood sugar will cause the baby to grow larger, thereby causing size-related difficulties at delivery. To prevent this, many women with GD are induced into labor with **Pitocin**—a synthetic form of the hormone oxytocin—earlier than their due date, before the baby has grown too large. A woman also has a greater chance of developing infection, preterm labor, gestational hypertension, or fetal abnormalities when she has GD.[61]

 BODYWORK PRECAUTIONS: A woman with GD may have an extra-large abdomen and be especially prone to low back pain, leg pain, and pelvic congestion. Proper abdominal support under the belly on the massage table is, as always, essential (see Figure 5.1). An abdominal support binder may be recommended.

Urinary Tract Infection

A **urinary tract infection** (UTI) increases the risks of preterm labor, kidney infection, and premature rupture of the membranes. Symptoms of a UTI may be mild, in which case the client may not perceive many discomforts, or the symptoms may be moderate with urinary urgency and frequency, low back pain, uterine contractions, pelvic pain, and fever.

 BODYWORK PRECAUTIONS: If your client has a UTI, ensure that she has been treated for this condition and is not having acute symptoms of pain, fever or chills, or preterm contractions during massage. It would be unlikely for you to see a client in this condition, unless the symptoms have only just begun to increase prior to the massage session. Avoid massage to the abdomen until a UTI is fully resolved.

High-Risk Complications of Pregnancy

Five percent of pregnancies develop complications that have the potential to seriously endanger the mother and/or baby during pregnancy, birth, or postpartum.[62] These complications occur only during pregnancy. They may contraindicate Type I massage or require specific and particular precautions. In most cases, a woman with these complications will be on a modified rest regimen, which might involve partial or total bed rest and the therapist will be making a house call. These conditions must be assessed for their severity to determine the type of precautions to be implemented. A medical release that describes necessary precautions or discussion with the client's PCP is important and strongly recommended before working with clients with high-risk conditions.

- Uterine and placental abnormalities
- Polyhydramnios
- Moderate to severe gestational hypertension
- Preeclampsia or HELLP syndrome
- Preterm labor

Women with these conditions should only be treated by massage therapists who have had significant practice in massage in the sidelying positioning and have confidence working with pregnant women. The risks of each condition should be fully understood and massage done in compliance with any medically indicated restrictions as described by the PCP.

Placental Abruption (Marginal or Partial)

Placental abruption is a condition in which the placenta begins to separate from the wall of the uterus before the delivery of the baby. It occurs in an average of 1 out of 150 to 200 pregnancies.[63] The placenta may separate partially, or there may be a complete abruption, in which case the placenta detaches entirely, leaving the maternal blood vessels open and bleeding at the site of placental attachment. Symptoms may include light or heavy bleeding, a hard, rigid abdomen with abdominal pain, or massive hemorrhage. Chronic high blood pressure is a primary risk factor for abruption, along with tobacco or cocaine use, premature rupture of membranes, and having had an abruption in a previous pregnancy.[33, 63-65] A full abruption is a medical emergency in which an immediate cesarean delivery is necessary.

With a partial or marginal abruption without heavy bleeding (determined by ultrasound), the mother may be restricted to bed rest until the bleeding resolves.

 BODYWORK PRECAUTIONS:
- *After recovery* from a partial abruption, once the mother is able to resume some of her daily activities (although they will likely be quite modified), massage can be done with gentle Type II work. *Avoid all abdominal massage and Type I stimulating massage.* Obtain a medical release prior to beginning bodywork to be certain the PCP approves of massage, and to alleviate concerns for the mother and yourself, as well as to ascertain other risks.
- Call 911 emergency services immediately if your client should develop symptoms of severe abdominal pain or sudden heavy vaginal bleeding during a session, as this could indicate another abruption.

Placenta Previa

When the placenta has implanted itself partially or completely over the opening of the cervix, it is called a **placenta previa** (Figure 4.10). This happens more frequently in women who have uterine fibroids or scarring from previous surgeries, as well as in smokers, women over 35 years old, and those who have had multiple pregnancies.[33] If the placenta is positioned low early in the pregnancy, it may still migrate upward and out of danger as the pregnancy progresses. If it does not, a cesarean section will be necessary at delivery, as the placenta will impede the vaginal delivery of the baby. There may be no symptoms

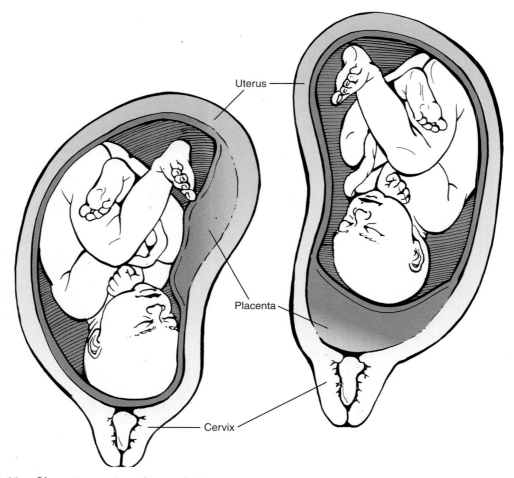

Uterus

Placenta

Cervix

FIGURE 4.10   Placenta previa and normal placenta.

Normally the placenta is positioned in the upper area of the uterus. With a previa the placenta is positioned over or very near the os, or opening, of the cervix. There is increased risk of bleeding with this condition and delivery must be by cesarean section. (LifeART image copyright 2009 Lippincott Williams & Wilkins. All rights reserved.)

manifested with a previa, and it may only be found by ultrasound. In other situations, there may be a small or large amount of bleeding as the uterus enlarges and pulls on the placental attachments. The danger of hemorrhage is extreme if the cervix dilates, pulling away from the placenta.

With a known complete previa, a woman is usually instructed to avoid heavy lifting, aerobic activity, and sexual stimulation and intercourse, which can stimulate the abdomen, cervix, and uterus.

 BODYWORK PRECAUTIONS: Gentle massage can be done, and will benefit a woman, but avoid abdominal massage. All Type I full-body stimulating massage is also contraindicated if the client has had any bleeding. A medical

release is highly recommended to be certain the PCP approves of massage, alleviate concerns for the mother and massage therapist, and to ascertain other risks.

Polyhydramnios

Polyhydramnios is a condition in which excessive amniotic fluid is produced in the uterus. It is associated with maternal shortness of breath, diabetes, preterm labor, and fetal anomalies.[38] With the increased fluid, there is an increased intrauterine pressure and impaired perfusion of blood between the uterus and placenta. This can lead to dangerous effects, such as sudden rupture of the uterus or placental abruption, irritable uterine contractions, preterm labor, or premature rupture of the amniotic sac. A woman may be treated with modified activity or restriction to lateral bed rest. Type II bodywork is beneficial.

 BODYWORK PRECAUTIONS: Precautions for this condition depend on the history of the problem and the current level of severity. Obtain a medical release to determine the need to restrict Type I massage or additional necessary bodywork restrictions. No abdominal massage should be performed.

Preterm Labor

Preterm labor, also known as premature labor, is defined as the onset of contractions *with changes to the cervix* (dilation, shortening, and effacing) before 37 weeks' gestation and with risk of the baby being born early. Preterm contractions do not always lead to preterm *labor*. A woman may have contractions that do not cause cervical change. She may also have cervical change without being aware of any contractions. Early contractions can be caused by simple things, such as dehydration or urinary tract infection—either of which can be easily treated. More serious preterm labor can be caused by other problems, such as issues with the health of the baby, a shift in hormones, rupture of the amniotic sac, or infection. Most often, the cause is unknown.

A woman with this condition may be restricted to lateral bed rest and may take medications to help prevent or decrease preterm contractions.

 BODYWORK PRECAUTIONS: Full body Type I massage is contraindicated for a client relegated to bed rest or restricted activity due to preterm labor, but localized Type I or general Type II massage can still be done. Obtain a medical release prior to beginning bodywork. Offer her a drink of water and encourage her to drink more than normal after receiving massage to minimize the effects of a massage-stimulated release of cellular waste into the circulatory system, which could potentially further irritate an already irritable uterus.

Gestational Hypertension, Preeclampsia, and HELLP Syndrome

Gestational Hypertension (GH) refers to high blood pressure that develops during pregnancy, usually beginning sometime between 20 weeks' gestation

and 1 week postpartum. Mild gestational hypertension is not necessarily dangerous, but up to 50% of women with GH are likely to progress into a condition called **preeclampsia**,[66] in which changes begin to develop in the organ systems, blood chemistry is altered, and blood pressure continues to rise. A woman might be relegated to bed rest to reduce stress and blood pressure, but as long as her blood pressure stays consistently below 140/90, there may be no restrictions, other than to have her blood pressure monitored weekly throughout the rest of her pregnancy.

The etiology of preeclampsia is unclear, but it occurs in 3% to 7% of pregnancies and occurs most commonly in first time pregnancies.[60,65,67] As it progresses, it can lead to premature births and increased risk of placental abruption. In 25% of pregnancies, preeclampsia first becomes evident in the postpartum period and her blood pressure can stay elevated for up to 6 weeks postpartum.[60]

Symptoms of preeclampsia may include sudden rapid weight gain, visual disturbances, such as spots before the eyes, epigastric pain similar to heartburn, increased blood pressure, nausea and vomiting, unrelenting headache, pitting edema of the extremities and face, along with abnormal lab tests. A woman with severe preeclampsia will be in the hospital on bed rest.

HELLP is an acronym for **H**emolysis, **E**levated **L**iver enzymes, and **L**ow **P**latelets. It is insidious and considered by some to be a variation of advanced preeclampsia. It is characterized by pain in the epigastric area or right upper quadrant of the abdomen, often accompanied by general malaise, nausea, vomiting, and headache.[65] Though rare, occurring in less than 1% of pregnancies,[68] it is easily confused with other conditions that cause malaise, and yet HELLP can be extremely dangerous. It more typically develops in the third trimester of pregnancy, but can occur in the second as well.[68]

 BODYWORK PRECAUTIONS: If your client has GH or preeclampsia with no activity restrictions, then no bodywork restrictions may be necessary. If the client has progressed into preeclampsia with modified activity, Type I techniques should be limited and a medical release is highly recommended. Many women are restricted to the left-sidelying position, which can provide increased blood and oxygen perfusion to the fetus and uterus. This must continue during a massage, with sessions performed with the client solely in the left lateral position.

Women with HELLP will be in the hospital for medical management of the condition. Type II bodywork may be supportive, but all Type I bodywork will be contraindicated.

 CAUTIONS: Be aware of insidious symptoms of HELLP, which can develop relatively quickly. If your client in the late second or third trimester has not been seen yet by her PCP for a recent development of headache, nausea, right upper abdominal pain, or general malaise, have her call her PCP before deciding to continue with a massage.

Case Study 4.2:
BLOOD CLOTS DURING PREGNANCY, II

Joan was a 34-year-old client at 35 weeks' gestation who came for a massage complaining of a mild headache, along with pain and cramping in her left calf that developed earlier that day. Joan also stated she was experiencing an increase in bilateral swelling of her feet and ankles since her last massage 2 weeks ago. The pain was moderate and increased when the left foot was dorsi-flexed with walking. It did not refer elsewhere. The therapist assessed the leg and found no signs of swelling, heat, or redness in the area of discomfort, but did note the edema of the foot. There was no obvious bruising, but the calf was painful with moderate palpation of the gastrocnemius. Joan had not done any recent physical exertion, nor changed to new shoes recently, but she had been having an increase in leg cramps at night.

The therapist asked about Joan's headache. Joan stated it had been low-grade, but constant, and that she had last seen her doctor 8 days ago, though her next appointment was scheduled in 2 days.

The massage therapist had several concerns. Noting the increase in edema, though minor and nonpitting, and the complaint of persistent headache, the therapist considered the possibility of early preeclampsia. Joan stated that her blood pressure had been normal until her last prenatal visit, when it had been slightly elevated, though her doctor had stated that there was nothing to worry about. The massage therapist was also concerned about the calf pain and swelling and the potential for blood clot, since she was unable to discern clearly whether the client's pain was only musculoskeletal. Because it was *bilateral* swelling,

Eclampsia

If left untreated, GH and preeclampsia are precursors to a more serious condition that develops when preeclampsia is not controlled, called **eclampsia**. This can lead to convulsions and even death. Preeclampsia and eclampsia are the third leading cause of pregnancy-related deaths in the United States.[69,71]

 BODYWORK PRECAUTIONS: Eclampsia and HELLP are life-threatening conditions and the woman will be in the hospital. In this case, all Type I bodywork is contraindicated. Type II

she thought it was unlikely to be a clot, but she had enough uncertainty that she felt it important that Joan be evaluated by her PCP.

Due to this uncertainty, the therapist informed Joan that she would be unable to do her standard massage at this visit but suggested that she call her prenatal clinic from the massage office and query whether she should be seen right away. Joan did this, and made an appointment for later that afternoon. Knowing Joan would be seen soon, the therapist then offered to do a Type II energy session with a head and neck massage to help her relax, if it did not interfere with the timing of Joan's appointment. She also gave Joan a medical release form to bring to her PCP to be signed before her next massage, after her condition was evaluated.

Joan returned to the massage therapist the following week with the medical release and explanation that no clot was found in her leg. The doctor had suggested that her discomfort might be residual from her frequent leg cramps, of which she had several the night before her last massage visit. Her headaches resolved with Tylenol, and she was told she would be monitored twice weekly for blood pressure changes, since her pressure had increased slightly again, yet was still not of significant concern requiring activity restrictions.

The therapist then felt comfortable massaging Joan's legs to help relieve tension from muscle cramping. Each subsequent visit she asked for an update on her client's blood pressure and any other medical concerns so that she would know if she would need to enact any restrictions to general massage.

bodywork for women with severe conditions requires a medical release.

Client Restricted to Bed Rest

For women with high-risk pregnancies, confinement to bed may be one of her prescribed treatments. Her prescription may vary from total bed rest, with use of a bedpan or bedside commode, to bed rest with 2- to 4-hour breaks during which she may be upright and move about the house minimally. These types of restrictions can lead to numerous complaints, including general muscle stiffness, aches, weakness, and atrophy; structural and postural changes that cause back pain; increased constipation due to immobility; emotional stress due to boredom, guilt, or anxiety about her condition; increased heartburn from horizontal positioning; and an increased risk of blood clots. Massage can be a life saver. If she works on a laptop computer in bed, she may have further problems related to poor posture and positioning, such as carpal tunnel syndrome and brachial plexus syndrome.

Bodywork Precautions

Working with bed-bound women necessitates communication with her PCP. Obtain a medical release for massage prior to beginning your work with your client. Requesting enough information about her condition to feel secure about what type of bodywork is appropriate. For most conditions, Type I work is

contraindicated for the full body, though it is useful in local areas such as the shoulders, neck, and arms. Your client is in bed to avoid excessive stimulation that might cause her either to lose her baby—such as in cases of preterm labor—or increase her risk of bleeding—such as with placenta previa or partial abruption. Therefore, abdominal massage will often be totally contraindicated. She may also be on bed rest to avoid increasing severe high blood pressure.

If uncertain what is appropriate, always err on the side of gentle, calming energy work, and decreasing stimulation. Incorporate calming visualizations and breathing practices in your work. Typically there are no restrictions to working on the head, neck, shoulders, arms, and upper back. You can have a huge effect merely by offering emotional support and gentle hands-on holding, if that is all you are able to do.

 CAUTIONS: A woman's risk for blood clots increases greatly when her activity level has been restricted. Maintain all precautions for blood clots with your client on bedrest, as described under "Massage to Adductors and Inner Thigh" earlier in the chapter.

Health Intake for Client on Bed Rest

A thorough health intake is mandatory for clients relegated to bed rest. In addition to the standard health questionnaire and intake, ask the following questions

Self Care Tips FOR MOTHERS:

Stress Relief for the Client Restricted to Bed Rest

For the client who is on bed rest, simple stretches and activities are recommended by PCPs to maintain muscular tone and blood and lymphatic circulation, reduce the risk of blood clots, improve mood and energy level, decrease muscular aches, relieve boredom, give a woman a way to engage in her care, and stimulate inspiration and respiration. Some of these stress-relieving methods are included here. The massage therapist might remind the client of these tools to diminish tension between massages.

Conscious breathing is a known stress reliever and can help minimize anxiety that develops for women on restricted activity.[72-74] When engaging in the following activities, attention to the inhalations and exhalations will help increase a woman's relaxation response. Breath-holding should be avoided, as it increases pressure and strain to the abdomen. If you or the client has any uncertainty about the appropriateness of these activities for her condition, she should contact her PCP. Practices 1 to 6 can be done with the client in any position. The others are best done in the semi-reclining position.

1. Deep abdominal breathing: Slowly allow the abdomen to expand as the breath slips in through the nostrils. After the belly fills, let the chest continue to fill, expanding the ribs out laterally. Pause for a moment before exhaling slowly through the mouth, allowing all the breath to be released. Pause between the exhalations and inhalations.
2. Arm stretch: Reach each arm out to the side, and over the head as far as possible, while inhaling deeply with each stretch. Exhale returning the arms to the side.

Reach forward on an exhalation with fingers extended. Make a fist and inhale as the arms are drawn back toward the torso, imagining bringing in healthy energy with the inhalation. Repeat several times. Try reversing the breath, inhaling as the arms reach out, exhaling when drawing into the body.

3. Shoulder shrugging and shoulder rolls: Inhale as the shoulders are shrugged up to the ears. Exhale as the shoulders relax. Raise the shoulders to the ears with an inhale and rotate them backwards and down on an exhale. Repeat, rotating the shoulders forward.
4. Hand stretches: Alternate between making fists and stretching open fingers. One hand can pull back on the fingers of the other hand to increase stretching.
5. Foot circles: Stretch the toes back and rotate the feet in circles in either direction.
6. Kegel exercises: On an exhalation, squeeze the perineal muscles. On an inhalation, relax them. (See "Kegel Exercises" in Chapter 3.)
7. Neck rolls: Allow the chin to fall to the chest on an exhale. Lift the head and allow it to fall back with an inhale. Roll the head from one side to the other.
8. Chest opener: Place hands behind the head, retract the scapula, pulling the elbows posteriorly on the inhale. Exhale and return the elbows to neutral or forward.
9. Leg press: On an inhalation, plantar flex the feet, pulling the toes back, tighten the buttocks, perineum and lengthen the back of the legs, pressing the knees toward the bed. Exhale and relax the legs.
10. Leg Roll: Roll the legs in and out, bringing the knees together and apart.

of your bed-bound client or her care provider before beginning bodywork. The information gathered will help you offer the type of touch most appropriate for each individual.

1. What is her diagnosis and what are her risks?
2. Has she had this experience with previous pregnancies or earlier in this pregnancy? What was the outcome?
3. What are her limitations with regard to positioning and being up out of bed? Can she get out of bed and onto a massage table?
4. Has she had any bodywork while on bed rest?
5. What limitations would the care provider recommend with regards to bodywork?

CHAPTER SUMMARY

Most women who receive massage will have a healthy, low-risk pregnancy. However, occasionally complications develop. The massage therapist who is educated about these conditions will be able to offer with confidence, the safest bodywork for her or his clientele. Most bodywork precautions for women with a risk condition during pregnancy involve using safe and proper positioning, avoiding excessive full body stimulation or abdominal massage, using gentle touch to the legs and avoiding all work on legs with multiple, severe varicose veins or known blood clots. By being aware of the necessary precautions, and empowered with the ability to ask appropriate and discerning questions, the therapist can determine when extra caution may be appropriate, and when a medical release or discussion directly with a client's PCP or office nurse is highly recommended. To enhance your understanding of particular pregnancy conditions, you may be able to access support and information through doctors' or midwives' offices, by attending midwifery conferences, using research libraries, or by contacting other pregnancy massage specialists. As you become more educated, your confidence will increase, and your clients will be able to relax more in the security of your hands.

CHAPTER REVIEW QUESTIONS

1. Name three dangers of improper positioning during pregnancy massage.
2. Describe the difference between Type I and Type II forms of bodywork according to this text, and in what situations their use would be inappropriate.
3. Name three health-related questions specific to pregnancy that should be included on a health intake.
4. What concerns would you have with a client at 14 weeks' gestation, who states that she has had three consecutive miscarriages just prior to this pregnancy? What kind of adjustments might you make to your bodywork with her, if any?
5. Name three bodywork techniques or modalities that are contraindicated during pregnancy and explain why they are contraindicated.
6. Give two reasons why the use of certain essential oils or scents would be contraindicated during pregnancy.
7. Explain why pregnant and postpartum women have a higher risk for DVTs than nonpregnant women.
8. Name two health-related circumstances where a medical release would be highly recommended before working with a pregnant client.
9. Describe two situations that demonstrate why a thorough health intake is important.
10. Name a triad of common symptoms that could indicate a dangerous condition that only occurs during pregnancy.

REFERENCES

1. Jones W. Safe Motherhood: Promoting Health for Women Before, During and After Pregnancy — At a Glance 2007. National Center for Chronic Disease Prevention and Health Promotion At a Glance Health Pamphlet. Centers for Disease Control and Prevention.
2. Ventolini G, Heard M. Keys to minimizing liability in obstetrics. Contemp Ob Gyn 2003;48:81–96.
3. Beers MH, ed. The Merck Manual of Medical Information—Second Home Edition Online Version. Whitehouse Station, NJ: Merck & Co, 2004–2005.
4. Dickerson VM. Statement Regarding Medical Liability Reform. March 15, 2005. ACOG News Press Release, Office of Communications. Found at http://www.acog.org/from_home/publications/press_releases/nr03-15-05.cfm.
5. Mayo Clinic Staff. Tools for Healthier Lives. Education pamphlet. 2006. Available online at http://www.mayoclinic.com/health/miscarriage/PR00097.
6. West Z. Acupuncture in Pregnancy and Childbirth. Edinburgh: Churchill Livingstone, 2001.
7. Johnson E. Shiatsu. In: Tiran D, Mack S, eds. Complementary Therapies for Pregnancy and Childbirth. 2nd Ed. Edinburgh: Harcourt Publishers Limited, 2000.
8. Budd S. Acupuncture. In: Tiran D, Mack S, eds. Complementary Therapies for Pregnancy and Childbirth. 2nd Ed. Edinburgh: Harcourt Publishers Limited, 2000.
9. Yates S. Shiatsu for Midwives. Oxford: Elsevier Science, 2003.
10. Wang B, Liu JY, Han Y, et al. [Study on effect of electroacupuncture at Hegu (LI 4) on the uterotonic time in parturients of uterus inertia]. [Article in Chinese] Zhongguo Zhen Jiu 2006;26(12):843–846.
11. Rabl M, Ahner R, Bitschnau M, et al. Acupuncture for cervical ripening and induction of labour at term — a randomized controlled trial. Wien Klin Wochenschr 2001;113(23-24): 942–946.
12. Deadman P, Al-Khafaji M, Baker K. A Manual of Acupuncture. Seattle: Journal of Chinese Medicine Publications, Eastland Press, 2001.
13. Acupuncture Research and Resource website. http://www.acuxo.com.
14. Gach MR. Acupressure's Potent Points: a guide to self-care for common ailments. New York: Bantam Books, 1990.
15. Yin Yang House: Acupuncture for the World. http:www.Yingyanghouse.com.
16. Stillerman E. Prenatal Massage: a textbook of pregnancy, labor, and postpartum bodywork. Mosby, 2008.
17. Dale RA. The contraindicated (forbidden) points of acupuncture for needling, moxibustion and pregnancy. Am J Acupunct 1997;25(1):51–53.
18. Rempp C, Bigler A. Pregnancy and acupuncture from conception to postpartum. Am J Acupunct 1991;19(4): 305–315.
19. Zotz R, Gerhardt A, Scharf R. Prediction, prevention and treatment of venous thromboembolic disease in pregnancy. Semin Thromb Hemost 2003;29(2):143–153.
20. Gherman RB, Goodwin TM, Leung B, et al. Incidence, clinical characteristics, and timing of objectively diagnosed venous thrombo-embolism during pregnancy. Obstet Gynecol 1999;94:730–734.
21. Soomro RM, Bucur IJ, Noorani S. Cumulative incidence of venous thromboembolism during pregnancy and puerperium: a hospital-based study. Angiology 2002; 53(4):429–434.

22. Warren SE. Pulmonary embolus originating below knee. Lancet 1978;2(8083):272–273.

23. McKinney ES, Ashwill JW, Murray SS. Maternal-Child Nursing. Philadelphia: WB Saunders, 2000.

24. Cao YN, Zhang Y, Liu Y, et al. [Effects of exposure to extremely low frequency electromagnetic fields on reproduction of female mice and development of off-springs][Article in Chinese] Zhonghua Lao Dong Wei Sheng Zhi Ye Bing Za Zhi 2006;24(8):468–470.

25. Li DK, Odouli R, Wi S, et al. A population-based prospective cohort study of personal exposure to magnetic fields during pregnancy and the risk of miscarriage. Epidemiology 2002;13(1):9–20.

26. Feychting M. Non-cancer EMF effects related to children. Bioelectromagnetics 2005;26(Suppl 7):S69–S74.

27. Ahlbom IC, Cardis E, Green A, et al. Review of the epidemiologic literature on EMF and health. Environ Health Perspect 2001;109(Suppl 6):911–933.

28. Lee GM, Neutra RR, Hristova L, et al. A nested case-control study of residential and personal magnetic field measures and miscarriages. Epidemiology 2002; 13(1):21–31.

29. Kinsella SM, Lohmann G. Supine hypotensive syndrome. Obstet Gynecol 1994;83:774–788.

30. Carbonne B, Benachi A, Leveque ML, et al. Maternal position during labor: effects on fetal oxygen saturation measured by pulse oximetry. Obstet Gynecol 1996;88(5):797–800.

31. Jeffreys RM, Stepanchak W, Lopez B, et al. Uterine blood flow during supine rest and exercise after 28 weeks of gestation. BJOG 2006;113(11):1239–1247.

32. Brock-Utne JG, Buley RJ, Downing JW, et al. Advantages of left over right lateral tilt for caesarean section. S Afr Med J 1978;54(12):489–492.

33. Cunningham FG, Gant NF, Levene KJ, et al. Williams Obstetrics. 21st Ed. New York: McGraw Hill Medical Publishing, 2001.

34. Pergament E, Stein Schechtman A, Rochanayon A. Hyperthermia and pregnancy. Illinois Teratogen Information Service Risk Newsletter, June 1997;5(6). Last accessed May 2007 at http://www.fetal-exposure.org/HYPERTH.html.

35. Milunsky A, Ulcickas M, Rothman KJ, et al. Maternal heat exposure and neural tube defects. AMA 1992;268(7):882–885.

36. Li DK, Janevic T, Odouli R, et al. Hot tub use during pregnancy and the risk of miscarriage. Am J Epidemiol 2003;158(10):931–937.

37. Ananth CV, Savitz DA, Williams MA. Placental abruption and its association with hypertension and premature rupture of membranes: a methodological review and meta analysis. Obstet Gynecol 1996;88(2):309–318.

38. Mazor M, Ghezzi F, Maymon E, et al. Polyhydramnios is an independent risk factor for perinatal mortality and intrapartum morbidity in preterm delivery. Eur J Obstet Gynecol Reprod Biol 1996;70(1):41–47.

39. Ananth CV, Oyelese Y, Srinivas N, et al. Preterm premature rupture of membranes, intrauterine infection, and oligohydramnios: risk factors for placental abruption. Obstet Gynecol 2004;104: 71–77.

40. Richter ON, Rath W. [Thromboembolic diseases in pregnancy.] [Article in German] Z Geburtshilfe Neonatol 2007;211(1):1–7.

41. Ninet J. [The risk of maternal venous thromboembolism disease. Synopisis and definition of high-risk groups] [Article in French] Ann Med Interne (Paris) 2003;154(5-6):301–309.

42. Gates S, Brocklehurst P, Davis L. Prophylaxis for venous thromboembolic disease in pregnancy and the early postnatal period. Cochrane Database Syst Rev 2002;2.

43. Lindqvist P, Dahlback Ba, Marsal K. Thrombotic risk during pregnancy: a population study. Obstet Gynecol 1999;94:595–599.

44. James AH, Tapson VF, Goldhaber SZ. Thrombosis during pregnancy and the postpartum period. Am J Obstet Gynecol 2005;193(1):216–219.

45. Thromboembolism in pregnancy. ACOG Practice Bulletin; No. 19. Washington, (DC): American College of Obstetricians and Gynecologists, 2000 Aug: 10p.

46. Hill DR, Smith RB. Examination of the extremities: pulses, bruits, and phlebitis. In: Walker KH, Hall DW, Hurst JW. Clinical Methods: The History, Physical and Laboratory Examination. 3rd Ed. London: Butterworth-Heinemann, 1990.

47. Urbano FL. Homan's sign in the diagnosis of deep venous thrombosis. Hosp Physician, March 2001. Available at: http://www.turner-white.com.

48. Bulger C, Jacobs C, Patel N. Epidemiology of acute deep vein thromboisis. Tech Vasc Interv Radiol 2004; 7(2):50–54.

49. Joshua AM, Celermajer DS, Stockler MR. Beauty is in the eye of the examiner: reaching agreement about physical signs and their value. Intern Med J 2005; 35 (3):178–187.

50. Lefor AT, Bogdonoff D, Geehan D. Critical Care On Call. New York: McGraw Hill Medical, 2002.

51. Levi M, Hart W, Büller HR. Ned Tijdschr Geneeskd. [Physical examination — the significance of Homan's sign] [Article in Dutch] 1999;143(37):1861–1863.

52. ACOG Education Pamphlet Item #AP090. Early Pregnancy Loss: Miscarriage and Molar Pregnancy. American College of Obstetricians and Gynecologists, 2002.

53. U.S. Pregnancy Rate Down from Peak; Births and Abortions on the Decline. Revised Pregnancy Rates, 1990–97, and New Rates for 1998–99: United States. NVSR;52(7), 15 pp. (PHS) 2004-1120. Last viewed on May 2007 at http://www.cdc.gov/nchs/pressroom/03facts/pregbirths.htm.

54. Wilcox AJ, Weinberg CR, O'Connor JF, et al. Early loss of pregnancy. N Engl J Med1988;319(4):189–194.

55. Kleinhaus K, Perrin M, Friedlander Y, et al. Paternal age and spontaneous abortion. Obstet Gynecol 2006;108(2):369–377.

56. Slama R, Bouyer J, Windham G, et al. Influence of paternal age on the risk of spontaneous abortion. Am J Epidemiol 2005;161(9):816–823.

57. National Institute of Child Health and Human Development, NIH, DHHS. Division of Epidemiology,

Statistics, and Prevention Research (DESPR), NICHD: Report to the NACHHD Council, 2001. Washington, DC: U.S. Government Printing Office. Last accessed on 9/08/07 at: http://www.nichd.nih.gov/publications/pubs_details.cfm?from=&pubs_id=128.

58. Rasch V. Cigarette, alcohol, and caffeine consumption: risk factors for spontaneous abortion. Acta Obstet Gynecol Scand 2003;82(2):182–188.

59. Tolstrup JS, Kjaer SK, Munk C, et al. Does caffeine and alcohol intake before pregnancy predict the occurrence of spontaneous abortion? Hum Reprod 2003;18(12):2704–2710.

60. Beers MH, Berkow R, eds. The Merck Manual of Diagnosis and Therapy, 17th Ed. Section 18, Ch 250. Whitehouse Station, NJ: Merck & Co, 1999–2005.

61. Gestational Diabetes Resource Guide. American Diabetes Association. http://www.diabetes.org/gestational-diabetes.jsp.

62. Pernoll ML. Benson & Pernoll's Handbook of Obstetrics & Gynecology. Columbus, OH: McGraw-Hill Professional, 2001.

63. Ananth CV, Smulian JC, Vintzileos AM. Incidence of placental abruption in relation to cigarette smoking and hypertensive disorders during pregnancy: A meta analysis of observational studies. Obstet Gynecol 1999;93(4):622–628.

64. Kramer MS, Usher RH, Pollack R, et al. Etiologic determinants of abruptio placentae. Obstet Gynecol 1997;89(2):221–226.

65. Wolf JL. Liver disease in pregnancy. Med Clin North Am 1996;80:1167–1187.

66. Management of Chronic Hypertension During Pregnancy. Summary, Evidence Report/Technology Assessment: Number 14. AHRQ Publication No. 00-E010, August 2000. Agency for Healthcare Research and Quality, Rockville, MD. Available at: http://www.ahrq.gov/clinic/epcsums/pregsum.htm.

67. Gofton EN, Capewell V, Natale R, Gratton RJ. Obstetrical intervention rates and maternal and neonatal outcomes of women with gestational hypertension. Am J Obstet Gynecol 2001;185(4):798–803.

68. Padden MO. HELLP Syndrome: Recognition and Perinatal Management. Am Fam Physician 1999;60(3). Online access: http://www.aafp.org/afp/990901ap/829.html.

69. Douglas KA, Redman CW. Eclampsia in the United Kingdom. Br Med J 1994;309:1395–1400.

70. Preeclampsia and eclampsia, while often preventable, are among top causes of pregnancy-related deaths. Fam Plann Perspect July/August 2001;33(4). Online at www.guttmacher.org/pubs/journals/3318201.html.

71. MacKay AP, Berg CJ, Atrash HK. Pregnancy-related mortality from preeclampsia and eclampsia, Obstet Gynecol 2001;97(4):533–538.

72. Kaushik RM, Kaushik R, Mahajan SK, Rajesh V. Effects of mental relaxation and slow breathing in essential hypertension. Complement Ther Med 2006;14(2):120–126.

73. Joseph CN, Porta C, Casucci G, et al. Slow breathing improves arterial baroreflex sensitivity and decreases blood pressure in essential hypertension. Hypertension 2005;46(4):714–718.

74. Mack S, Steele D. Complementary therapies for the relief of physical and emotional stress. In: Tiran D, Mack S, eds. Complementary Therapies for Pregnancy and Childbirth, 2nd Ed. Edinburgh: Harcourt Publishers, Ltd., 2000.

CHAPTER 5

GENERAL MASSAGE FOR PREGNANCY

LEARNING OBJECTIVES

After reading this chapter, you should be able to:

- Describe common bodywork needs of pregnant clients.
- Arrange a massage office space to meet the special needs of pregnant clients.
- Describe the specific concerns of each trimester and relevant bodywork precautions.
- Explain how to position clients for optimum comfort and safety for both client and practitioner.
- Utilize appropriate draping for the sidelying position.
- Implement bodywork techniques useful for a general pregnancy massage.
- Describe positioning methods appropriate to a client's trimester and size.

Certain themes apply to nearly every massage during pregnancy. For instance, a woman will generally have an increased need for nurturance. She will benefit from stretching and muscular work that elongates the areas that are shortening and compressing as pregnancy progresses. For optimum well-being, she will also benefit from attendance to postural adaptations to her changing weight, as discussed in Chapter 3. She will expect her massage therapist to be educated and vigilant about precautions and contraindications throughout pregnancy, to create an environment safe for herself and her unborn child. And she will most commonly expect that receiving

bodywork will diminish discomforts and help her feel more grounded and at ease in her body.

While a treatment-oriented, technical medical massage model is appropriate for a variety of clients, during pregnancy the need for a distinctly nurturing touch often becomes greater. This need mirrors the growing nurturing energy that is often arising within women as the time draws nearer to nurture a new baby. Receiving compassionate touch does more than help a growing mother feel good; studies have shown that women who receive this caring touch during pregnancy have a greater capacity to attend to their infants with an increased devotion of nurturing energy.[1]

In addition to the increasing need for *nurturance*, once a woman has reached the late second and third trimester, she will benefit the most from a touch that helps to create *length* and *space* in her body, defying the forces of gravity that may be causing a collapse in her chest, tension in her neck, constriction in her groin area, and tightness in her low back. During a massage, think about the ways you can help your client relax, release, and find renewal as she discovers space and freedom in areas of her body that have been compressed. Whatever type of touch you use, ask your client to help facilitate easier releases by breathing fully into the tight areas, imagining her breath helping to expand and open the spaces that are being freed by your touch.

Since a woman's posture changes drastically throughout pregnancy, the bodywork practitioner should be sure to take time before a session to observe the client's posture, help bring her awareness to the ways she can make adjustments to it, and then address the related muscular stresses with bodywork. This postural attention is an important link in addressing a pregnant woman's complaints.

Pregnancy poses a variety of massage concerns, as there are risks and considerations that are not encountered with the standard nonpregnant massage client. This is true regarding the general office set-up and massage practice for pregnant women as well; for instance, lateral positioning is necessary through at least half of a woman's pregnancy, and the therapist needs to learn how to work competently in this position. Different questions are asked on a health intake and different practicalities are taken into consideration when setting up your office.

This chapter will look at these issues, as well as considerations based especially on the stage of a woman's pregnancy. First, we will consider how to set up your office to meet the needs of pregnant clients, including what equipment you will need. Then, we will review treatment guidelines and precaution reminders for each trimester of pregnancy. Positioning for bodywork is addressed next, with a look at sidelying, semi-reclining, prone, and supine positions and how each position can be adapted for work with a pregnant client. Finally, bodywork techniques adapted specifically for pregnant clients are presented, including techniques for the whole body and for each body region.

Before we begin, however, let us review some of the basic practical aspects that are a part of any massage. These include the following:

- *Safe Environment:* Create a workspace that encourages clear communication and feedback channels between the client and the therapist.
- *Relaxing Touch:* Use slow, even, and consistent strokes that encourage relaxation.
- *Proper Body Mechanics:* Use proper body mechanics and client positioning to ensure that neither the giver nor the receiver experiences muscular strain during the bodywork.
- *Breath:* Use breath attunement to facilitate deeper relaxation. (The cultivation of an association between breath and relaxation during pregnancy will become a powerful ally during birth.)
- *Hydration:* Offer a large glass of water after every massage to help flush cellular waste released during massage, thereby avoiding dehydration. This is especially important in pregnancy, as dehydration can lead to premature uterine irritability and contractions.
- *Avoid Heartburn:* Encourage your client to wait at least 2 hours after eating a meal before getting a massage. Heartburn is a common complaint during late pregnancy.
- *Avoid Boney Pressure:* Avoid pressure directly on bones, except in the case of the sacrum, where direct pressure can be beneficial during late pregnancy.

PREPARING FOR MASSAGE

As with any type of massage, it is essential to make proper preparations before actually beginning your work. You must make sure that your office is arranged to meet the needs of pregnant clients, as well as conduct a thorough health intake with each client, as discussed in Chapter 4, to understand her unique needs or restrictions.

Office Considerations

Certain aspects of office setup and practice are different when working with pregnant women. Below is a list of these considerations.

- *Baby activity:* The baby may become very active during massage, making it more difficult for the mother to relax. Be prepared to help the client change position to the other side if necessary to try to settle the baby.
- *Music:* Suggest that your client bring her own music CDs to the massage sessions if she plans to use music during labor. As she associates touch and relaxation with particular music, she may find herself automatically relaxing when she hears it during labor.
- *Body fluids:* Pregnant, laboring, and postpartum women may leak body fluids such as amniotic fluid, breast milk, or blood. Have gloves available to practice universal precautions if you do encounter these fluids on your sheets.
- *Fan:* Many pregnant women suffer from sinus congestion due to increased blood volume and dilated blood vessels. Try using a fan to blow fresh air across her face during a massage, temporarily alleviating sensations of stuffiness.
- *Restroom:* A restroom should be easily accessible and offered to the client before, in the middle, and after a massage. Pressure from the baby on the bladder increases urgency, incontinence, and frequency.
- *Scents:* Pregnant women are often sensitive to smells. Do not use heavily scented oils, aromatherapies, or incense without having the

client determine first that she can tolerate the scent.

- *Temperature:* Pregnant women are generally warm due to changes in hormones, body weight, and blood volume. Consider lowering the office temperature slightly if you tend to keep it warmer for other clients. Some women may also prefer to have their feet exposed from under sheets.
- *Time:* Allow extra time in your scheduled sessions for pregnant women to undress, get positioned, use the bathroom, and address health concerns.

Additionally, accessories as described in the following list, are necessary for optimum comfort for pregnancy sidelying positioning:

- *Sheets:* A full- or queen-size flat sheet is necessary. A single flat sheet will usually *not* be adequate.
- *Breast drape:* A small towel or pillowcase can be used as a breast drape for belly rubs or if offering breast massage.
- *Pillows:* At least five to seven pillows are necessary, as follows: one head pillow, one arm pillow, one belly pillow (a small rolled towel, wedge, or thin pillow), and two to three firm, flat, long bolsters or pillows for supporting the leg. Alternatively, use a long body pillow or the Body-Support Systems, Inc., four-piece contoured bodyCushion. This will provide support under the belly, back, head, and leg and eliminate the need for extra cushions, and is especially versatile during pregnancy.
- *Oil:* Use unscented oils unless you are trained in aromatherapy and are aware of the prohibited essential oils during pregnancy, labor, postpartum.
- *Stepstool:* A stepstool will be necessary to help a mother get onto the raised table, and to help the practitioner access parts of her body that are higher than normal.

TRIMESTER CONSIDERATIONS

Each trimester of pregnancy poses different experiences for a mother and new opportunities for the therapist to offer comfort and healing. Knowing what part of pregnancy your client is in will help guide you in choosing techniques, noting precautions, and providing optimum positioning. The following are basic suggestions and precautions to be aware of during each trimester.

Suggested Guidelines and Precaution Reminders for Each Trimester

The pregnancy massage therapist has several angles from which to approach a session with a pregnant client, depending on her needs, and also depending on the stage of her pregnancy. Each trimester implies guidelines and presents precautions specific to that stage. The following precautions have been addressed at various points through the previous chapters. They are discussed briefly again here as a reminder and listed in Table 5.1.

Throughout pregnancy, regardless of trimester, the following reminders apply:

- Do a thorough health intake prior to the first massage with a client, and update the information at each session.
- Observe and use precautions for varicose veins and deep vein thrombosis.
- Avoid contraindicated acupressure points until 38 weeks, and take note of precautionary points, which are contraindicated with those at high risk for miscarriage or preterm labor as discussed in Chapter 4.
- Teach the client early the proper body mechanics for pushing up from supine positioning while avoiding abdominal strain and help establish this method of sitting up as the pregnancy progresses (see Figure 3.5).

First Trimester

In the first trimester, when the embryo is becoming a fetus and developing its core neurological system, gentle, nurturing bodywork is often more appropriate than deep manipulations. Risk of miscarriage is highest in this trimester, so avoid deep abdominal massage and do a thorough health intake at each visit. Generally the client can be positioned prone and supine if comfortable, otherwise, consider the sidelying or semi-reclining position, especially when she has tender breasts or nausea.

Remind the client, if she complains of feeling fatigued, that resting regularly is quite appropriate, and allows her body to devote its energy to the primary task at hand: creating life. For many women, generating life and giving birth will be the most powerful and creative experience of their lives.

Second Trimester

In the second trimester, the belly becomes more apparent with the growth of the baby. The highest risk of miscarriage has passed and women who

DISPELLING MYTHS:
Avoiding Massage in the First Trimester

Some massage therapists are taught to avoid massaging the pregnant client during the first trimester because it is believed to be dangerous. There are thoughts that massage could be disruptive to the baby's development, concerns that it could harm the placenta, or that women experiencing fatigue, nausea, or ambivalence about their pregnancy will find massage uncomfortable in some way. Many are concerned about causing or being associated with a miscarriage that might occur, since the first trimester is known to be the time of greatest risk for miscarriage. All of these concerns are unfounded.

The first trimester is a time when a woman often experiences enormous fatigue, confusing emotions, and a flood of new sensations as her body surges with hormones. Massage can actually be a wonderful tool to help your client feel more unified and grounded in her experience of pregnancy. Acupressure points, energy work, and massage can help decrease a woman's nausea and increase her sense of grounding and vitality. Massage can

support the woman's physiology, improving hormonal function and supporting the healthy development of placenta and baby. Bodywork is not a cause of placental dysfunctions or fetal anomalies.

While miscarriages do occur frequently in the first trimester, it is rarely a reason to avoid massage. As discussed previously in this text, it is appropriate to use precautions if a mother has a history of three or more consecutive miscarriages in the first trimester or is currently having miscarriage risks. In this case, while a full-body Type I massage might be contraindicated, nurturing energy work and soothing, gentle Type II massage can still be beneficial. A medical release is highly recommended for clients with this type of history.

First trimester bodywork has some other considerations to keep in mind. A health history is always important to obtain. Deep abdominal work is contraindicated. But for the majority of women, nurturing touch and manual therapy during the first trimester can offer wonderful musculoskeletal and circulatory benefits as well as comfort, reassurance, and relaxation that should not be missed!

previously experienced miscarriage in the first trimester, now breathe a sigh of relief. Avoid supine positioning if the client becomes uncomfortable. After 22 weeks, use it only for short duration for specific

techniques and only if the client tolerates it well. Begin using sidelying positioning after 22 weeks, when the belly is visibly protruding, or anytime the mother is more comfortable that way.

Traditional Birth Practices:
Uterine Massage

*I*n many cultures, midwives massage the pregnant uterus through the abdomen, starting in the second trimester. With their hands, they can feel the baby's position and activity, reposition as needed, and have a good sense of its health. Rosita Arvigo is a Napropath (a specialist in evaluation and treatment of musculoskeletal conditions related to connective tissue, using manipulations and mobilizations) who has learned uterine massage techniques from Mayan midwives. She teaches abdominal massage to align the uterus before, during, and after pregnancy. While not within the scope of this book, Arvigo's uterine massage work is well worth investigating further if you wish to specialize in pregnancy massage (see Appendix B).

Third Trimester

In the third trimester, mothers often feel vibrant and enthusiastic initially, but as delivery becomes imminent, some begin to experience, perhaps for the first time, some common complaints. This is an excellent time to receive massage; many women come for their first massage in this trimester.

Positioning will only be in the sidelying, semi-reclining, or left-tilt positions. Supine positioning can be used only for very short durations of 3 to 8 minutes for specific therapeutic techniques, and only if client is comfortable. Focus on creating length and space in the woman's body. Short belly rubs in the third trimester can help the client attune with the baby, feel comfortable with abdominal sensations, and relax when touched on her abdomen, a touch which may be useful in alleviating some types of contraction pain during birth. Offer labor supportive techniques in the last 1 to 2 weeks of pregnancy, as discussed in Chapter 7.

Table 5.1	Bodywork Considerations by Trimester

Treatment Guidelines for First Trimester

Teaching	• Develop skills for decreasing varicose veins, heartburn, leg cramps, low back pain, hemorrhoids. • Instruct in abdominal strengthening techniques. • Encourage prenatal exercise. • Suggest client empty bladder before beginning massage. • Suggest beginning Kegel exercises.
Assessment	• Assess for increased risk of nausea and position accordingly. • Assess for diastasis recti if had previous births. • Assess for increased miscarriage risks. • Collect health update and intake information at each visit to assess for increased pregnancy-related risks.
Bodywork	• Use nurturing touch that supports the growth and development of embryo and fetus. • Use standard massage work in prone and supine positioning usually through all of first trimester. • Encourage relaxation and renewal.
Precautions	• Limit sauna, hot tubs to 5–10 minutes if over 102°F. • Avoid hot packs longer than 5 minutes over 100°F to abdomen or low back. • Avoid electric heating pads on massage table. • Use blood clot and varicose vein precautions. • Avoid acupressure on contraindicated and precautionary points. • Avoid scents, passive range of motion, rocking if client has nausea. • Avoid deep abdominal massage.

Treatment Guidelines for Second Trimester

Teaching	• Use methods for decreasing varicose veins, heartburn, leg cramps, low back pain, hemorrhoids. • Make postural adjustments and awareness as needed. • Suggest client empty bladder before beginning massage. • Instruct in abdominal strengthening techniques. • Suggest beginning Kegel exercises. • Teach proper methods for sitting up and repositioning on table.
Assessment	• Assess for diastasis recti if client had previous pregnancy, or has large baby in this pregnancy. • Assess and address postural changes and maladaptations. • Collect health update and intake information at each visit to assess for increased pregnancy-related risks.
Bodywork	• Use massage and stretches to create length and space in client's body. • Focus on areas of primary stress based on client info and postural assessment.
Precautions	• Use diastasis symphysis pubis precautions. • Avoid prone and supine positions if client uncomfortable, breasts too sore, nausea, or visible belly. • Use blood clot and varicose vein precautions. • Avoid acupressure on contraindicated points. • Avoid prone positioning and limit supine positioning once belly is showing or after 22 weeks' gestation.

Treatment Guidelines for Third Trimester

Teaching	• Use methods for decreasing varicose veins, heartburn, leg cramps, low back pain, hemorrhoids. • Make postural adjustments and awareness as needed. • Suggest client empty bladder before beginning massage. • Give perineal massage instructions in last 6 weeks of pregnancy. • Encourage continuation of Kegel exercises. • Teach proper methods for sitting up and repositioning on table.
Assessment	• Assess and address postural changes and mal-adaptations. • Assess for increased risk of heartburn and position accordingly. • Collect health update and intake information at each visit to assess for increased pregnancy-related risks.
Bodywork	• Use massage and stretches to create length and space in client's body. • Focus on areas of primary stress based on client info and postural assessment. • After 38th week, offer labor preparation techniques, including possible use of previously contraindicated acupressure points. • Offer belly rubs for relaxation and connection to the baby.
Precautions	• Use blood clot and varicose vein precautions. • Avoid acupressure on contraindicated points until 38th week. • Avoid prone positioning and limit supine positioning to 3–8 minutes.

POSITIONING TECHNIQUES

In the first trimester, prone and supine positioning can be used as long as it is comfortable for the client. During the second trimester, sidelying is generally used. Semi-reclining is also an option and a comfortable position to use when sidelying is not optimal.

Sidelying Positioning

Sidelying positioning is used for two important reasons:

1. To prevent pressure on the abdomen and breasts, as occurs with prone positioning.
2. To prevent pressure on the large blood vessels in the abdomen, as occurs with supine positioning.

Sidelying is a very restful position that allows access to one side of the body at a time and enables the practitioner to provide full shoulder and hip mobilizations. Varied pillows and bolsters are necessary for optimum comfort and are used to support the body under the neck, hip, belly, and the superior leg and foot.

When to Use the Sidelying Position

During pregnancy, the sidelying position is most frequently used after 22 weeks' gestation, when the baby is about 1.5 to 2 pounds, or when the abdomen is visibly protruding, with the top of the uterus at or above the navel. It may also be used at any time during pregnancy if it is more comfortable for a client for any reason. Some situations indicating the need to position sidelying include the following:

- Hypotension when in supine position
- Obesity
- Difficulty breathing when prone or supine
- Breast tenderness causing discomfort when prone
- When good verbal communication is more important than prone positioning
- Extreme nasal congestion, which becomes worse with prone positioning
- Back pain aggravated by prone or supine positioning

Table Height

To work effectively with good body mechanics from *behind* sidelying clients, as opposed to *over* them, as with supine or prone positioning, the therapist must raise the massage table higher than normal. An easy way to assess the proper table height is to stand next to the table and have the table top reach the level of your anterior superior iliac spine or the level of your wrist when your arms are relaxed and extended straight down. Play with the table height until you find the best level for your body. On average, it may be 2 to 4 pegs higher than normal.

Alternatively, some people prefer to keep the table low. In this case, the practitioner may sit in a chair when working on the client's back. When standing, the practitioner will have access to the hip and leg without need for a stepstool as described for when the table is higher. Find the table height for which you can most easily utilize proper body mechanics and avoid strain. This book describes most work with a higher table height.

Client Positioning in Sidelying

Note on terminology: Here I use the term "superior" to refer to the client's side that is *up* and accessible. The side *on* the table I refer to as the "inferior" side.

Proper positioning in sidelying involves supporting every arch and space to prevent strain on musculature or ligaments (Figure 5.1). All muscles should be

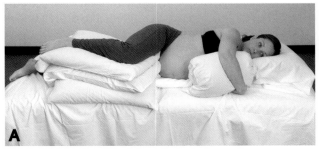
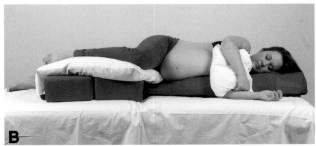

FIGURE 5.1   Supportive sidelying positioning.
(A) All body arches are supported with pillows. Spine is 2 to 4 inches away from and parallel with edge of table. Extremities are supported on pillows and parallel to tabletop, with muscles in neutral position. Protruding belly is supported with small wedge, rolled towel, or thin pillow. (B) A bodyCushion offers optimal support in sidelying. Notice the angling support under the torso, which prevents compression in shoulder joint.

in a relaxed and supported position, unless a stretch is intentional. There should be no pressure from bone on any other part of the body; therefore, one pillow should be placed under the arm and two to three pillows should support the superior leg and foot.

All body parts should be horizontal and parallel to the table—pillows should be placed such that the superior leg is flexed with the knee and thigh horizontal and supported and parallel to the tabletop. The lateral hip rotators should be in a relaxed position. The lower leg should be extended straight. Some women find it more comfortable and natural to have both legs flexed with pillows in between. This arrangement is acceptable if necessary; however, the position can make it more difficult to work on both the superior and inferior leg and can cause some restriction to venous blood flow in lower leg.

The neck pillow should support the crook of the neck. Avoid having her inferior shoulder rest on the pillow, as this will cause compression in the shoulder and neck. Keep the cervical spine horizontal—parallel with the table.

The superior arm should be supported by a pillow, with the humerus nearly horizontal and the rhomboids and upper back musculature relaxed; this helps to avoid breast compression from the weight of the arm.

The spine should be straight and aligned with the edge of the table, rather than angled across the table or rolled forward or back. Once the belly is visibly protruding, a soft wedge, rolled towel, or small pillow can be placed under the belly to prevent gravitational, downward pull on the uterus, causing strain to uterine ligaments. If desired, a small rolled cloth can be placed behind the client under her inferior hip and waist. This can give her added posterior support and security, although there can be a tendency for this roll to slide out when rocking or doing joint mobilizations.

Draping in the Sidelying Position

It is a good idea to practice sidelying draping several times before using new draping for the first time with a client. Though simple, there is a skill to draping smoothly, securely, and effectively for a client in the sidelying position. Sheets do not "stay put" as naturally as they do with prone and supine clients, and draping the upper leg without exposing the belly and lower leg often requires a little extra time before some practitioners are comfortable. It may be helpful to use a bath towel to help hold the sheets in place after exposing the back or upper leg and gluteals, or to use a clothespin or hairclip to hold them bunched together. The use of the towel can be seen in Figure 5.2 and Figure 5.3.

Case Study 5.1:
PAIN RELIEVED BY POSITIONING

At 38 weeks' gestation, Tawny came to her massage therapist, Trina, with complaints of shoulder and neck aches that developed 1 month earlier. It hurt worse in the morning and improved with activity during the day, but the discomfort returned again every morning. Her doctor said it was muscular strain, probably due to the size of her growing breasts. She pointed to her rhomboid area as the site of primary discomfort. The therapist asked how she was positioned when sleeping, and Tawny stated she slept on her side, with one pillow between her knees. Trina noted that Tawny has some collapsing of her upper chest as her shoulders internally rotated.

Trina gave Tawny a massage, and included some pectoralis and subscapularis stretches. Afterwards, Tawny said that she had never slept with a pillow under her arm before, and noted that as she lay on her side on the massage table, the pain in her shoulder was relieved. Her superior arm had been well supported with a thick pillow, and she determined to try that now at home in bed. She also stated that the stretches felt good, and was surprised to find that her pectorals were sore, as she had only been aware of her upper back. Trina described how the weight of the superior arm falls forward when unsupported by a pillow, and not only compresses the breasts, but puts the rhomboids in a stretch position and shortens the pectoralis and subscapularis all night long. Trina suggested Tawny explore strengthening exercises for the rhomboids, and external shoulder rotators, and stretches for the internal rotators.

Tawny returned a week later excited that her shoulder pain was now almost totally relieved by using a pillow under her arm in bed. Trina suggested she also work with her posture. She helped Tawny become aware of how she sank inward in her chest and how that, too, would contribute to upper back pain. Trina also suggested that Tawny get help to find a well-fitting, supportive bra that she could use for nursing as well. Since her breasts would get even larger once her milk came in, that too would affect her posture and increase back pain.

During pregnancy, a full- or queen-size sheet is necessary for adequate draping of the lower leg and foot, abdomen, and breasts. This is due to the number of supportive pillows used, and the size of the abdomen in later pregnancy, both of which require extra coverage with the sheet.

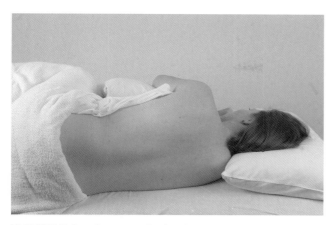

FIGURE 5.2   Draping the back.

The arm pillow is on top of sheet to prevent the sheet from falling forward and exposing the breasts. Angle sheet so superior hip is partly exposed, but maintaining coverage of gluteal cleft. Tuck sheet under inferior hip. A bath towel over her superior hip adds extra security if desired.

Draping the Back (Figure 5.2)

Note: Before exposing the back, ensure that the arm pillow is on top of the sheet, as it will help prevent the sheet from falling forward and exposing the breasts.

1. Standing behind the client, pull the side of the sheet up from the tabletop and over the edge of her superior waist and scapula, laying the sheet along her superior side.
2. While holding the sheet securely against the superior hip near the trochanter, pull the lower edge of the sheet slightly cephalically, exposing the superior hip, while covering the gluteal cleft.
3. Tuck the sheet in under the inferior waist. The sheet should now be at an angle with the lowest corner at the superior trochanter, and the upper corner at the inferior waist.
4. Lay a heavy bath towel, if desired, on the sheet over her superior hip for extra security.

Draping to Expose the Gluteals and Superior Leg

1. Stand on the client's anterior side at the foot of the table holding that corner of the sheet.
2. With that corner in hand, pull the sheet up behind the thigh of the client's superior leg, just proximal to the knee.
3. Tuck the corner you are holding beneath the posterior side of the superior leg's thigh, toward the client's belly (Figure 5.3A). Pull it several inches out on the anterior side, just above the knee from posterior to anterior. There

will be slack and bunching of excess sheet at the posterior leg. *Do not* pull it all the way through, as if doing a "diaper" drape (Figure 5.3A).
4. Pull some extra sheet from the abdomen area and toward the anterior side of the superior leg's thigh with one hand and, with the other hand, pull the excess sheet up along the posterior thigh toward the trochanter. Essentially, your hands are both holding the sheet and sliding up the client's leg on either side of her superior thigh at once (Figure 5.3B).
5. Slide over the trochanter and continue until the entire superior gluteals are exposed. Tuck the abdomen side of the sheet under the mid or lower anterior thigh (Figure 5.3C).
6. Roll the sheet up tightly over the back of the gluteals to keep it in place.
7. For extra security, if desired, place a bath towel over the rolled up section of sheet at the gluteals, either tucking it in with the rolled sheet or laying it across the rolled sheet.

Draping to Expose the Inferior Leg   When ready to work on the inferior leg, slide the sheet from the edge of the table over the inferior leg.

Draping to Expose the Belly

1. For easy access to the abdomen in the sidelying position, remove the belly support first.
2. Lay a drape, such as a long pillowcase or thin folded towel, across the client's breasts on top of the sheet and secure it under her superior arm.
3. Ask her to hold the breast drape while you pull the sheet out from under it, exposing the belly.
4. Push the sheet down below her belly, and secure it at her back, under her inferior hip. (See draping used in Figure 5.17.)

Common Comfort Problems in Sidelying

Sidelying can be a very satisfying and extremely comfortable position, but without adequate cushioning or good adherence to positioning details, some discomforts can arise.

Sore Hips   Without having the option to change positions to supine or prone during the second and third trimesters, women's hips may become sore from sleeping and lying on their side when at rest. For optimum comfort on a massage table, use a foam mattress pad or a thick sheepskin cover for extra cushioning.

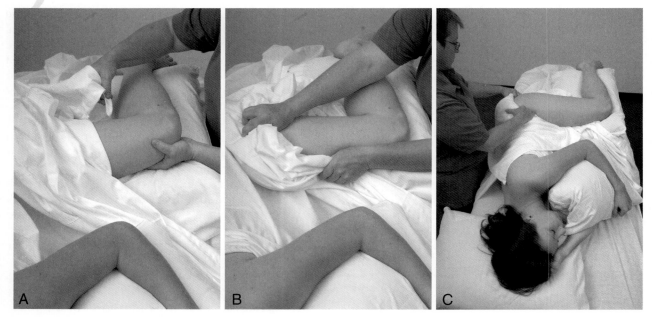

FIGURE 5.3   Draping to expose the gluteals and superior leg.
(A) Step 1: Stand on client's anterior side holding the foot-end corner of the sheet. With smooth movement slide sheet up behind client's superior thigh, tucking corner under posterior thigh. *(B)* Step 2: Pull extra sheet from abdomen area toward thigh while pushing up excess sheet along posterior thigh toward the trochanter. *(C)* Step 3. Tuck the abdomen side of sheet under mid or lower anterior thigh. Roll sheet up tightly to keep it in place. A bath towel over her superior hip adds extra security if desired.

Shoulder Compression   During a sidelying massage, some women will experience compression in the shoulder joint or brachial plexus, developing numbness or discomfort in the arm and hand. Extra padding on the table can help to avoid this. Also, ensure that her inferior shoulder is pulled slightly forward out from under her, as opposed to having her rolled over the top of her shoulder.

A foam triangular wedge placed under the client's hip and ribs, tapering from about 4 inches at the shoulder to 1/2 inch at the hips gives a space for the shoulder and alleviates compression. The Body-Support Systems, Inc., four-piece contoured bodyCushion offers ideal support, holding under both the waist and abdomen, alleviating compression on the shoulder joint, giving a soft cushion for the hips, and eliminating a few extra pillows. It is an excellent choice for practitioners with regular pregnant clients or who work often with clients in the sidelying position.

Instability   Throughout the massage, ensure that the client stays positioned directly on her hip and side and that her limbs are horizontal to the tabletop. Her back should be parallel to the tabletop. The superior trochanter should be stacked directly over the inferior, so a vertical line could be drawn

between them. Avoid having her rotate forward, twisting her spine or being pushed forward into the table when you apply pressure to her back. If she does fall forward frequently when you work on her posterior side, she probably needs to adjust her inferior hip more anteriorly. The inferior shoulder should be pulled forward slightly to help maintain her position. The top leg pillow should be angled slightly across the table and between the client's legs, as this will allow for more stability, as opposed to having every pillow parallel with the edge of the table. This can be seen in Figure 5.1.

Practitioner Comfort   Until you are accustomed to the sidelying position, you may find yourself straining as you work from different angles and with different leverage. If this is the case, investigate the following to help improve your body mechanics:

- Ensure that the table is the appropriate height and that the client's back is aligned with and positioned close to the working edge. You can help her position well by placing your hands on the edge of the table and having her inch back until her back is close to your arms or until her hips and head are within 2 to 4 inches of the edge of the table.

- Good therapist body mechanics are critical to avoid strain. Rather than working above a client with downward pressure, as with someone in supine position, you will be working from a horizontal gliding position and moving your hips often. Keep your body moving as you work, swaying from one bent knee or lunge position to the other and initiating the effort from your belly, not from your hands or arms.

Changing Sides   After working on the mother's superior side, you will want to access her other side. Women with large bellies will have more difficulty moving from side to side. Remove all pillows first, except the head pillow, and ask the client if she needs to use the bathroom before repositioning. Pregnant women frequently have pressure on the bladder and may need to use the restroom in the middle of a session.

If she is ready to roll over, she may find it easier to sit up, using proper body mechanics as described in Chapter 3, or she may choose to get on her hands and knees to switch sides. Whichever is easier for her is fine, however, in the hands and knees position, be aware that her breasts will be more exposed in the front. The therapist should therefore stand closer to her hips to hold the sheet.

For client safety, position yourself on the side of the table her back will be facing, making certain that she does not lie down too close to the edge of the table. Once she is positioned, replace all the pillows, including the wedge for her belly.

Semi-Reclining Positioning (Figure 5.4)

Semi-reclining is an excellent position for certain situations and is sometimes preferred by clients who are having difficulty finding comfort in sidelying due to hip problems, nausea, or heartburn, or who just want an alternative to sidelying. Bodywork in this position is similar to standard supine massage for nonpregnant clients, but a step stool may be necessary to access behind the client's head and back more easily.

When to Use the Semi-Reclining Position

The semi-reclining position is useful in a variety of situations:

- When the client is uncomfortable in sidelying.
- When a client is close to her due date and would like to receive bodywork in a position she expects to deliver in. (Many women in hospitals deliver in a semi-reclining position.)
- When a client experiences excessive heartburn, nausea, or nasal congestion when in a lateral position.

MASSAGE THERAPIST TIP   *Making Your Table Comfortable for Pregnancy*

It can be difficult for a pregnant women to find a position where she can rest comfortably. If she is able to find comfort on the massage table, it will provide at least one arena where she can rest deeply. She will appreciate a foam pad to soften the pressure of her hips on the table. Firm pillows supporting the legs will be less likely to collapse under the weight of her knee and will create more stability. Having a variety of pillow sizes and shapes will offer more flexibility for positioning each individual client. Using an angled foam wedge under the torso can help to prevent shoulder compression. A belly wedge using a rolled towel or thin, soft, small pillow can feel supportive for some women.

Even after you have acquired various pillows, bolsters, and cushions, you may still be unsure of how comfortable your table will be. Get on the table yourself with the supports you will be using, and rest there for 10 minutes or so. Better yet, get a massage from a peer who can use your table and pillows. Notice how your body is aligned. Notice how your hips are pressing on the table. Notice the compression of your shoulder.

Within 10 to 15 minutes, if changes need to be made, you will begin to become aware of areas that do not feel as comfortable as they could. You will also get an indication as to whether you will have problems with your pillows being too full and therefore unstable after some time, or too fluffy and sinking down after the weight of your leg compresses them. If you start to feel shoulder compression, your pregnant client will also; reposition yourself, try a wedge under the upper torso, obtain a body cushion, or put a thicker foam pad on your table. Along with getting feedback from your clients, lying on the table yourself will help you discover how to create optimum comfort.

- When the therapist chooses to do a belly rub, in which easy access to the entire belly at once is needed.
- When the therapist desires full access to both sides at once of the head, neck, and shoulders.
- When the therapist desires to work more directly on the legs and quadriceps and perform passive stretching of the hip adductors.

Table Height

When doing the entire massage with the client in the semi-reclining position, the table height will need to be lower than for sidelying and possibly lower than for regular massage. Determine the proper height by considering first which body areas you expect to work on longest and at what height you will have easiest access to those areas with the least stress to your body. Have a stepstool available for reaching behind the client's head, neck, and back if needed.

Note: If you are only using semi-reclining position for a belly rub at the end of a sidelying massage, the table height need not be adjusted, but you will likely need to use a stepstool for easier access to her belly and back.

How to Position Comfortably in Semi-Reclining

To position the client, use a triangular wedge or an arrangement of firm pillows that allows the client's back to rest at a 45-degree angle or greater to the table, as seen in Figure 5.4. Ensure that her low back is well supported with pillows and is not curving onto the table. Her knees and hips should be flexed using a firm knee bolster. Her neck should be well supported to prevent hyperextension.

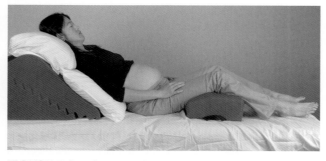

FIGURE 5.4   Semi-reclining positioning.
Semi-reclining position is useful in special situations. Use a triangular wedge or an arrangement of firm pillows that allows the client's back to rest at a 45-degree angle or greater. Ensure that low back is well supported with pillows. Knees and hips should be flexed using a firm bolster. Her neck should be well supported to prevent hyperextension.

Supine Positioning

Supine positioning is inappropriate after the middle of the second trimester, anytime the belly is visibly enlarged with the top of the uterus at or above the navel, or anytime a mother is uncomfortable in the position. As discussed in Chapter 4, supine positioning causes the weight of the baby, uterus, placenta, and amniotic fluid to fall directly onto the large maternal blood vessels along the anterior spine, depending on the position of the baby. This compression reduces blood and oxygen flow to both the baby and the mother and can cause initial "uneasy" feelings, followed by maternal dizziness, shortness of breath, fainting, and eventually, when unresolved, can lead to unconsciousness, along with a reduction in the fetal heartbeat. No extended work should be done in the supine positioning after the middle of the second trimester.

Brief periods of 3 to 8 minutes can sometimes be appropriate, dependent on the baby's positioning and a mother's comfort. If the baby does not lay in such a way as to put pressure on the inferior vena cava, the mother can be comfortable in the supine position. As long as you are both observing for signs of unease or dizziness, specific work such as passive stretches of the psoas and hip rotators or assessment of diastasis recti can be done without problem. A pregnant woman is able to discern when she needs to roll off her back, but always maintain good communication during this type of work to ensure no client discomfort is developing.

Left Tilt Positioning

In some situations you may wish to work more in-depth on the neck, do traction of the spine, or do cranial-sacral type work in the supine position. A left tilt position can be used, if comfortable for the client. Place a pillow or foam wedge behind the client's right hip, tilting her toward the left slightly. This shifts the weight of the uterus and prevents compression of the large blood vessels along the spine. This position can be used occasionally, but be aware that it is generally not ideal for more than 15 minutes, as the spine is slightly twisted, which can lead to compensatory tightening in other areas of the body.

BODYWORK TECHNIQUES

While Chapter 6 describes specific techniques for some of the common complaints of pregnancy, this section describes basic general relaxation techniques in sidelying positioning. These are useful during a

DISPELLING MYTHS:
The Safety of Prone Positioning

Pregnancy massage "tables" and "pregnancy cushions" are sold with cut-outs designed for pregnant bellies and large breasts, so that women can lie, presumably safely, in the prone position. Some practitioners have found these beneficial as it enables them to work with their clients in the prone position throughout pregnancy, rather than sidelying. Some women have found this a wonderful relief from their otherwise regular sidelying positioning at home. Other women report that they enjoyed the position initially, and yet within 5 to 10 minutes they developed an uneasy feeling about being positioned face-down and essentially lying on their baby.

While these tables might be comfortable and safe for resting in for short periods of time, there are several valid reasons why prone positioning is *not appropriate* for longer than several minutes when receiving massage in the third trimester.

- Size: Cut-out holes in tables are one size. A smaller woman will be supported differently than a larger woman. Some women's hips essentially sink through the hole or are minimally supported, increasing lumbar stress and ligamentous strain.
- Lumbar lordosis: Applying repetitive pressure downward on the back during a massage, when a mother is in the prone position, exacerbates lumbar lordosis, a condition already exaggerated during pregnancy.
- Breast compression: Prone positioning, along with added pressure from the massage therapist, compresses the breast tissue, which is often sore, sensitive, and developing glandularly during pregnancy.
- Uterine ligament strain: It is possible that after an extended period of prone positioning, the uterosacral ligament will spasm or be strained as it tries to support the weight of the forward-dangling uterus.
- Intrauterine pressure: Applying pressure downward on a prone client increases pressure in the uterus. A small percentage of women have

undetected problems with the placenta; if this were the case, it is possible that this increased pressure could unintentionally cause harm to the placenta or the baby.
Note: There is no documentation of this having occurred during massage, but since it is a risk, prudence would dictate avoidance.
- Congestion: Nasal congestion is a common complaint during pregnancy due to vascular and hormonal changes. Positioning prone aggravates this condition.
- Client education: Positioning prone sidesteps the opportunity to help a woman learn how to help herself find comfort in the sidelying position at home. Many women have been thrilled to discover at their massage session that the use of a few more pillows and cushioning creates comfort in the sidelying position, which heretofore had been causing distress.
- Communication issues: Many clients are uncomfortable telling their practitioner that something does not feel right. In these situations, basic body cues, such as facial grimacing, help make the therapist aware of a client's discomfort. When the client is prone, communication pathways are decreased and these cues may be lost. If a mother is experiencing uncomfortable sensations, her ability to share verbally or nonverbally will be more limited. In addition, general feedback about pressure, desired changes, or arising emotions are not easily conveyed by the client when face-down.

If a client with a low-risk pregnancy requests prone positioning, it can occasionally be acceptable for short periods up to 5 to 10 minutes at a time as a "treat," but only if you have a pregnancy table or cushion manufactured for this purpose. For the majority of situations, and for optimum comfort and safety, sidelying or semi-reclining positioning should be used throughout the latter half of pregnancy, leaving prone positioning behind until postpartum, or for a rare, occasional 5-minute treat, if a mother requests and enjoys it.

full-body relaxation massage or as a prelude to more focused therapeutic work.

Note: For simplicity of instruction only, all of the following techniques start with the client lying on her right side, unless otherwise described. All sidelying techniques can, and usually should, be done on both sides.

Breathing and Connecting

Massage during pregnancy is an excellent time for a mother to focus on herself and to devote attention to deepening her connection with her baby. Conscious and intentional breathing practices are a way to facilitate this focus by helping her relax physically and

MASSAGE THERAPIST TIP	Positioning for a Client With Hip Pain

*I*n general, if your client has hip pain or discomfort when lying on one side, begin the massage with her positioned with the painful hip up. If she cannot be repositioned to the opposite side, the massage can be modified to do all massage from one side. Alternatively, position her in the semi-reclining position.

ease emotional tension. Each breath she takes nourishes the baby inside with increased oxygen flow through the placenta. Each breath can reinforce an association between relaxation, nurturing touch, and pain relief. Begin each massage by encouraging the client to take slow, full breaths into her belly.

Visualizations of inspiring imagery can facilitate even greater relaxation. During labor, visualization combined with breathing is an excellent tool to ease and help carry a mother through her discomforts or fears during birth— but she must be familiar and comfortable with them before labor begins!

There are numerous ways to incorporate visualization and conscious breathing techniques to help build this familiarity and comfort. Visualization techniques are discussed in more detail in Chapter 7. Two ideas are described here.

Belly Breathing

According to Suzanne Yates, author of *Shiatsu for Midwives*, the kidneys send energy to the uterus.[2] Help encourage this flow by standing behind the sidelying client's back and placing one hand gently on her belly, over the sheet. Place a second hand on her back at one kidney area. Encourage her to inhale through her nose into her belly. Allow the abdominals to move outward with the inhalation, lifting the baby away from her body. Help her to visualize each breath as full of oxygen, nourishing her baby. On the exhalation, encourage her to tighten the abdominals lightly, pulling the baby back to the center of her body, hugging the baby with her belly muscles. You might help her imagine herself to be like the ocean, gently floating her baby on the receding and advancing, rising and falling waves. As she inhales, she lifts the baby up and away on a small wave, and as she exhales, the baby sinks back into union again with the ocean.

Light Breath

Place one hand on her sacrum and the other as support between her scapulas. Direct the client to draw a slow breath down her spine to your hand at her sacrum, imagining the breath as a column of light filling her whole body and circulating around the bowl of her belly. This light brings health, vitality, and love to the mother's baby and increases her body's capacity to nurture life. Encourage the exhalation to be full and relaxed.

General Full-Body Relaxation: Sacral Compression and Unwinding

Benefits: Opening a massage with a full-body relaxation technique can help to set the mode and pace for the massage to come. It allows the mother's body to more readily receive your touch and encourages the breath to become full and natural. It also brings a client's attention to the sensations throughout her body.

One effective technique to use with your pregnant client for full-body relaxation is sacral compression and unwinding. This unwinding helps lengthen her spine, release the sacrum, and balance and soothe the nervous system.

Position: Sidelying. Stand facing the client's back,

Technique
1. *Note:* Work without oil and over the sheet. Place your left hand flat on her sacrum, fingers pointing caudally (toward her toes). Place your right hand under her occiput using a C-clamp position, with your thumb on one side and the other fingers on the other side of her vertebrae.
2. Apply slight traction with the occipital hand and ask the client to inhale deeply.
3. On her exhale, very slowly and gently begin tractioning between your two hands, leaning into the sacrum. Ninety percent of the pressure is on the sacrum. The sacral hand directs energy slightly anteriorly, but is primarily focused caudally. Brace the elbow of the sacral arm against your body above the anterior superior iliac spine, and lean your body weight into it to increase pressure. Do not push the client forward; she should not need to resist your force but should be able to relax as her spine lengthens (Figure 5.5). If she does roll forward easily, she may be positioned too far forward in general. Ask her to reposition her hip more directly beneath her or slightly

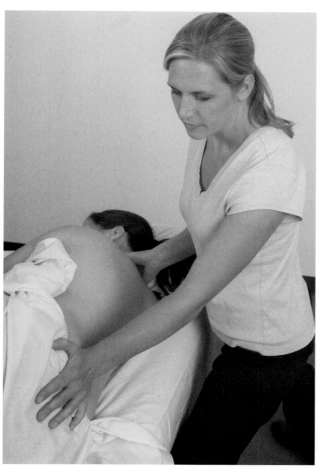

FIGURE 5.5   Sacral compression and unwinding.
Brace elbow of sacral hand against your body and increase pressure by leaning into it. Right hand under occiput applies only gentle traction with light fingers. Focus pressure in direction of client's toes, lengthening the spine, rather than pushing forward.

How the Partner Can Help
Sacral Compression and Unwinding

*S*ometimes clients or partners and support people ask about simple techniques that they can do to beneficially touch the pregnant woman. The sacral compression and unwinding technique is one that falls into this category. It can often bring immediate relief to back pain, offer a sense of nurturing care, and encourage the woman to breathe deep and lengthen her spine. For the giver, it is easy to learn, does not demand a great deal of dexterity in the hands, and can be done on a bed or couch if both parties can find comfortable positions. Help the partner use appropriate body mechanics to avoid strain to her or his own body, while encouraging sensitivity in the hands to feel for the release and unwinding of the pelvis, spine, and neck. Even if the subtle energy too difficult to sense, as long as a firm sacral pressure in a caudal, anterior direction is used, and the client is reminded to breathe slowly and deeply, the effect will still be one of relieving pressure on the sacrum, and encouraging relaxation.

anterior. The occipital hand traction is very gentle, more than actually pressing. Imagine stretching her tailbone to her heels.

 CAUTION: Your hand placement must be exactly aligned on the sacrum to avoid pushing a hypermobile sacrum out of alignment.

4. While performing the traction, suggest that your client envision her breath flowing from her head down to her coccyx, noticing the connection between her head and her sacrum as her spine lengthens.
5. Increase sacral pressure gradually, holding until you feel an unwinding and release in sacrum (usually at least 1 to 2 minutes). Release sacral pressure very gradually. Do not repeat.

Head and Neck

Benefits: Relaxation of the head and neck will help relieve headaches, improve insomnia, and help a client become more aware of her postural stresses. Below are several techniques effective for the head and neck.

Position: Sidelying.

Techniques: Petrissage, Slide-Compression, and Palming

1. Stand at the client's back facing her head. Warm the oil in your hands first, then wrap your left hand around her shoulder anteriorly. Traction slightly caudally.
2. Place the right hand palm at the base of the occiput and push slightly cephalically, increasing the traction of the neck.
3. Use palmar compressing pressure down the neck from occiput to shoulder.
4. With the right forearm or hand on the neck just above the left hand, (which is still wrapped around the shoulder and tractioning down), slide up the neck and rest your hand at the base of the head, providing slight gradual traction to head with the heel or palm of your hand and creating a stretch for the

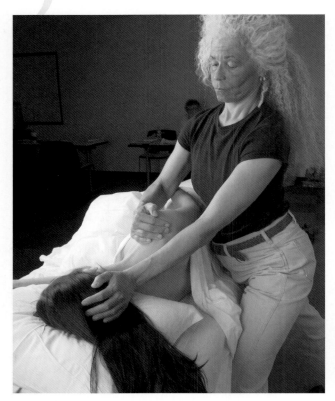

FIGURE 5.6   Alternating traction and sliding compression on neck.
Holding traction with one hand on shoulder, other hand slides up neck to occiput, creating slight traction with heel of hand or forearm.

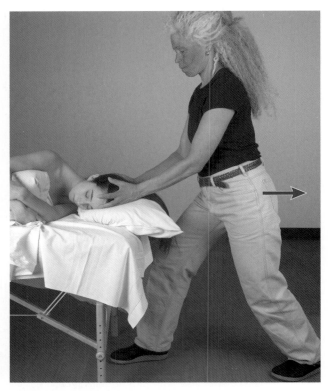

FIGURE 5.7   Occipital traction.
Standing at the head of the table, place one hand under client's occiput in a "C-clamp" position-fingers and thumb encircling under the occipital ridge. Place your other hand on forehead, fingers spread across eyebrows. Cervical spine should be parallel to the table and slightly flexed. Apply slight traction to the head and neck.

neck between the two tractioning hands (Figure 5.6).

5. Slide down the neck with compression to replace the left hand on the shoulder with the right, while the left hand slides up and over the right hand to traction gently at the occiput.

6. Repeat as a continuous movement, hand-over-hand, the left sliding up to apply occipital pressure, while the right tractions at the shoulder, and then the right sliding up as the left comes down to traction. As the right hand slides up, use the right thumb to stroke along the levator and trapezius muscles to their attachments at the base of the occiput and press into the attachments under the occiput.

Occipital Traction

1. Standing at the head of the table, place your left hand under the client's occiput in a

C-clamp position, with your fingers and thumb encircling under the occipital ridge.

2. Place your right hand on the forehead, fingers spread across the eyebrows. Be sure the cervical spine is positioned parallel to the table and slightly flexed (Figure 5.7).

3. On the client's exhalation, apply slight traction to the head and neck.

4. Hold for several moments and slowly release.

Occiput and Eyebrow Points

1. After the occipital traction above, continue standing at the head of the table. Press your left fingertips into the muscular attachments under the occipital ridge, starting from the spine and moving laterally toward the mastoid process.

2. Simultaneously, with your right hand fingertips, press up into and hold points just under the eyebrow ridge, starting from the bridge of

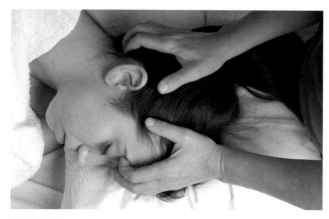

FIGURE 5.8   Occiput and eyebrow points.
Press fingertips into muscular attachments under occipital ridge, starting from spine and moving laterally toward mastoid process. Simultaneously, press up into and hold points just under eyebrow ridge, starting from bridge of the nose and moving toward ear.

the nose and moving toward the ear. Press one point per breath (Figure 5.8).

3. As you reach the lateral edge of the eyebrow with one hand and the end of occiput with the other hand, slide the two hands together at the jaw to apply gentle circular effleurage to the masseter region.

Shoulders and Chest

Benefits: With the extra weight of the growing breasts and postural changes, the chest often collapses inwardly, stressing the rhomboids as the pectoralis and subscapularis shorten. Massage helps to stretch the muscles that are pulling anteriorly, release trigger points, and improve posture and breathing. Effleurage, petrissage, and traction are three strokes that are effective for working in this area.

Position: Sidelying. Stand behind the client facing her back.

Technique:

1. Perform general effleurage and petrissage to the shoulder. Use deep tissue work on the trapezius, levator scapula, and supraspinatus.
2. Drag the fingertips, hand-over-hand, across the shoulder and down the back to the hips.
3. Place the client's arm straight on her side or draped over your left arm. Place both of your hands on top of the shoulder and traction down gently toward her feet, while mobilizing, stretching, rocking, and rotating the shoulder (Figure 5.9A).

4. Place the client's arm, with palm out, behind her hip. Mobilize the shoulder while you apply friction to tight points behind the scapula, at the rhomboid attachments (Figure 5.9 B).

Back

Benefits: The erector spinae work hard to maintain a mother's erect posture during pregnancy while a heavy anterior load pulls her forward. Back massage will help to alleviate this general stress. Holding pressure on either side of the spinal vertebrae brings a mother's awareness to her spine, helps you locate areas of particular tension, and releases tension with the relaxing touch and compression on areas of restriction. These points are also the location of acupressure points on the Bladder meridian.

Below is a description of applying massage to the back in the sidelying position. A second technique is described in the box, "Complementary Modality: Acupressure for Back Release."

Position: Sidelying. Stand Behind the client.

Technique: Effleurage and Petrissage to the Back

1. Apply oil to the back and shoulders. Stroke down either side of the spine, across the trapezius to the sacrum.
2. Make small circles with your thumbs, working firmly down either side of the spine, moving caudally. Direct pressure toward the toes rather than anteriorly, so as not to push the client forward.
3. Stroke from the head toward the tailbone, rather than up her spine to the head, which increases lumbar lordosis.
4. Standing on the client's anterior side and using a stepstool, reach over her superior side and petrissage more deeply into the erector spinae of the superior back (Figure 5.11).

Lateral Hip Rotators and Gluteals

Benefits: As relaxin loosens all the body ligaments, the hips and sacroiliac joint often become misaligned and sore. The lateral hip rotators are often tightened as a mother's hips externally rotate and her stance widens to better support the additional weight. Massage to the area can help relieve hip aching and improve posture. Fanning, compression, and thumb pressure are useful techniques here.

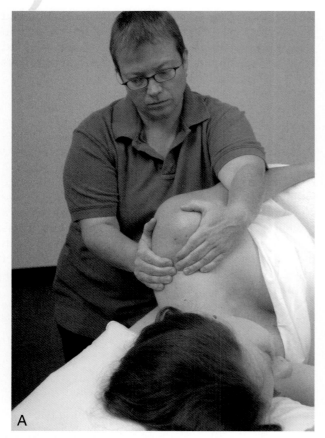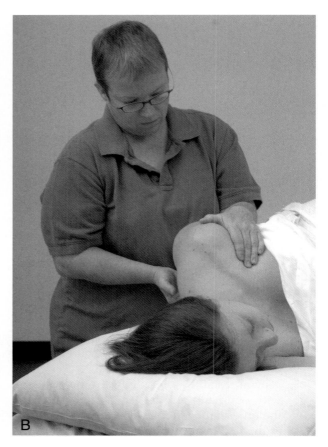

FIGURE 5.9   Opening the chest.
(A) Place client's arm straight on her side or draped over your left arm. Place both your hands on top of shoulder and traction caudally while mobilizing, stretching, rocking, and rotating the shoulder. (B) Place client's arm, with palm out, behind her hip. Mobilize shoulder while applying friction to rhomboid attachments.

Position: Sidelying.

Technique:

1. Drape to expose the superior leg.
2. Fan with the thumbs toward or away from the trochanter attachments of the gluteals and lateral hip rotators (Figure 5.12). Use your fingers, forearm, or a gentle elbow, depending on the depth needed, to compress entirely around the trochanter.
3. With the heel of your hand, press and slide from the iliac crest toward the trochanter. Slide and compress back toward the sacrum.
4. Make small circles with your thumbs along the sacroiliac joint and just below the crest of the ileum.
5. In the third trimester, press gently and directly into the sacral foramen and just lateral to the foramen.

 CAUTION: Do not use deep stimulating pressure directly into the sacral foramen when there are high risks for miscarriage or preterm labor. Acupressure points Bladder 31 and Bladder 32 in the sacral foramen have potentially stimulating effects to the pelvis and uterus. As well, strong stimulation of the sacral nerves, which pass through the foramen, could theoretically also be stimulating to an already irritable uterus. General effleurage and broad compression to the sacrum are different techniques which are *not* contraindicated.

Arms and Hands

Benefits: During the mid to latter part of pregnancy, many women experience edema of the wrists and hands and sometimes temporary carpal tunnel syndrome.

Complementary Modalities:
Acupressure for Back Release

*A*ccording to the acupressure system, each Bladder point along the spine correlates with a specific organ system. Bringing energy to each of these points can help to renew the entire body. Use the following method for stimulating the Bladder meridian as you work down the back.

1. Standing behind the client, feel for the space between the transverse processes of the vertebrae around T-1.
2. Using your thumbs, press into this space on either side of the spine while the client exhales (Figure 5.10).
3. As she inhales, release pressure and move to the next space, moving toward the sacrum. Repeat down the spine to the sacrum.

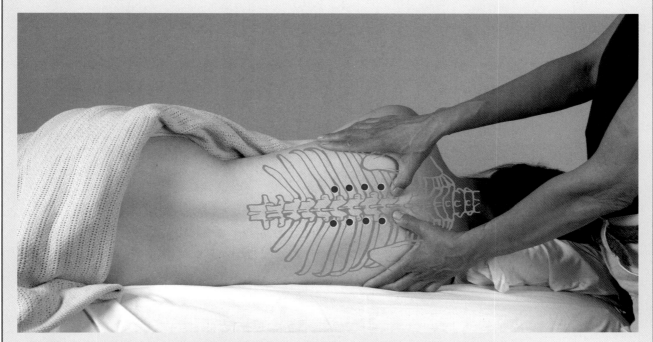

FIGURE 5.10   Erector spinae/bladder meridian acupressure points.
Standing behind client, feel for the space between the transverse processes of the vertebrae around T-1. Using your thumbs, press into this space on either side of the spine while client exhales. As she inhales, release pressure and move to the next space moving toward the sacrum. Repeat down the spine to the sacrum.

Massage to the hands and arms, along with arm stretches that open the upper chest shoulder area, can help alleviate general discomfort. Hand edema techniques are addressed more specifically in Chapter 6.

All general massage techniques to the hand are beneficial.

Position: Any position with access to the hands.

Technique:

1. Spread open the client's palm with your thumbs, sliding and compressing across the palm.

2. Manipulate the wrist with circular range of motion, flexion, and extension.
3. Fan the wrist on the ventral and dorsal sides.
4. Squeeze the fingers from the fingertips toward the hand with incremental movements.
5. Using the flat of your thumb, strip the arm extensors and flexors from the wrist toward the humerus.
6. Apply general petrissage to the deltoid, biceps, and triceps.

 CAUTION: Avoid directed, intentional acupressure into the acupoint Large Intestine 4,

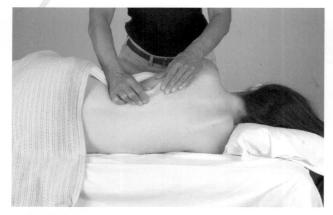

FIGURE 5.11   Petrissage to back from client's anterior side.
Stand on step stool on anterior side of client's body. Reach over her to access superior side of her spine with petrissage.

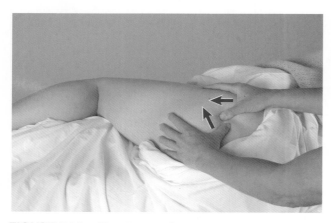

FIGURE 5.12   Fanning trochanter attachments.
Fan with the thumbs toward or away from the trochanter attachments of the gluteals and lateral hip rotators.

(Figure 4.3), which is contraindicated during pregnancy. General effleurage and petrissage are different techniques and are not contraindicated.

Legs

Benefits: Women's legs often feel achy from carrying the weight of pregnancy. Calf cramps are not uncommon, and both the quadriceps and hamstrings may be tight as they help balance the weight of the belly. Massage can help reduce the occurrence of cramps and relieve general discomfort.

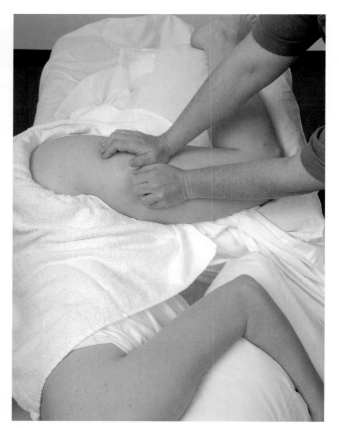

FIGURE 5.13   Kneading thigh.
Begin close to trochanter, and knead tissue, pushing cephalically. Gradually slide down leg, always kneading toward hip, but working incrementally toward the knee.

Position: Sidelying

Techniques:

 CAUTION: Avoid deep work on the inner thighs, where deep vein thrombi are more likely to occur. Avoid direct work on varicose veins.

Kneading the Thigh
1. Stand on a stepstool so that you are above the client and working on the flexed superior leg from the client's anterior side.
2. Use your palm and the heel of your hands to compress and slide up the quadriceps and hamstrings, beginning close to the gluteals at the upper lateral thigh. Knead the tissue in the direction of the heart, while working the hands down toward the knee. Alternate the hands, as if kneading bread, squeezing upward, then sliding down a palm-length and repeating (Figure 5.13).

3. Perform general massage to the iliotibial (IT) band, hamstrings, and quadriceps.

Compression of Thighs and Iliotibial Band
1. Stand on the stepstool so that you are above client and working on the flexed superior leg. Press with the back of the extended fingers against the IT band.
2. Compress into the IT band and slide around the leg (Figure 5.14A).
3. Squeeze and slide from under leg, back up to IT band again. Move toward the knee with each new compression (Figure 5.14B).
4. Fan on the IT band and quadriceps tendons just superior to the knee.

Calf
1. Stand on the client's anterior side. Reach over the leg and grasp the gastrocnemius and soleus with both hands. Squeeze and slide the hands, sliding the cephalic hand toward the feet and the caudal hand toward the head and then back again. Slide up and down the calf with a squeezing, kneading and compressing motion. Use a hip motion in your body to aide your hands, so that the force comes from your full body movement, as opposed to entirely from arm and hand effort.

Inferior Leg
1. While the client is in the sidelying position, you can work lightly with gentle effleurage on the inferior leg if there are no known or visible varicose veins.

Feet
1. Dorsiflex and rotate the feet.

 CAUTION: *Do not* plantarflex the feet. This can stimulate calf cramping.

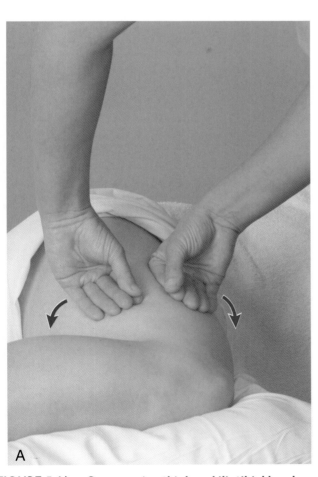
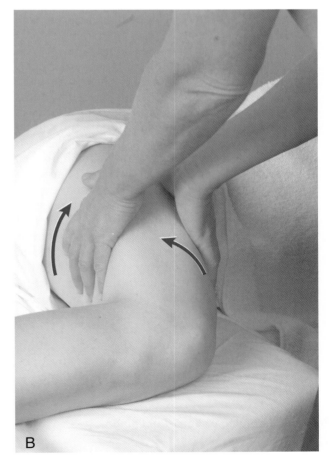

FIGURE 5.14   Compressing thigh and iliotibial band.
Stand on stepstool to allow for vertical compression onto iliotibial band with flat backs of fingers. Press down slowly onto lateral thigh, compressing around thigh, (A) then switching fingers to slide back up, squeezing leg between open fingers and palms (B).

2. Fan the dorsal and plantar sides of the feet with firm pressure.
3. Squeeze the points between the toes, where the toes meet the main body of the foot at the metatarsal-phalangeal joint.

Belly Rubs (Second and Third Trimesters Only)

Benefits: Belly rubs offer time for the client and therapist to connect with the baby. They can be wonderfully relaxing and nurturing and help a mother feel more united in her body, as both the belly and back can be massaged simultaneously. Both sidelying and semi-reclining positioning are excellent for giving and receiving belly rubs. Be aware of a few basic conventions regarding belly rubs in pregnancy:

- Treat the belly as if you are approaching sacred ground—with respect and care. Always ask permission before touching the abdomen. After permission is obtained, slowly and gently place the palms on the belly. Attune with and say hello to baby before you begin to rub. Remember, you are massaging two people!
- In general, your pressure should be firm, with a solid palmar touch, rather than feather-light. Very light touch is irritating to many women. Ask for feedback about the pressure. Most practitioners are fearful of pressing too hard, consequently working much too lightly to be satisfying to the mother.
- Do not do belly rubs for more than 5 minutes, unless intentionally attempting to support contractions for labor. The client may experience mild uterine contractions or tightening and releasing of the uterus during abdominal massage. This can be normal in the third trimester and does not necessarily indicate she is going into labor! However, if labor is not due and more than 1 to 2 contractions are felt during the belly rub, stop. Five to ten minutes of belly massage will not cause a woman to begin labor, even if a couple contractions are felt. However, if the uterus is particularly contractile under your touch, it would be inappropriate to continue stimulating the abdomen if labor is not due.

Position: Sidelying or Semi-Reclining

Techniques:

Honoring Honor the belly and help your client relax by telling her exactly what you are about to do. Place your hands gently, palm down on her belly and

breathe together with her for at least 3 to 4 breaths, or until her belly softens under your touch. As she begins to trust your touch in this vulnerable area, she will relax more.

Always work slowly and with respect for emotions which are often held firmly in the belly and which sometimes come to the surface when touched in a caring way. If the client is reluctant to have touch directly on her skin, she may welcome touch through her clothes or sheet.

Below are two belly rubbing procedures, one for the sidelying position and one for the semi-reclining position.

Sidelying Belly Rub
1. Stand at the mother's back, facing her back.
2. After honoring the belly, as described above, apply oil to your hands and spread the oil in a very slow, firm circle around the entire globe of her belly.
3. From behind her, reach over her belly to the underside and slide back up and over the belly, making hand-over-hand raking strokes toward the upper side of her belly (Figure 5.15).

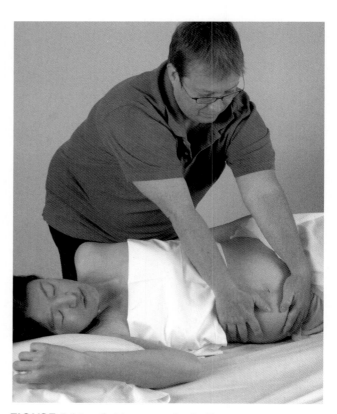

FIGURE 5.15   Raking over the belly.
From behind client, reach over to underside of belly and slide back up and over, making hand-over-hand raking strokes toward the superior side of her belly.

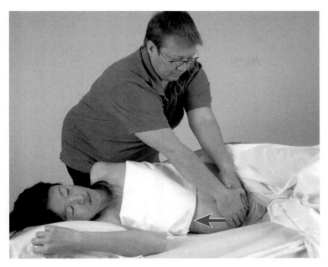

FIGURE 5.16   Lifting from groin.
Make lifting strokes from the groin area toward the navel, hand-over-hand, imagining lifting the weight of the belly and relieving pressure on the groin.

4. Make lifting strokes from the groin area toward the navel, hand-over-hand, imagining lifting the weight of the belly and relieving pressure on the groin. (Figure 5.16)
5. Position yourself in a lunge position, facing the client's feet.
6. If she is on her right side, place your right hand on her belly and your left on her back. Mirror your hand-motions as you make circles on her belly while applying strong pressure on her low back/sacrum simultaneously (Figure 5.17A). When both the hands meet at the superior hip area, smoothly rotate on your heels to change the position of your feet so that you are facing her head and your hands so that your right hand is on her back and your left hand is on her belly.
7. Continue circling, this time circling high on her belly while mirroring circling pressure on the mid-back (Figure 5.17B).
8. Change your direction every circle or two.

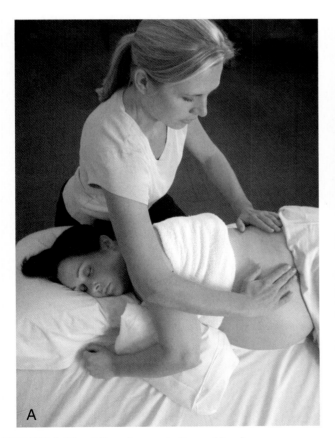
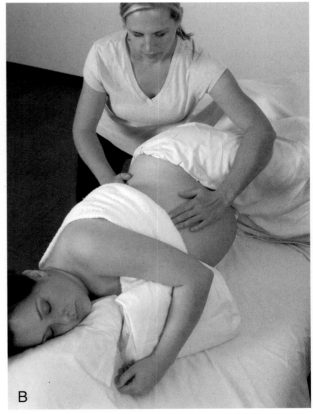

FIGURE 5.17   Mirroring on belly and back.
(A) Position yourself facing client's feet. Place cephalad hand on her belly, and caudal hand on her back. Mirror your hand-motions as you make circles on her belly and applying strong pressure on her low back/sacrum simultaneously. When both hands meet at the superior hip area, change your position so that you are facing her head. (B) Continue circling, this time high on her belly while mirroring circling pressure on the mid-back.

Semi-Reclining Belly Rub

Note: You may need to use a stepstool to reach adequately around the client's back from her anterior side.

1. Position the client semi-reclining, drape the breasts, and expose the belly in standard fashion. Proceed with honoring the belly first, as described above.

2. Warm the oil in the hands and spread it slowly in large full circles around the belly.
3. Spiral out slowly from the navel until the circling includes the waist area.
4. Make smooth raking strokes from one side to the center, reaching across the belly with hand-over-hand motions. Repeat on the opposite side.

MASSAGE THERAPIST TIP — Choosing the Position for a Belly Rub

A wonderful belly rub can be done in either sidelying or semi-reclining positions. Both have advantages and disadvantages. In general, do a belly rub in sidelying position when you do not want to disturb your client with repositioning, or when you have a client who might feel overwhelmed with the therapist proximity during a semi-reclining belly rub, or who needs limited repositioning due to hip and back complaints. Also use it with someone who is much larger than you. Generally semi-reclining belly rubs are used more during the third trimester, and are useful with clients who are more comfortable in semi-reclining, or when you or the client wants to be more engaged with talking or sharing about the baby, or visualizing the belly and baby.

Sidelying Advantages

- Relaxing: If a full massage has been done in the sidelying position, a belly rub in sidelying allows the woman to continue relaxing without having to change position again.
- Back Access: In sidelying, it is easier to massage both the back and belly at once, creating more unity in the client's body.

Sidelying Disadvantages

- Disturbs Final Relaxation: If the client is deep in a quiet internal space at the end of a massage; making the effort to move her body and wait for you to reposition all the pillows can disturb that reflective space.
- One-sided: As with the rest of the massage in sidelying, you can only access one side of the body. While most of the work is done anteriorly and posteriorly with a belly rub, the lift from the side can only occur on the one side at a time. Usually a belly rub in sidelying is only done from one

position; the client is not asked to roll over to have the belly rub repeated on the other side.

Semi-reclining Advantages

- Belly Access: In this position, you can see the belly and visualize more clearly the baby's position, body parts, and movements. You have access to the entire belly and back and the massage will feel more evenly dispersed across the belly.
- Client engagement: When upright in the semi-reclining position, the client may be more alert after a massage and might share more about the baby and her experiences of getting to know him or her through kicks and responses to external stimuli. The client can watch how you do the belly rub, and be more easily engaged in giving feedback about what kind of pressure or touch feels good.
- Repositioning: Moving out of the sidelying position will be a relief for a client who is getting uncomfortable on her side. She may be able to breathe more deeply and enjoy the belly rub more.

Semi-reclining Disadvantages

- Physical Proximity: In semi-reclining position, you may have closer contact with the client than she feels comfortable with. To reach the back of a woman who has a large belly or who is much larger than you, you must nearly embrace her belly. This may feel awkward or invasive for some women.
- Repositioning: It takes time and energy to reposition a client. If you are short on time, or don't want to disturb her, don't reposition.

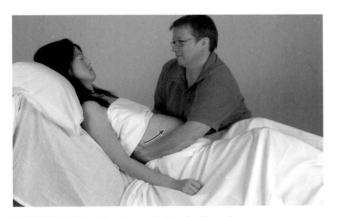

DISPELLING MYTHS:
Touching the Pregnant Belly

Massage therapists have sometimes been taught to avoid any touch to a woman's belly throughout pregnancy. This is generally based on uncertainty about what is appropriate or not, as well as on fear that pregnancy is a fragile condition, and additionally on a legitimate desire to avoid causing harm. However, it is a broad-based rule that fails to define the actual risks and when and how to avoid them while still offering gentle and nurturing abdominal work. Of course, deep abdominal work to the psoas or internal organs is contraindicated throughout pregnancy. However, belly rubs for comfort and baby-connection are beneficial and desirable, especially during the third trimester.

In the first trimester, the risk for a miscarriage is high; it is therefore standard practice to advise massage therapists to avoid touching the abdomen to avoid association in anyone's mind between massage and a possible miscarriage. After the first trimester, however, and assuming the therapist does a thorough health intake and ascertains that there are no further obvious or known risks for preterm labor or miscarriage, belly rubs are a wonderful way to share with a growing mother and her child. Belly rubs do have the capacity occasionally to stimulate temporary contractions; to avoid this, restrict belly rubs to a duration of no longer than 5 minutes until the last couple weeks of pregnancy, when longer rubs may be desirable to support labor.

FIGURE 5.18   Semi-reclining belly rub.
Use stepstool if necessary to reach around client's back and pull up into erector spinae before sliding around to front again. Be aware of client's comfort level as it may feel invasive to some.

CHAPTER SUMMARY

To safely and optimally provide pregnant clients with bodywork, the massage therapist must attend to the specific needs of the population. This includes preparing the office setting with a comfortable table, pillows and supports, using appropriate-sized sheets that will drape her securely, moderating the climate for clients who may be warmer than nonpregnant clients, and having a step stool and unscented oils or lotions available. Additionally, the massage therapist must be skilled at positioning methods appropriate to the client's trimester and size, knowledgeable enough to do a thorough health intake, and adhere to relevant precautions and contraindications. Following these steps, combined with conscientious draping and caring touch, the massage therapist will have met the client's most essential needs during a massage for safety, respect and nurturing.

5. Make smooth strokes with the fingers, lifting up from the area toward the navel.
6. Stand facing the client's face. You may need to stand on a stepstool.
7. Start with both hands at the navel, and slide around to the belly and waist to reach to the spine. Press into the erector spinae, pulling toward you slightly as you slide again to the belly (Figure 5.18).
8. Repeat, reaching to different areas along the spine, rubbing there momentarily before sliding back to the belly and circling again.

CHAPTER REVIEW QUESTIONS

1. Name two reasons why you might choose to schedule longer sessions with your pregnant clients.
2. Name three extra items you might have available in your office set-up to provide optimum comfort for yourself and/or your client.
3. Describe how you would set up your massage table specifically for pregnant clients in the side-lying position. Name three alterations to your standard set up.

4. Explain how you would position a client who is 15 weeks pregnant and complains of breast tenderness and nausea and why you would choose that position.

5. If a client complains of numbness or tingling of her hand on the side she is lying on, describe changes you might implement to improve her comfort.

6. Describe three adjustments you might try to improve your body mechanics if you are feeling strain in your back while working with a client in the sidelying position.

7. Describe how you would direct a client to change positions from one side to the other on the massage table.

8. Explain what you would do if a client became uncomfortable in sidelying positioning after starting a massage. What other position might be tried? What other positioning techniques?

9. Discuss the pros and cons of prone positioning after 22 weeks' gestation. Describe the dangers of supine positioning after 22 weeks.

10. Your new client of 32 weeks agrees to a belly rub. Describe what positions you could do this in, and what considerations would help you choose.

REFERENCES

1. Field TM, Hernandez-Reif M, Hart S, et al. Pregnant women benefit from massage therapy. J Psychosom Obstet Gynaecol 1999;20(1):31–38.

2. Yates S. Shiatsu for Midwives. Oxford, UK: Elsevier Science, 2003.

CHAPTER 6

COMMON COMPLAINTS DURING PREGNANCY

LEARNING OBJECTIVES

After reading this chapter, you should be able to:

- Describe 10 common complaints of pregnancy and their common causes.
- Identify simple massage techniques to address common complaints of pregnancy.
- Describe the use of facilitated stretching to help address specific musculoskeletal discomforts.
- Identify the benefits, concerns, and contraindications of breast massage during pregnancy.
- Identify the need for self-care client education to help prevent or alleviate discomforts.
- Understand the limitations of massage to address common pregnancy complaints.

$\mathcal{M}$any women sail through their pregnant months feeling healthier and happier than ever before. Others are plagued with one to a number of discomforts. Doctors and friends may minimize these complaints with common comments such as, "You're pregnant, what do you expect?" or "Don't worry, it will go away after you have the baby." Because of this, women often find themselves suffering needlessly through a pregnancy with annoying or sometimes painful conditions which bodywork techniques may relieve.

This chapter addresses common complaints and describes massage techniques along with self-care tips for your client that may aid in alleviating her discomforts.

 CAUTION: Before you address any of the following complaints, be certain to study the precautions and contraindications for pregnancy massage in Chapter 4.

Note: For simplicity of instruction only, all of the following techniques start with the client lying on her right side, unless otherwise described. All sidelying techniques can, and usually should, be done on both sides. I use the term "superior" to refer to the client's side that is *up* and accessible. The side *on* the table I refer to as the "inferior" side.

BACK PAIN: LOW

By the end of pregnancy, a woman is making many adjustments to compensate for the increased weight of the pregnant uterus, baby, amniotic fluid, placenta, and breasts. It has been estimated that two thirds or more of pregnant women experience back pain, most frequently in the low back. It most commonly begins by the sixth month of pregnancy and can last for up to 6 months after delivery.[1-4] The pregnant woman who is particularly at risk for musculoskeletal low back pain (LBP) is one who:

- has history of chronic back pain or back injury prior to this pregnancy

- is now pregnant with her second or subsequent child
- has had back pain in previous pregnancies
- works in a job that involves physical exertion or strain.

Cause

There are a variety of causes of LBP in pregnancy, some of which can be addressed with massage. The most common causes include poor posture, hormonally induced ligament laxity, and diastasis recti. Other causes of aching or pain in the low back may include constipation, uterine contractions, and occasionally, with more severe pain, kidney infection. Each of these are addressed briefly below:

- *Posture*: Postural changes are a very common cause of LBP in pregnancy due to the extra anterior weight of the breasts and enlarged uterus, the anterior rotation of the pelvis, increased lumbar lordosis, and contraction of the lateral hip rotators, quadratus lumborum (QL), and iliopsoas muscle.
- *Hormones*: The hormone relaxin causes the ligaments in the hip, symphysis pubis, and sacroiliac joints to become more flexible. Sometimes these hypermobile joints can become misaligned, causing discomfort that may be felt in the low back or across the buttock, or which may manifest as sciatica.
- *Diastasis recti*: Weak and untoned abdominal muscles can cause the abdominal contents and uterus to fall forward, putting undue strain on the lumbar vertebrae, spinal muscles, and abdominal wall. If the abdominal muscles separate, in a diastasis of the recti, the lack of abdominal support will increase back pain further (see Chapter 3).
- *Constipation*: A dull, low ache in the back may be due to the displacement of the intestines and resultant constipation.
- *Contractions*: For some women, uterine contractions may be felt as LBP rather than as tightening in the abdomen.

⚠ CAUTION: If your client is in her 37th week of gestation or less and has recently begun to experience intermittent aching in her low back, be sure to ask if she has seen her prenatal care provider to ensure that preterm contractions are not the cause of the back discomfort.

- *Kidney infection*: Sharp back pain on one side below the ribs could indicate a kidney infection, which is not an uncommon occurrence in pregnancy. Once an infection develops, it is often accompanied with fever and nausea or vomiting. A client who complains of increasing, constant or sudden sharp pain in the kidney area should be referred to her prenatal care provider.

General Treatment

Stretches and general massage are effective as general treatment for musculoskeletal LBP.

- Stretches: For LBP related to postural and structural stress, encourage your client to practice self-care with muscular strengthening and stretches to help adjust her posture and enable her to relieve her own discomforts. Pelvic tilts, abdominal strengthening, hip rotator and QL stretches are a few that can ease LBP.
- General massage: Perform massage on the QL, spinal muscles, multifidi, gluteals, and quadriceps. Include effleurage and petrissage to the erector spinae, and apply deep warming strokes toward the sacrum and radiating out across the waist and lumbar area.

Specific Bodywork Techniques

Below are a few bodywork techniques that address low back pain caused by a tight QL and psoas, or by sacral tension. Before beginning this deeper focused work, warm up the back with effleurage and petrissage.

Quadratus Lumborum Compression Points

Benefits: Helps release a tight QL that has become shortened and strained due to attempts to stabilize the pelvis and support the ever-increasing abdominal weight.

Position: Sidelying.

Technique
1. Stand at your client's back facing her head.
2. Warm up the QL area by using your palm or forearm for effleurage, sliding from the iliac crest to the lower border of the ribs.
3. After the QL has been warmed, wrap the hand closest to your client's hips around her iliac crest and traction the hip caudally. With the thumb or fingers of the opposite hand, slowly apply static, ischemic pressure onto the lateral edge of the QL, just lateral to the erector spinae (Figure 6.1). Move up from the

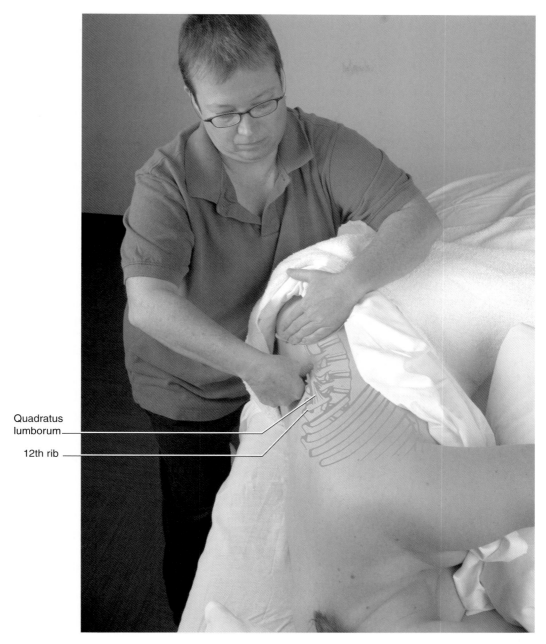

FIGURE 6.1 Quadratus lumborum compression points.

Tractioning the hip caudally from the iliac crest while slowly applying static pressure onto the lateral edge of the QL.

iliac crest incrementally, holding each point for at least 2 to 4 of the client's breaths as the tissues release. When you feel a particularly tight spot or trigger point, press carefully into that point, using a pain-rating scale with your client. Ask her to rate discomfort on a scale of 0 to 10 (0 is painless, 10 is excruciating, and 6 is the maximum tolerable discomfort while still being able to relax with focused breathing). Hold at a level of 6, if that is comfortable for her, for at least 15 to 20 seconds or 4 to 5 client breaths.

4. Encourage the client to inhale into the area, envisioning a softening and stretching as she breathes. Maintain pressure, feeling the tension release under your thumb. When the client says the pressure feels like a 3 or 4 or less, increase the pressure until it is again at a

6 and repeat if necessary, or move to the next tight spot.

> **CAUTION:** The QL can be very sensitive. Work slowly and ask for feedback to ensure an appropriate level of pressure.

Quadratus Lumborum Release

Benefits: Same as for the Quadratus Lumborum Compression Points above.

Position: Sidelying, with the client's upper arm extended over her head. To increase this stretch, if necessary, ask the client to extend and drop her top leg behind her bottom leg. She may need to bend her bottom leg to stabilize balance. For greater QL stretch, place a rolled pillow or foam wedge beneath her waist on the table to arch her superior side more laterally as demonstrated later in Figure 6.2A.

Technique

1. Stand on the client's posterior side, facing her back. Cross your hands and place one palm on your client's posterior iliac crest and the other on the superior lateral edge of the QL, on or just inferior to the lowest ribs. Ask her to inhale as you press in opposite directions with both hands, lengthening the QL between the hip and ribcage. Hold for several relaxing breaths as the fascia unwinds. Slowly release pressure as the client exhales and relaxes (Figure 6.2A).
2. Move the leg pillows out of the way. Ask the client to flex her bottom knee slightly to support her body. Have her drop her top leg behind her bottom leg, and even off the side

of the table if comfortable. From here, as she exhales, press on the lateral calf of the dropped leg and have her push vertically up against the resistance of your hand with 1/4 of her effort, activating the QL from a slightly stretched position (Figure 6.2B). Hold for 8 seconds. Have the client inhale and relax, and then repeat 1 to 2 times.

Quadratus Lumborum Extension

Benefits: Activates and stretches the QL; lengthens the compressed space in the waist.

Position: Sidelying, with the client's top arm extended over her head.

Technique

1. Stand at the client's feet. Have her extend her top leg. Hold this leg above her ankle with two hands and lean back gently to apply traction to her hip, lengthening her side and the QL. Hold for 10 seconds, then ask her to dorsiflex her foot, pressing her heel down while hoisting her hip up toward her head, activating the QL from a slightly stretched position (Figure 6.3).

Full Body Stretch

Benefits: Creates length and space in the compressed waist area.

Position: Sidelying.

Technique

1. Stand at the client's head and bring her left arm up over her head into full extension, with her arm hooked over yours at her elbow.

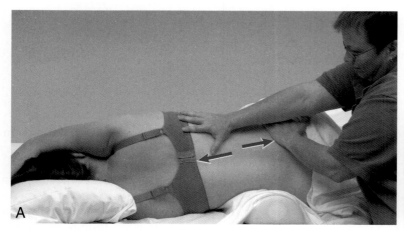
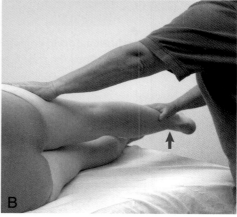

FIGURE 6.2 **Quadratus lumborum release.**
(A) *Lengthening the QL between the hip and ribcage. (B) Pressing on the lateral calf of the dropped leg as the client resists isometrically.*

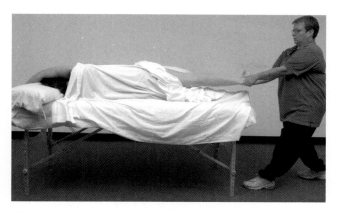

FIGURE 6.3   Quadratus lumborum extension.
Gently applying traction to the hip while the client dorsiflexes her foot and presses into her heel.

2. Place your left hand on her iliac crest and push caudally, maintaining traction of her arm as in Figure 6.4. Instruct the client to breathe deeply to extend the stretch.

Sacral Rub

Benefits: Increases circulation and brings warmth to the sacrum and pelvis; relieves sacral and low back discomfort.

Position: Sidelying.

Technique
1. In the late second or third trimester, stimulate the sacral fascia, sacral multifidi, and attachments of the gluteus maximus with brisk fingertip friction, cross-fiber friction, and skin rolling for up to 1 to 2 minutes or more, bringing heat to the area.

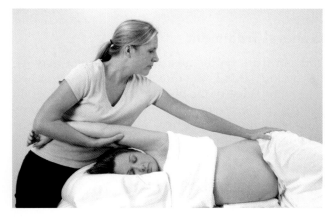

FIGURE 6.4   Full body stretch.
Extending the arm and pushing caudally on the iliac crest to stretch the torso.

2. Press into the sacral foramen gently.

Assisted Psoas Stretch

Benefits: Releases tight psoas; helps alleviate low back pain.

Position: For this stretch, the client lies supine with the ischial tuberosities near the table edge. The leg with the tight psoas is extended and hanging relaxed. The other leg is flexed and held toward the belly. The low back is flat on the table. Do this with the client dressed, after the massage.

Technique
1. Before assuming the above position, first assess psoas tightness and the need for this stretch, by having the client start several inches further up on the table than described above, so that her hamstrings are *on* the table. Assess whether the hamstrings of the extended leg touch the table or are held in the air. With a tight psoas, the extended leg will not lie flat on the table. If one or both sides are tight, do the following stretch on the tight side(s) after repositioning as described in "Position" above.
2. Ask the client to push the heel of the extended leg toward the floor, to lengthen the psoas.
3. Place your hand on the extended leg, just superior to the knee and ask the client to push her knee up isometrically against the resistance of your hand with one quarter of her effort as she exhales (Figure 6.5). Maintain clear communication and remind her to stop immediately if she feels discomfort.
4. Hold for 8 seconds. Release. Press down *slightly* on the leg to extend the stretch. Release slowly and *help her* bring her extended leg back into flexion.
5. Repeat on the other side if necessary.
6. To get up from this position, help the client to either roll to her side and stand from the end of the table, or have her pull both heels in close to her buttocks, to rest on the table edge and push herself with her heels further up on the table. She can then roll to the side to push up with her hands.

 CAUTION: Do not do psoas stretch with pubic diastasis.

BACK PAIN: MID AND UPPER

While LBP is quite common during pregnancy, mid-back and upper back pain can also cause complaints.

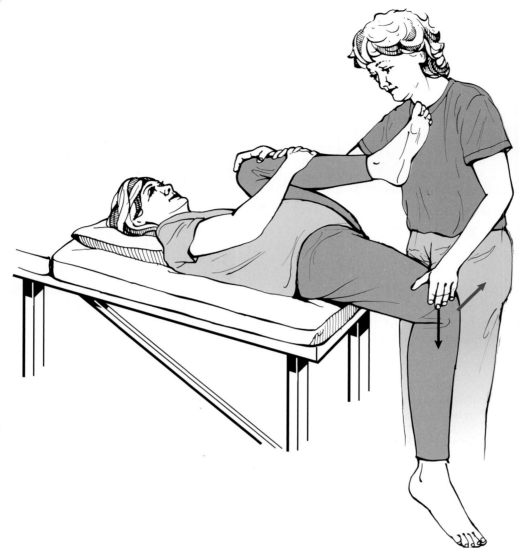

FIGURE 6.5   Assisted psoas stretch.

With the therapist's hand on the client's extended leg, the client pushes isometrically against the hand with the knee.

This discomfort can often be managed with a proper-ly fitted, supportive bra; postural awareness; support-ed positioning when sidelying in bed or on the massage table, as well as with stretches and massage to alleviate tension and trigger points.

Cause

Upper back pain is often caused by improper posture while adjusting to changes in balance. The weight of the enlarged breasts pulls the upper torso forward, causing the muscles that internally rotate the shoul-der to become shortened. Pain then develops in the upper midback, in the chronically stretched rhom-boids, and in the posterior neck musculature.

General Treatment

You can work on the area where the client may feel discomfort, such as the rhomboids. However, to help relieve the cause of the discomfort, you will generally need to perform stretches and petrissage, compres-sion, friction, and cross-fiber friction on the anterior-pulling, internally rotating muscles, such as teres major, subscapularis, latissumus dorsi, and pectoralis major.

Specific Bodywork Techniques

Below are bodywork techniques to address midback and upper back pain in specific muscles or regions.

Self Care Tips FOR MOTHERS:

Decreasing Low Back Pain

*R*emind your client of the following suggestions to help relieve low back pain (LBP):

- Sleep on the side, with knees bent and the top leg supported on a pillow.
- When standing, have a stepstool or block to rest one foot higher than the other.
- Keep the knees flexed and higher than the hips when seated for long periods.
- Learn and practice postural awareness.
- A pregnancy abdominal binder helps support the weight of the pregnant belly, reducing LBP.
- Low heeled, comfortable shoes prevent LBP that occurs with higher heels.
- All practices that strengthen the abdominals, stretch the psoas, lengthen the low back, and stretch the hip rotators can be helpful.

The following stretches and strengtheners can be taught beginning in early pregnancy to relieve LBP and continued after delivery to help regain appropriate non-pregnancy posture.

Quadratus Lumborum Stretch

Stand with the left side next to a wall, one arm width away. Extend the right arm to the side and place the hand on the wall. Cross the left leg close behind the right leg. Raise the left arm over the head, pushing the left hip laterally away from the wall and arching toward the wall with the head and left arm. Hold and breathe, feeling the stretch in the left QL area (Figure 6.6). Repeat with the right leg crossed behind the left leg, stretching different fibers on the QL. Turn around and repeat on the opposite side. This can also be done from a kneeling position if there is concern for losing balance (Figure 6.6).

Psoas Stretch

A weakened, short psoas is common in pregnancy and can be a direct cause of LBP. From the hands and knees position, bring the right knee forward and place the foot flat on the floor, directly below the knee. Extend the left leg further back, sinking into the extended left hip and stretching the groin and psoas. Bring the torso upright to increase the stretch. Repeat on the other side.

During the third trimester, you may lunge while sitting in a chair. Sit with the right hip in the chair, right leg forward. Stretch the left leg behind, for a modified lunge. Sink into the left hip, extending the leg back to extend the stretch.

Pelvic Tilt

Pelvic tilts help to lengthen the low back. Some tilts can strengthen the abdominal muscles, lengthen the psoas, and soften the QL. There are several positions in which to practice pelvic tilts, depending on how far along the pregnancy is.

Lie supine, with both knees flexed, feet flat on the floor. Adjust the low back by lifting the buttocks slightly and curling the tailbone between the legs, then lying down flat again—this lengthens and flattens the back before beginning. Contract the abdominal muscles, as if pulling the navel down through the belly toward the floor and flatten the low back against the floor. Hold for 3 to 10 seconds, breathing steadily and relaxing the body. Do not lift the buttocks off the floor, and as much as possible, attempt to use the abdominal muscles and the iliopsoas, rather than the leg or gluteal muscles, to flatten the back.

This can be practiced standing by pressing the low back against a wall. Once familiar with the action, it can also be done when standing freely, sitting, sidelying, or on hands and knees. A larger pelvic tilt can be done by intentionally lifting the buttocks off the floor into the air and arching the back.

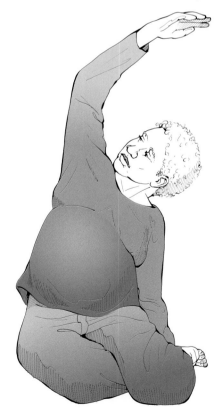

FIGURE 6.6 Kneeling Quadratus lumborum stretch.

Chest Opening

Benefits: Helps the client expand the chest against the gravitational pull of heavy breasts and poor posture; stretches the pectoralis.

Position: Sidelying with the client's arm extended with the palm out, behind the hip.

Technique

1. Stand on the client's posterior side, facing her head. Place your left hand on her anterior shoulder over the head of the humerus and the acromion process. Place the other hand on her scapula.
2. On the client's exhalation, have her envision her chest opening and expanding as she allows her shoulder to drop backward toward table with the gentle encouragement of your hands.
3. Apply slight pressure to the shoulder with the left hand to assist expansion as she widens her upper ribs with her breath.
4. Stroke laterally from the sternum toward the head of the humerus with firm fingertip pressure along the subclavius and the superior border of the pectoralis to encourage release and opening, still supporting behind or under the scapula.

 CAUTION: Avoid rotating her shoulder to such a degree that her low back begins to twist or strain.

Pectoralis Stretch and Resistance

Benefits: Stretches the muscle that internally rotates the humerus.

Position: Sidelying.

Technique

1. Stand behind the client. Grasp the humerus just proximal to the elbow, bring her arm straight up toward the ceiling. While supporting it, allow it to drop posteriorly with the elbow slightly bent. Allow the chest to roll

slightly posterior also. To avoid positioning in a way that overstretches or strains, ask the client herself to place her arm in a position that stretches the upper fibers of the pectoralis muscle (Figure 6.7).
2. Place your left hand on the hip/gluteals at the same time to stabilize the back and to increase expansion and rotation.
3. Do resistance stretches, asking the client to push forward isometrically against the resistance of your arm with one quarter of her effort

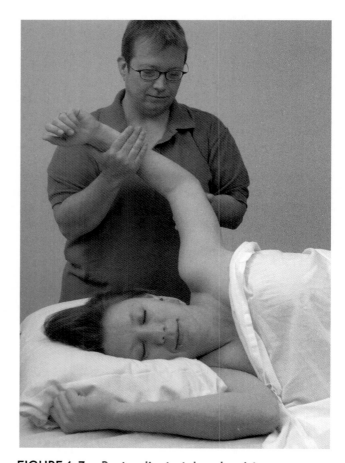

FIGURE 6.7   Pectoralis stretch and resistance.
The client pushes anteriorly isometrically against the therapist's arm to stretch the pectoralis.

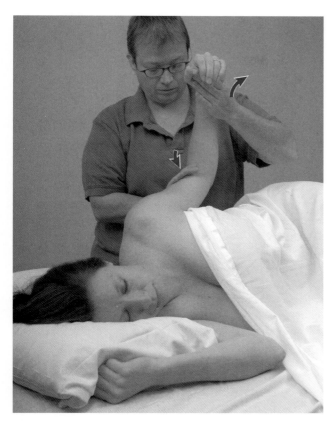

FIGURE 6.8   Subscapularis stretch.

As she exhales, the client isometrically pushes her forearm medially against the therapist's hand.

for 8 seconds during exhalation (Figure 6.8). Repeat, increasing the stretch slightly. Relax.

Subscapularis Stretch

Benefits: Stretches the muscle that medially rotates the shoulder.

Position: Sidelying with the upper arm extended straight down on her side.

Technique
1. With her arm extended down to her side, have the client flex her elbow to 90 degrees, palm facing anteriorly.
2. Stabilize her elbow and bring it slightly anterior with one hand, and with the other hand bring her forearm posteriorly, pushing carefully at her wrist.
3. Holding the elbow anteriorly, ask her to slowly push her hand and forearm anteriorly against your upper hand isometrically, using one quarter of her effort and holding pressure for 8 seconds.
4. Relax the resistance, and increase the stretch. Repeat the resistance as above. Relax.

BREAST TENDERNESS

As soon as a woman conceives, her breasts, nurtured by an increase in production of estrogen and progesterone, begin to enlarge and prepare for mothering. Estrogen enlarges the ducts that transport milk, and progesterone stimulates the development of the glandular tissues. Breast massage can help reduce discomfort associated with the development of lactating breasts, and can help women feel more at ease with the new sensations.

Cause

Breasts are often tender early in pregnancy due to hormonal influences and swelling glands, along with a 30% to 40% increase in blood supply. A woman may feel tenderness and sore nipples in the first trimester and initially become aware of her new pregnancy based on breast changes. Later, a woman may experience aching or discomfort as the breasts enlarge.

General Treatment

In the first trimester, avoid prone positioning if your client complains of breast tenderness or place a pillow under her ribs just below her breasts, to avoid compression of the tender tissue. In the sidelying position, be sure to place a pillow between her superior arm and breasts to prevent arm compression on the breast tissue.

Specific Bodywork Techniques

Below are bodywork techniques to address specific muscles or regions related to breast tenderness.

Breast Massage

Benefits: Breast massage can mobilize lymph, help a mother connect more fully with her changing body, and relieve breast aching.

Contraindications
There are several contraindications for breast massage. These are explained below.

1. State law: Whereas in Europe breast massage is considered a normal and expected part of a therapist's training and practice, in the United States, each state massage board has particular legislation regarding the practice and legality of breast massage. Research the laws governing massage in your own place of practice. If it is illegal in your state, or if your client is uncomfortable with receiving breast massage, you can teach her the benefits and

methods of massaging the breasts herself, if she is interested.

2. Infection: If a woman has a breast infection, direct massage to the affected area is contraindicated.

3. Other physical reasons: If there is any undiagnosed lump(s) or abscess or problems with implants, breast massage is contraindicated.

4. Lack of good rapport or consent: If you do not have good communication or rapport with your client, or if she does not wish to receive breast massage, it is contraindicated.

5. Nipple contact: Touch to the nipples is contraindicated during a professional massage. In addition to being inappropriate and prohibited by state massage legislation, it is important to realize that nipple stimulation during pregnancy causes the release of oxytocin, the hormone that causes uterine contractions. This hormonal release is triggered specifically by nipple stimulation, such as when a baby is nursing. However, if a client has a particular risk for preterm labor or miscarriage, *all breast massage* will be contraindicated due to the slight chance that a hormonal increase could occur due to general breast stimulation.

6. Deep tissue, heavy pressure, or kneading: Small Cooper's ligaments that support the breast can be damaged by deep pressure. Breast tissue is not muscle; the breasts lie on top of muscles, which can be accessed around and under the breast tissue. Breast massage is primarily concerned with lymphatic drainage, increased circulation, and for a nursing mother, promoting lactation.

Position: Sidelying, at times with her superior arm extended over her head. This can also be adapted for semi-reclining position.

Technique

1. Stand behind the client's back. Use a breast drape if desired. Undrape one breast at a time. With unscented lotion or oil, place your flat fingertips at the lateral superior edge of the sternum just under the clavicle, and slide laterally above the breast tissue, toward the axilla. Repeat several times.

2. Make small circles medially back to the sternum and then down the sternum.

3. Place the heel of one hand inferior to the breast, and the other low and lateral to the breast. Use a scooping motion with the heels of the hands toward the breast. Work your way, hand-over-hand toward the sternum,

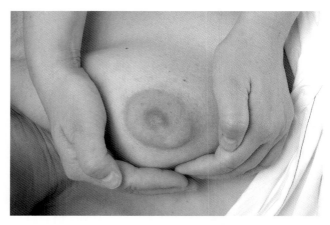

FIGURE 6.9   Scooping under the breast.

Place the heel of one hand inferior to the breast, and the other low and lateral to the breast. Use a scooping motion with the heels of the hands sliding into the breast tissue toward the nipple (but don't go to the nipple). Always scooping hand-over-hand toward the center of the breast, gradually work your way from the lower border of the breast toward the sternum.

scooping toward the center of the breast. You may need to cup the breast tissue at the sternum in one hand as you slide with the other (Figure 6.9).

4. Place flat fingertips at the lateral edge of the sternum, just inferior to the clavicle. Scoop or press with very light pressure, as if stroking a baby's lips or eyelid, moving all strokes toward the client's head. Incrementally move the hand lower into the breast tissue. Gradually move laterally toward the axilla as well, and then repeat down the lateral edges of the breast stroking toward the axilla (Figure 6.10).

5. Place one palm above the breast, just lateral to the sternum. Place the other palm inferior to the breast. Slide the sternum hand toward the axilla and the inferior hand toward the lower sternum. The hands will cross each other above and below the breast. Repeat several times.

Lymph Pump

Benefits: Mobilizing the lymph can help relieve some of the tenderness due to general swelling and restriction of circulation.

Position: Sidelying

Technique

Standing behind the client, hold her humerus just proximal to the elbow and lift the arm straight toward

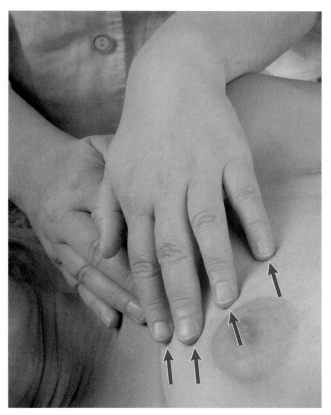

FIGURE 6.10   Light stroking from the breast toward the axilla.

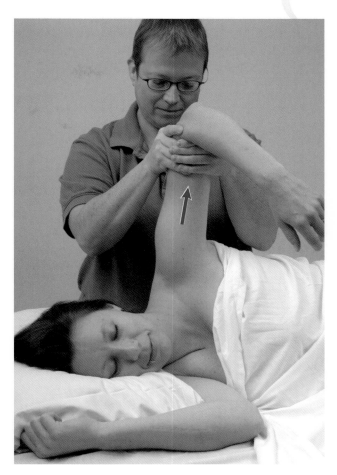

FIGURE 6.11   The therapist raises and lowers the client's arm to stimulate axillary lymph flow.

the ceiling. Raise the arm up and down, as if pumping water with a hand pump (Figure 6.11).

BREECH BABY

The most common and optimum position for a baby to be in for birth, is with its head down in the mother's pelvis. This is known as a **vertex** presentation. When the baby is positioned with the head up and the feet or buttocks down in the mother's pelvis, it is considered a **breech** presentation. This is shown in Figure 9.1C. This occurs in 3% to 4% of full-term pregnancies in the United States.[5] Frequently babies are breech earlier in pregnancy, but most turn to vertex before labor begins. If the baby is still breech at the time of labor, it can sometimes pose a more difficult or dangerous delivery. Many doctors choose to deliver breech babies by cesarean section because of this concern.

Cause

There is no known specific *cause* for a baby to position breech. Possibly breech and posterior positions

(when the baby's face is toward the mother's abdomen) are more comfortable for babies whose mothers sit frequently in chairs, such as in office jobs. There seems to be a lower incidence of breech births in cultures where women frequently squat, rather than sit in chairs. However, in many of these cultures, midwives also massage the pregnant woman's abdomen throughout pregnancy to ensure a vertex positioning.

General Treatment

Massage therapists are likely to encounter clients whose babies are breech. Abdominal massage, when used in conjunction with other practices, can encourage the baby to move. However, abdominal massage toward this outcome should only be done with the support and guidance of a client's prenatal care provider. Several traditional birth practices are also commonly used to help move a baby.

Traditional Birth Practices:
Breech Baby

In many cultures, traditional midwives massage a pregnant woman's belly beginning in the second trimester to prevent the baby from positioning breech. If the baby is found to be breech in the third trimester, there are some practices that may help the baby move into a more optimal position for vaginal birth. Midwives will often teach a mother to lie upside down on a board leaned against a couch for 10 minutes at a time, while massaging her belly and talking to the baby.

Some women put a soft ice pack on the top of the belly and apply a warm compress to the lower belly several times a day while envisioning the baby moving. This may encourage the baby to turn its head away from the cold and reposition itself.

According to herbalist and Naprapath, Dr. Rosita Arvigo, in Belize midwives washed a baby duck and put it on the pregnant woman's solar plexus. The duck walking over the belly helped the baby to turn.[5]

Acupressure point Bladder 67, located on the lateral side of the little toenail, is very frequently used to help encourage a baby to move from breech position. Acupuncturists stimulate the point with a needle or use moxibustion, a technique of burning dried mugwort plant on or close to the skin to stimulate a particular point. In one Chinese study, 130 women of 33 weeks' gestation with breech presentation were given 7 days of daily moxibustion treatment, followed by 7 more days of treatment if the baby had not moved yet to vertex. By the end of the 2-week period, 75% of the babies in the treated group had shifted to the head-down position, as compared with 47% of the 130 women who did not receive treatment.[6]

EDEMA

Edema is the accumulation of fluids in the interstitial spaces, and often develops in the hands and feet during late pregnancy.

Cause

Some swelling of the hands and feet is normal during pregnancy due to the rise of estrogen and progesterone, the relaxation and dilation of the blood vessels, and the general increase in blood volume. Pelvic pressure from the weight of the uterus also compresses major blood vessels as they pass through the groin, decreasing circulation in the lower extremities and forcing the slowed blood to release fluids into the tissues faster than they can be removed.

Mild nonpitting edema increases as pregnancy advances and is most prevalent in the third trimester and in hot weather, especially for women who stand for many hours. Massage can help stimulate resorption of excess fluids.

 CAUTION: Any edema that persists for more than 1 day or is pitting (i.e., after pressing a finger firmly into the swelling for 5 seconds, an indentation remains) (see Figure 4.6), should be reported to the client's PCP. A recent development of pitting edema, unrelated to hot weather or to restriction in the inguinal region, is one symptom associated with preeclampsia. Listen for reports of other preeclamptic symptoms as well: gaining more than 2 pounds per week, edema unrelieved after having legs elevated for 45 minutes, headaches, epigastric pain, blurring vision, or spots before the eyes. If your client reports any of these symptoms, be certain she has been evaluated by her PCP.

General Treatment

Lymphatic drainage, mobilization of the pelvis and hips, and abdominal binders that lift the weight of the uterus off the groin are helpful treatments for edema. Cool hydrotherapy to the areas of swelling can also ease discomfort. Women who exercise regularly generally have fewer problems with edema.

The left sidelying position helps relieve pressure, aids the body in resorption of fluids, and can be used exclusively if edema is excessive or annoying.

According to Traditional Chinese Medicine, edema during pregnancy can be caused by dietary factors, overwork, and worry, which all can lead to stagnation of the vital life force or qi.[7] This is not uncommon during the latter part of pregnancy when the body is becoming exhausted from supplying energy for two people and coping with daily stresses. Women who are pregnant in their late 30s or in their 40s may have a greater tendency toward edema and general qi depletion.

Specific Bodywork Techniques

Below are specific bodywork techniques to address edema.

Edema Reduction

Benefits: Massage can help improve circulation, thereby supporting the body's ability to process excess fluids and wastes.

 CAUTION: When working with edema, all massage techniques should move toward the heart. Do not use any techniques deeper than lymphatic massage on pitting edema, as tissue may be damaged with deep pressure.

Position: Semi-Reclining or Sidelying Position

Technique

For legs, begin at the proximal thigh; for arms, in the deltoid region. This description is for legs, but can be applied to arms and hands as well.

1. Beginning at the proximal end of the thigh, do light and medium pressure effleurage and petrissage toward the trochanter, working your way toward the knee using upward moving strokes.
2. Make long sliding compression strokes with the palms all the way from the knee toward the groin, trochanter, and ischial tuberosity. This helps improve circulation in distal areas before working closer to edematous areas.
3. Open the lower leg: Effleurage and petrissage the lower leg. Begin just inferior to the knee, with strokes working toward the heart, gradually moving toward the feet, so that the proximal areas are opened first. Use light effleurage strokes on the ankles and feet, still stroking toward the knee. Alternate thumbs crossing over thumbs to help move excess fluid.
4. Apply light effleurage to edematous areas at the ankles.
5. Facing the feet, use the flats of the fingers to make light, scooping, alternating strokes from the proximal area of edema up toward the knee (Figure 6.12). Advance toward the ankles and feet, always stroking up. Imagine that you are moving the fluid up the leg and back into the primary circulation a little at a time. You have to move the proximal fluid before you can move the distal!
6. When you have worked one small area with numerous short, light strokes, complete and connect the strokes by making a C-clamp with your hand around the lower leg and compressing and sliding up toward the knee, and even into the thigh.

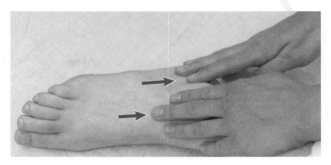

FIGURE 6.12   Edema reduction.
The therapist makes light, scooping, alternating strokes from the proximal area of edema toward the ankle, advancing incrementally into the edema, and always stroking toward the torso.

7. Rotate the ankles and feet in slow circles.
8. Repeat all the above techniques on the arms and hands if necessary, always pushing fluid up and out of the extremity and into the main circulation.

Myofascial Hip Opening

Benefits: A gentle fascial release that helps create space for improved blood circulation.

Position: Sidelying. Stand at the client's back, by her hip. The top leg may be extended for extra opening, but the therapist should lean into the client's body to prevent her from rolling backward with the therapist's hand pressure. This technique may also be done in a low semi-reclining position.

Technique

1. Standing behind the client, cross your arms, place your left hand on the client's hip bone or anterior superior iliac spine (ASIS). Place your right hand firmly on the rectus femoris and vastus lateralis just distal to their origins.
2. Press securely onto the ASIS while applying a gradual melting traction to the quadriceps, slowly opening the inguinal area for increased blood flow (Figure 6.13).

GROIN PAIN AND ROUND LIGAMENT PAIN

The round ligament is a primary uterine ligament that supports the uterus anteriorly, attaching into the pubic and vaginal areas (see Chapter 3). Pain from round ligament spasm is often experienced as sharp, sudden pain in the groin area and most commonly occurs in the last months of pregnancy.

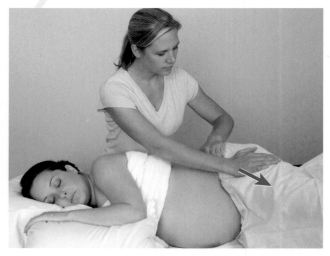

FIGURE 6.13   Myofascial hip opening.
The therapist applies a gradual melting traction to the quadriceps, slowly opening the inguinal area for increased blood flow.

The discomfort can persist for moments or days. Many women are surprised by the intensity of the discomfort and often are not certain of its origin, until assessed by their PCP.

Cause

Groin pain is often caused by spasms of the uterine round ligament as it stretches. Sometimes spasms occur due to improper body mechanics when lifting and carrying, or commonly by "jackknifing" up to a sitting position from horizontal. Labor contractions, as well as vaso-congestion in the pelvic area, can also create aching in the groin. Rather than assuming it is ligament pain, a client should have any undiagnosed pain evaluated first by her PCP.

General Treatment

Proper support for the laterally positioned client is an important element in preventing ligament stress. When positioned in sidelying, be sure to put a small pillow or foam wedge under a large belly to prevent the belly from sagging over to one side and pulling on the ligaments. Most importantly, teach your client proper ways of sitting up from lying down, encourage good body mechanics when moving and lifting, and demonstrate ways to relieve the discomfort when it occurs, as instructed in Chapter 3. Applying moist warm compresses to the affected area can also bring some relief.

Specific Bodywork Techniques

Below are specific bodywork techniques to address groin and round ligament pain. See the myofascial hip opening technique under "Edema" above for an additional treatment for this complaint.

Lifting Effleurage

Benefits: Helps alleviate tension and discomfort related to groin pressure and ligament pain.

Position: Semi-Reclining or Sidelying.

Technique
1. Use hand-over-hand strokes to gently lift up and away from the groin toward the belly. Imagine lifting the pain away (Figure 5.17).
2. Make light, slow, small circles along the groin.

Compression and Cross-Fiber Friction

Benefits: It is possible to help release a pulling or spasmed ligament by working on muscular attachments on and near the pubic bone.

Self Care Tips FOR MOTHERS:

Improving Circulation and Reducing Edema

The following tips can be shared with your client as ways to improve circulation and reduce edema.

- Walk at least 1 mile every day.
- Elevate legs regularly through the day.
- Lie in left sidelying position for at least 30 minutes twice a day to improve circulation.
- Wear loose fitting clothing, without restriction in the groin, legs, abdomen, or arms.

- Rotate the ankles in circles to the left and right. Extend the legs and dorsiflex the feet. Use varying hamstrings stretches to increase circulation in the feet.
- Resting on the hands and knees, with forearms to the floor and buttocks up in the air, helps relieve pressure from sitting on the buttocks and decreases pooling of blood in the pelvis.

ertain essential oils stimulate and tonify the circu-latory and lymphatic systems, relieving edema. This includes all citrus oils and geranium.

 CAUTION: Some people have skin sensitivities to citrus. Test the diluted oil on a patch of skin and wait 24 hours, watching for rash, before applying to the whole body.

Aromatherapy is an in-depth study and science. If you choose to make your own mixture, undertake a course of study that will guide you in appropriate mix-tures for pregnancy. However, the following is a specific blend of essential oils that is safe to use during *the last trimester* of a low-risk pregnancy only in this dilution (or in a lesser dilution). To help reduce edema while doing your massage of the extremities, add 4 drops each of geranium (Pelargonium graveolens//odorantissimum) and lavender oil (Lavandula officinalis; L. angustifolia) to 2 tablespoons of unscented massage oil. Shake well, and use this for massage.

Even without massage, immersing the extremities in cool water can be helpful; the pressure of the water can help the body to reabsorb some of the interstitial fluids. Four drops of either rosemary (*Rosmarinus offic-inalis*) or lemon (*Citrus limonum*) can be added to a footbath to help reduce edema. Mix the oils in the water well before immersing the feet, by splashing the surface of the water with your hand.

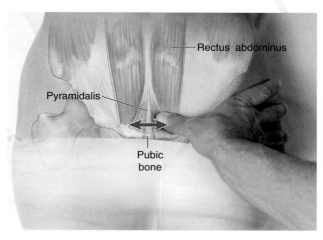

FIGURE 6.14   Compression and cross-fiber friction.
The therapist presses onto the superior edge of the pubic bone and the abdominal and pyramidalis attachments. She then moves across the bone laterally, with firm fingertip or thumb compression and cross-fiber friction until the tissue releases. (From Clay JH, Pounds DM. Basic Clinical Massage Therapy, 2nd Ed. Philadelphia: Lippincott Williams & Wilkins, 2008.)

until you feel a release of tissue. Continue lat-erally until just before entering the inguinal area of veins, arteries, and nerves. Encourage feedback from the client regarding your pres-sure in this area, as it can be very sensitive and vulnerable (Figure 6.14).

3. Use light circling effleurage to soothe the area after focused work.

 CAUTION: Avoid pressure on the external iliac and femoral veins in the groin where you feel strong pulsing.

LEG CRAMPS

Many pregnant women get cramps in the gastrocne-mius and soleus of the calf, often in the middle of the night. Women quickly learn methods to cope with them, as they are very painful and disturbing to the sleep.

Cause

Cramping may be the body's way of saying it has had a long day of poor circulation or overzealous exertion, with fatigue to the calf muscle, compression of the nerves, and a build-up of lactic acid in the muscle tissue. It may also be related to an imbalance of

Position: Semi-Reclining. This work can be done through the sheet, or clothing, to help maintain a sense of privacy and diminish ticklish feelings experi-enced by some women.

Technique
1. Communicate with the client first to ensure she is comfortable with touch in the area of the pubic bone and inguinal area. Ask the client to place her fingers on her pubic bone to indicate its location, and then place your own there. Press onto the superior edge of the pubic bone, holding fingertip or thumb pres-sure on the abdominal and pyramidalis attachments.
2. Move across the bone laterally, with firm stat-ic fingertip pressure and cross-fiber friction

---

Self Care Tips FOR MOTHERS:

Relieving Groin Spasm

For immediate relief of groin spasm, instruct your client and/or help her to do the following:

1. Bring the affected leg up toward the abdomen and hold, breathing slowly into the abdomen.
2. Bend at the waist toward the affected side.
3. Apply slow, direct pressure with the fingertips onto the painful area, usually in the inguinal area or on the pubic bone.
4. Use slow, focused breathing during a spasm.

Other practices can help prevent or reduce the occurrence of spasms. Remind the client to do the following stretches or practices:

- Psoas stretch (see Self-Care Tips for Mothers: Decreasing Low Back Pain)

- Pelvic tilt (see Self-Care Tips for Mothers: Decreasing Low Back Pain)
- Use care when getting up from lying down: roll to the side and push up with the arms and hands
- Change positions slowly to allow ligaments time to stretch
- Avoid long periods of standing or sitting
- Wear an abdominal support wrap

---

phosphorus, calcium, or magnesium. Unsupportive shoes, high heels, or poor posture can also become a cause of calf cramping during pregnancy.

General Treatment

Preventative massage treatment should include general effleurage and petrissage to the calves, improving circulation through the groin area, instruction in proper posture, and stretch-resistance work on the gastrocnemius, soleus, pronators, and supinators.

The most common treatment if a cramp occurs during a massage, is to slowly push or pull client's foot of the affected leg into a dorsiflexed position, pulling the toes and sole of the foot up toward the head. Hold this position, until the cramp releases. It is more effective to do this to the client as a passive stretch, rather than having her activate her own leg muscles to move the foot. When the cramp has passed, gently shake or rock the calf muscles.

 CAUTION: Do not plantarflex the foot during massage, as this can activate cramping. Support the feet well on the massage table to prevent dangling, which can also lead to leg cramps. Do not petrissage a calf that is currently or just recently spasmed, as this may worsen or restimulate the cramping.

Specific Bodywork Techniques

Below are specific bodywork techniques to address leg cramps.

Circulatory Massage

Benefits: Circulatory massage to the legs will increase blood flow, reducing lactic acid and interstitial fluid buildup in the lower legs, and work out muscle tension developed from poor posture or unsupportive shoes.

Position: Sidelying

Technique
1. Any effleurage, petrissage, compression, stripping, or friction at muscular attachments, trigger point erasure, or myofascial and lymphatic work to the legs as performed in any standard massage will be helpful.

Inversion, Eversion, and Dorsiflexion Stretch-Resistance

Benefits: Stretches muscles of the lower leg.

Position: Semi-Reclining or Sidelying

Technique
1. Dorsiflex the client's foot.
2. Ask her to plantarflex her foot against your hand with about one quarter of her effort.

Self Care Tips FOR MOTHERS:

Preventing Leg Cramps

A mother can explore the following options for helping to reduce tension in the gastrocnemius/soleus muscles and decreasing the occurrence of leg cramps related to muscular stress.

- Do foot rotations and dorsiflexions on a daily basis, especially when standing or sitting for long periods. Stretch the toes up toward the head, spreading them apart. Stand up on the toes. Shift weight regularly.

- Do a runner's stretch of the calf by standing and leaning forward against a wall with one leg stretched back. Attempt to bring that heel toward the floor.
- Walk 1 mile every day.
- Improve posture to help increase lower extremity circulation.
- Elevate legs frequently through the day above the heart.
- Wear low-heeled shoes.

---

3. Hold 8 seconds, then ask her to relax her pushing, while maintaining the flexion. Then repeat step #2, dorsiflexing further.
4. Repeat on the other foot.
5. Invert the client's foot, turning the sole of her foot medially. Press against the lateral side of her foot and ask her to evert her foot, pushing it outward against your hand. Resist her effort initially for 8 seconds, allowing for a stretched isometric contraction. Then allow her effort to move your hand away, in an isotonic contraction.
6. Repeat with the client's foot everted, and ask her to invert her foot against your pressure on the medial edge of her foot.
7. Relax. Repeat two more times. She can do this herself holding a towel or strap over her foot as she explores different stretching, movement, and resistance with her feet.

SCIATICA AND SACROILIAC PAIN

The sciatic nerve, the largest nerve in the body, is a combination of nerves from the lumbar region and the sacral spine that connect to become one nerve in the buttocks and then travel down the back of each leg, dividing into two nerves in the lower leg. **Sciatica** is pain caused by compression of this nerve. Sciatic-like pain can also be caused by broad ligament spasms, or by misalignment of the sacroiliac (SI) joints. This may be accompanied with other discomforts such as sharp pain in the SI joint area, aching in the hip or low back, pain in the pubic symphysis area, or a general sense of being "out of alignment" in the hip. These discomforts are fairly common during pregnancy.

Cause

Sciatica may occur as the lateral hip rotators tighten with advancing pregnancy. The piriformis muscle can sometimes compress the sciatic nerve if the nerve passes between its fibers. The majority of "sciatica" during pregnancy is rarely true nerve compression, but more often a referred pain from psoas tightness and uterine ligament pain. However, the sensations of sharp shooting pain, vague numbness, or dull aching discomfort down the back, front, or sides of the leg or in the buttocks feel similar to sciatica.

The SI joints are held together by ligaments that soften under the influence of the pregnancy hormone relaxin. Because of this laxity, combined with the increased pressure of the baby's head against the pelvis and poor posture, the SI joint is at high risk for becoming misaligned. Sometimes one ileum may rotate forward or back, causing sharp pain in one joint. In addition, the sacrum itself can twist, causing dysfunction and pain in the SI joint. The associated pain may radiate down to the knee or calf, like sciatica.

General Treatment

Stretching the hamstrings, low back, gluteals, lateral hip rotators, and psoas, as well as *strengthening* the psoas, abdominals, and hip adductors can help relieve or prevent sciatica. For acute pain, applying ice to the lateral hip rotators can help numb nerve transmissions. Specific stretches are useful to encourage the SI joint to find its natural alignment. Chiropractic attention from one specialized in working with pregnant women can also be useful.

 CAUTION: If any exercise or massage increases pain, stop at once. Do not do deep compression, vibration, or tapotement to the hip adductors where potential clots may be located.

Specific Bodywork Techniques

The following five techniques are also helpful for low back pain, and descriptions can be found in the low back pain section.

- sacral rub
- QL compression points
- QL release
- assisted psoas stretch
- QL extension

Hamstring and Lateral Hip Rotator Releases

Benefits: Stretching the hamstrings and lateral hip rotators helps re-align the sacrum and pelvis and relieve sciatic nerve compression.

Position: Supine or low semi-reclining position, with the knee of the non-painful side flexed toward the chest.

Technique

 CAUTION: This technique requires the client to lie supine for 5 to 8 minutes. Maintain good communication throughout the technique to ensure she is comfortable. Discontinue if the client complains of dizziness, uneasy feeling, nausea, or general discomfort *Do not do the following techniques with known separation of the symphysis pubis or if the client complains of pain in that area when doing the resistance.*

1. Flex the knee and hip of the nonpainful side up toward the same side of her belly to a comfortable flexion. Hold for 10 seconds. This will be considered the active leg.
2. Place your superior hand on her shoulder of the same side as the flexed leg, stabilizing the upper body. Place your inferior hand on the lateral aspect of her raised knee. Push her knee across her torso, above or below her belly (depending on the size of the belly and on her comfort), but try to keep the hip flexed at least 90 degrees, as opposed to more extended. Ask the client to push laterally very slightly with her knee against the resistance of your hand. Hold for 8 seconds while she exhales slowly, then increase the stretch slightly across her body and hold again. If the client complains of groin discomfort, reposition the knee higher or lower being certain to stabilize her shoulder on the side of the leg being stretched, or discontinue the stretch.
3. With the knee midway across her body, place one hand on the lateral ankle of the flexed leg and one hand on the lateral knee. Externally rotate the hip, bringing the knee caudally. Slowly push the foot toward her head. Ask her to tell you when she feels a stretch in her hip rotators, and hold there as she breathes for relaxation. You may need to bring the knee more to midline of the torso for her to feel the stretch.
4. Extend the active leg and shake it loose.
5. Flex the hip of the active leg to at least 90 degrees with the knee flexed as well. Rest the lower leg on your shoulder.
6. Wrap one hand around the quadriceps of the active leg. Holding there, have the client extend the knee of the active leg as much as possible while contracting the quadriceps and iliopsoas. Place your other hand just proximal to her active ankle, to support the leg and assist with the stretch. Ask her to dorsiflex her foot, extending into her heel to stretch the hamstrings. Hold the stretch for 10 seconds.
7. Ask the client to exhale as she pushes against your ankle-hand with the active leg just slightly as if flexing the knee, activating the hamstrings.
8. Rest the leg on your shoulder again. With your fists, push into her biceps femoris, and semitendinosus (avoiding pressure on the semimembranosis closer to the medial thigh). Ask her to push into your pressure with her leg, while extending her knee and into her heel to increase the hamstring stretch. Work with your fists from just proximal of the back of the knee toward the muscle attachments at the ischial tuberosity.
9. Repeat the whole sequence on the painful side.
10. Apply ice to the lateral hip rotators after the work, and encourage the client to ice the affected area for 20 minutes every hour, if the pain is acute.

Self Care Tips FOR MOTHERS:

Reducing Sacroiliac Joint Pain

*W*hen a client experiences SI joint pain, suggest the following self-care tips:

1. If she is able, she can lie down immediately in supine position, with knees bent and feet flat on the floor. As she breathes slowly for 5 minutes and envisions her whole body relaxing, her ilium may more easily realign. Sometimes the support of a hard surface can help the hip to rotate back to alignment.
2. Do lateral hip rotator stretches.
3. Perform a psoas stretch (see Self-Care Tips for Mothers: Decreasing Low Back Pain).

Lateral Hip Rotator Attachments

Benefits: Helps release spasms and constriction of the sciatic nerve.

Position: Sidelying

Technique

1. Standing at her back, press firmly to support under the ischial tuberosity with the inferior hand, ensuring that you do not pull the gluteals apart or uncomfortably spread the client's gluteal cleft. Simultaneously, use melting compression and slide inferiorly and laterally with the superior hand from the iliac crest to the hip rotator attachments at the trochanter.
2. Slide around the trochanter in circles with the heel of the hand to touch on all the muscular insertions on the trochanter.
3. Perform cross-fiber friction on the attachments of the hip rotator muscles.
4. Perform effleurage and petrissage on the QL, gluteal muscles, hip rotators, hamstrings, and quadriceps.

Trochanter and SI Joint Traction

Benefits: Helps realign the SI juncture and release compression in the SI joint.

Position: Sidelying

Technique

1. Stand on the client's posterior side and place the palm of your right hand against the lateral aspect of the trochanter. (You can feel this if you slide the heel of your hand across her buttocks from the sacrum toward her trochanter. You will feel a lump or rise when you come across the trochanter.)

2. Place the other hand on the sacrum, and slide laterally with fingertips or thumb to press into the superior end of the SI joint, medial to the posterior superior iliac spine.
3. Gently push away with slow traction on the trochanter as you push into the SI joint, subtly tractioning the hip away from the SI joint (Figure 6.15). Focus on the SI joint and imagine the space opening, as you apply the traction to the trochanter. Hold for at least 30 seconds. This is a subtle movement, which should not push the client anteriorly.
4. Release slowly and reposition your SI joint thumb, moving slightly inferiorly in the joint and repeat the traction.
5. Repeat, sequentially moving distally along the SI joint.

Sacroiliac and Pelvic Rebalancing

Benefits: Provides potential immediate relief of SI joint pain; helps to realign hip bones, stretch and relax hip abductors/adductors, and realign the pelvis. If one hip has rotated slightly forward or back, resistance exercises can help it to realign.

Position: Supine with both knees bent and feet flat on the table spaced 2 to 4 inches apart. If the client cannot lie on her back at all, these techniques can be done one leg at a time in the sidelying position. In the semireclining position, the hips may not realign as easily, but the adductors will relax with this exercise.

Technique

This is a three-step process, involving isometric contractions in flexion, abduction, and adduction of the hip.

 CAUTION: Do not do the following techniques with known separation of the symphysis pubis

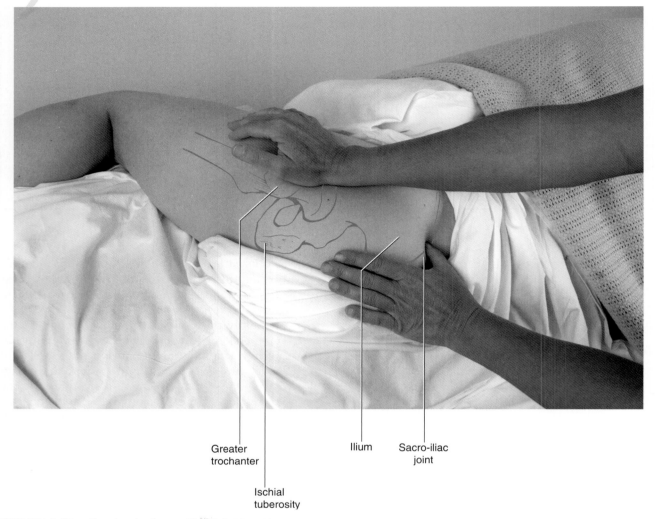

Greater trochanter

Ischial tuberosity

Ilium

Sacro-iliac joint

FIGURE 6.15   Trochanter/sacroiliac joint traction.

With one hand on the client's trochanter and the other on the sacrum, the therapist slowly tractions the hip away from the SI joint.

or if the client complains of pain in that area when doing the resistance. All of these techniques should be done cautiously, slowly, and carefully to avoid any risk of contributing to a diastasis of the symphysis pubis.

Step 1:

1. From the initial position above, instruct the client to bring one knee up to the chest, wrapping her hands around it. You can do this for her also, bringing her knee up and pushing it toward her chest or to the side of her belly.
2. Ask her to hold the flexion, breathing, and allowing the sacrum to relax. *Note: If this movement causes more pain, try flexing the opposite knee to the chest, flexing less, or stopping altogether.*

3. After she has relaxed a moment in this position, ask her to push her knee up slightly against your hands or against her own, isometrically attempting to lengthen the leg.
4. Repeat on the other side. One side normally will feel better than the other. Do not continue on a side if it increases pain. Do the isometrics three times on the least painful side.

Step 2:

1. Still in the initial position, place a hand on the lateral side of each knee. On the client's exhale, ask her to *abduct* isometrically—push out with her knees—against the resistance of your hands. Start slow to ensure there is no pubic pain that might indicate a separation of

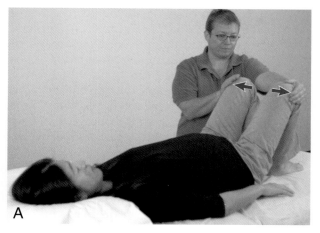 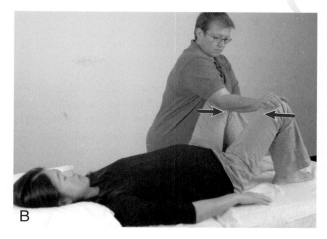

FIGURE 6.16 **Sacroiliac and pelvic rebalancing.**
(A) The client abducts her hips, pushing out with her knees against the therapist's hands. *(B)* The client adducts her hips, pressing in against the therapist's hand and elbow.

the symphysis pubis. Increase the pushing to her full strength for 10 seconds if there is no pain. If it hurts, stop (Figure 6.16A).

2. Place your forearm between the client's knees, with one hand against the medial aspect of the knee and your elbow region against the other knee. On the client's exhale, have her *adduct* isometrically against your resistance with the same care as above, gradually increasing in strength if it is comfortable for the client (Figure 6.16 B).

3. Rub firmly down the outside and tops of the thighs to help relax and soothe after this exercise. Extend the legs.

Femur Traction and Mobility

Benefit: Helps mobilize the hip joint, flattens the sacrum, and can relieve SI joint compression.

Position: Semi-reclining or supine with knees bent and feet flat on the floor. You need to be above the client to lift her upper leg easily. Use a stepstool.

Technique

1. Place your forearm, not your hand, under the client's knee and lift the leg without squeezing with your fingers into the thigh.

2. Use the femur like a lever, lifting up and out from the hip joint with traction (Figure 6.17).

3. Hold the traction as the client breathes and relaxes.

4. Push down into the hip joint, flattening the sacrum.

5. Work into the acetabulum, mobilizing the hip joint in small circles, and repeating traction.

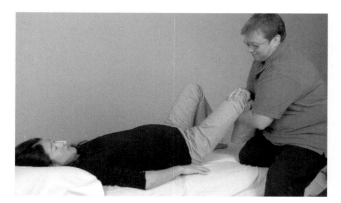

FIGURE 6.17 **Freeing the hip using the femur as a lever to work into the acetabulum and flatten the sacrum.**

SHORTNESS OF BREATH

Many women in late pregnancy experience the difficulty of getting a full, satisfying breath. If a woman has not been physically active before now and has a large belly and significant extra weight in pregnancy, she is likely to experience even more shortness of breath due to the extra workload.

Cause

Sensations of shortness of breath can arise from common pregnancy-related nasal and sinus congestion, anemia, as well as from the growing uterus and baby pressing up into the diaphragm and ribs. When the baby drops into the pelvis at the end of the pregnancy (called "lightening"), the mother is usually able to breathe more freely.

General Treatment

If shortness of breath is associated with the position of the baby, educate the client about correct posture and offer stretches that can help increase thoracic space, such as expanding the arms out, extending the upper spine, and stretching the internal shoulder rotators. Position the client in a semi-reclining position if it is uncomfortable for her to lie on her side. Often, having the head higher than the torso makes breathing easier. General massage to the scalenes, pectoralis minor, and the intercostals, and anything to help create *opening, lengthening,* and *space* in a woman's body will help to improve respiratory capacity.

Specific Bodywork Techniques

Below are specific bodywork techniques to address shortness of breath. Three more techniques, listed here, are presented in detail above, in the low back pain and midback and upper back pain sections.

- full body stretch
- chest opening
- pectoralis stretch and resistance

Shoulder Mobilization

Benefits: Opens chest, expands breathing.

Position: Sidelying

Technique
1. Stand at the client's back. Grasp the humerus firmly just proximal to the elbow. Encourage her to keep her arm heavy and to continue relaxation breathing.
2. Gently traction the arm straight up. Lift with your whole body and belly rather than just with your arms.
3. Holding the arm in gentle traction, rotate it in a circular motion, seeking the full range of motion.
4. Repeat in the opposite direction.

Rib Raking and Trigger Point Release

Benefits: Relieves shortness of breath, heartburn, and tension in the intercostals.

Position: Sidelying

Technique
1. Standing at the client's back, slide your fingers across the client's superior lateral side to

place your fingertips in the intercostal spaces of ribs 8, 9, and 10 (Figure 6.18). Apply firm pressure into the intercostal space and drag your fingers laterally, from anterior to posterior, following the ribs to the vertebrae. Shift your fingers superiorly into the next intercostal space on the anterior side and repeat. Continue moving up the ribcage. When nearing the breast tissue, stay lateral or work on the posterior side only. You can work into the intercostal spaces from the sternum toward the breast tissue if that is comfortable for your client. You may need to hold her breast tissue out of the way as you do that work in the sidelying position.
2. Areas that feel tight can be worked more specifically, one rib at a time. Apply pressure to trigger points and allow the tissue to relax under your fingers.
3. Reaching over the sheet, feel for the inferior edge of the costal margin just lateral to the xyphoid process. Sink the fingertips in against the cartilage and diaphragm attachments with gentle compression, releasing abdominal and diaphragmatic tension while

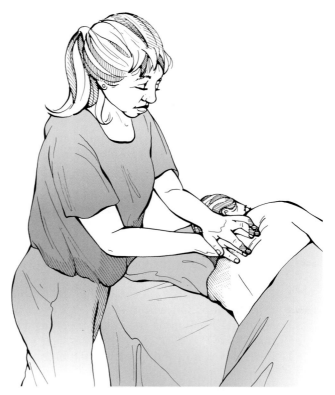

FIGURE 6.18   **Rib raking by sliding fingers through the intercostal spaces.**

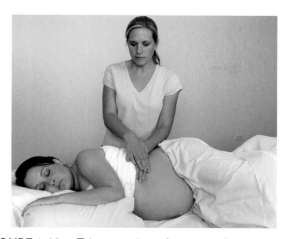

FIGURE 6.19   Trigger points along costal margin.
The therapist applies careful firm fingertip pressure along the inferior edge of the costal margin, starting medial and moving laterally.

moving laterally (Figure 6.19). Ask for clear feedback regarding pressure when working in this tender and vulnerable area.

Note: Rather than work over the sheet, you may choose to use a breast drape and expose the belly for work on the costal margin.

CHAPTER SUMMARY

Massage therapists commonly encounter particular physical complaints from their pregnant clients. General full-body massage can be used to enhance relaxation, which will help diminish some discomfort, but specific techniques are more useful for addressing specific concerns. The techniques discussed in this chapter are simple and can be incorpo-

---

Self Care Tips FOR MOTHERS:

Stretches to Increase Respiratory Capacity

*E*ncourage the client to do stretches that help expand the chest and lengthen the body. The following stretches may be helpful to her:

- *Arm Raise:* Sit against a wall, with legs extended. Raise the arms out to the side, palms against the wall, and walk them up the wall over your head while inhaling. Turn your palms out when necessary and relax.
- *Yoga Chest Opener:* This pose opens the chest, relieves pressure under the ribs, and increases lung capacity. From sitting or kneeling erect, raise one arm over your head, and with your elbow straight in air and close to your ear, reach your hand down the middle of the back. Place the other hand behind the back, bending the elbow, and reach up with it toward the top hand. Clasp your hands if you are able. Hold a scarf between your hands to help them connect, if necessary. Hold and breathe, filling the lungs and expanding the ribs (Figure 6.20).
- *Standing Arm Raise:* Stand and raise your arms up and out to the side with inhalation and the over your head until the hands are palm to palm. Exhale, bringing the arms down, curling your head down, tensing your hands into fists, and bringing them in toward the chest. On the inhale, extend your arms out, extend the fingers, and bring your arms over your head again. Repeat several times.

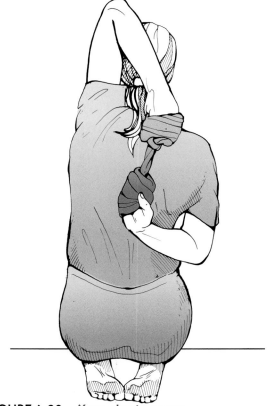

FIGURE 6.20   Yoga chest opener.
The mother can use a scarf between the hands if she cannot reach to grasp her hands behind her back.

Case Study 6.1
ADDRESSING A COMPLAINT OF SHORTNESS OF BREATH

Suzanne had seen her client several times during her pregnancy. Now Beth was in her 37th week and came for a massage complaining that the baby was kicking her in the ribs and pushing up into her diaphragm, making it feel difficult to get a full breath. She also stated that she was having sinus congestion and occasional nose bleeds.

Suzanne observed Beth's posture before positioning her on her left side on the massage table. She noted that Beth's breasts were quite large and that she was internally rotating her shoulders, collapsing somewhat in her chest. She spent some time helping Beth become aware of how she could expand her breathing capacity with some simple postural adjustments—lengthening her spine and lifting in her chest to externally rotate her shoulders. They also discussed the benefits of supportive bras during pregnancy, to help alleviate some of the anterior pull of the breasts.

Suzanne first ensured that Beth was positioned comfortably and had the fan blowing lightly toward her face. She then warmed Beth's back with effleurage and petrissage, and subsequently spent a significant amount of time working intercostally, releasing trigger points and encouraging Beth to breathe deeply to expand her ribs against Suzanne's finger pressure. She applied friction to and stripped along the attachments on the inferior edge of the clavicle and across the superior edges of the pectoralis. She worked briefly with compression on subscapularis. Suzanne then extended Beth's superior arm and did a full body stretch, encouraging Beth to breathe deeply. Suzanne worked similarly on the right side and then suggested repositioning to the semi-reclining position.

Before she changed position again, Beth wanted to use the restroom. As she shifted to sitting from lateral lying, and attempted to stand up, she suddenly felt lightheaded. She sat again on the edge of the table, and Suzanne stood by her, to ensure stability. Suzanne guessed it was a momentary episode of orthostatic hypotension, and apologized for forgetting to suggest that Beth wait a moment in a sitting position before attempting to stand. The lightheadedness passed quickly and Beth was fine after that.

Once back on the table and in the semi-reclining position, Suzanne reached around Beth's belly, and pressed into the multifidus and other spinae erectors on either side of the lumbar spine, pulling forward with enough pressure to arch Beth's back just slightly. She slid her hands anteriorly around the belly and repeated several times, adjusting the position at different areas of the lumbar spine region.

She then had Beth cross her arms over her chest and applied pressure anteriorly on both her arms while Beth pushed her arms out against the resistance during an inhalation. Suzanne had Beth raise both her arms up, flexed at the elbows. Standing behind her, Suzanne placed her hands on the anterior sides of Beth's elbows and inner arms, pulling slowly posteriorly until Beth felt some stretching in her chest. Beth then pushed anteriorly for 8 seconds against Suzanne's resistance, stretching fibers of the pectoralis. After a moment of relaxing the resistance, they increased the stretch and repeated the steps above.

At the end of the session, Suzanne remembered to instruct Beth to change positions slowly, but since she had already been in semi-reclining position, as opposed to lateral, she did not have an orthostatic hypotensive episode. Suzanne then taught Beth some stretches to open her ribcage and chest.

---

rated into a standard relaxation massage. Alternatively, an entire massage can be focused on a particular complaint. For instance, to help increase thoracic space and improve sensations related to respiratory capacity, a full massage session may be focused on warming up the upper chest and back adequately, releasing the pectoralis and subscapularis, extinguishing trigger points in the intercostal spaces, and utilizing the shoulder mobilizations and chest opening techniques. The choice of focus is dependent on the type of work you offer, and the client's preferences and needs.

Specific techniques that you like to incorporate in your work with *nonpregnant* clients can usually be adapted for work in the sidelying position for application with your pregnant clients as well.

MASSAGE THERAPIST TIP — Stretch Marks

*M*any women complain about stretch marks and ask their massage therapist for a cream or salve that can prevent them or make them go away. Stretch marks sometimes develop from the excessive skin stretching that can occur with twins, with an especially large baby, or after several pregnancies, but more often they are caused by hormonal and hereditary factors and cannot be prevented. Nourishing the skin with moisturizer cannot hurt, usually feels good, and can help maintain healthy skin tone, but will not prevent stretch marks from developing or make them go away. Perhaps, rather than thinking of stretch marks as disfiguring, a mother may think of them as her baby's unique story, written in the lines of her body. It is she and this child's unique and natural body art. They represent motherhood and are a sign shared by many women. Red marks during pregnancy generally become silvery and much less noticeable after pregnancy.

For general skin condition and care to the abdomen, add Vitamin E or wheat germ oil to your massage oils. The client may perform a daily moisturizing belly rub with any of the following oils known to be healing to skin: olive oil, cocoa butter, wheat germ oil, avocado oil, and vitamin E and A. Certain essential oils also aid skin healing and can be used in the second or third trimester. The following is a safe mixture that can nourish the skin and can be used with a low risk pregnancy *in the last trimester*: Add 4 drops of lavender and 3 drops of neroli, or 3 drops frankincense and 3 drops tangerine to 2 tablespoons of massage oil. Aromatherapy is an in depth study and science. If you choose to make your own mixture, undertake a course of study that will guide you in appropriate mixtures for pregnancy.

CHAPTER REVIEW QUESTIONS

1. Name two reasons why low back pain is so prevalent during pregnancy. Describe four maternal self-care tips and two bodywork techniques for decreasing low back pain during pregnancy.
2. Explain what might be a possible cause of mid-back pain developing as pregnancy progresses into the third trimester.
3. Determine whether breast massage is legal in your state and explain the social issues surrounding breast massage. Why should it be avoided with a client with a high risk of preterm labor?
4. Describe techniques you might use with a client who is 39 weeks pregnant and has a history of preterm labor and two previous consecutive miscarriages. She is now is complaining of upper back pain and breast tension.
5. Name three conditions for which use of an abdominal binder might be appropriate.
6. Discuss what problems may be avoided by having a client learn proper mechanics for sitting up from lying down.
7. Discuss whether the massage therapist has a responsibility to educate a client on body mechanics, postural awareness, and self-care. How could this benefit both massage therapist and client?
8. If a client experiences sharp pain in her groin, what might you suspect as a possible cause? Name two tips you could teach her as a method of addressing that cause.
9. Name three conditions discussed in this chapter that are often caused by poor posture or improper body mechanics during pregnancy.
10. Discuss your perception of stretch marks. What might you suggest to a client who has concerns about their development and asks for massage to reduce them?

REFERENCES

1. Pennick V, Young G. Interventions for preventing and treating pelvic and back pain in pregnancy. Cochrane Database Syst Rev. 2007 April 18;(2):CD001139.
2. Wang SM, Dezinno P, Maranets I, et al. Low back pain during pregnancy: prevalence, risk factors, and outcomes. Obstet Gynecol 2004;104(1):65–70.
3. Colliton J. Back Pain and Pregnancy: Active management strategies. Phys Sportsmed 1996;24(7). Last accessed online September 4, 2007. http://www.postgradmed.com/issues/1996/07_96/colliton.htm.
4. Kristiansson P, Svardsudd K, von Schoultz B. Back pain during pregnancy: a prospective study. Spine. 1996;21(6):702–708.
5. Arvigo R. Notes from lecture at Maya Abdominal Massage Professional Training, Massachusetts, 2002.
6. Cardini F, Weixin H. Moxibustion for correction of breech presentation: a randomized controlled trial. JAMA 1998; 280(18):1580–1584.
7. West Z. Acupuncture in Pregnancy and Childbirth. Edinburgh: Churchill Livingston, 2001.

CHAPTER 7

BODYWORK IN PREPARATION FOR BIRTH

LEARNING OBJECTIVES

After reading this chapter, you should be able to:

- Describe integrative bodywork techniques that can encourage relaxation prior to labor.
- Describe bodywork techniques that facilitate physical and emotional preparedness for labor.
- Practice the use of visualization and affirmations in conjunction with bodywork.
- Describe elementary acupressure techniques for supporting labor preparations.
- Have the resources to teach perineal massage techniques to a client's partner, and to know when that is and is not appropriate.
- Describe the massage therapist's role in supporting a client having an emotional release during a massage session.

*L*abor has a life, energy, and direction of its own, which, for a laboring woman, can be experienced as joyful, hard work, painful, and utterly transformative. In whatever way it is experienced, the process of inviting another life into the world through one's body is a rite of passage that is unpredictable and powerful. Nurturing and supportive touch can empower a woman to undergo it with trust in her body wisdom.

Massage can help women prepare for birth by releasing muscular and emotional tension, both of which can delay labor. Reducing muscular tension can help a woman "go with the flow" of labor more easily

and increase her vitality and endurance. Releasing emotional tension will decrease production of stress hormones and allow beneficial hormonal releases to promote labor. Massage will give her a focused opportunity to practice relaxing with gentle touch while envisioning and practicing surrendering to the process of birth.

In the last 2 weeks of pregnancy, your client may wish to begin focusing on physical preparations for her birthing time. Specific massage techniques, acupressure points, breathing, affirmations, and visualizations all can be helpful. If your client is past her due date and is growing concerned about a possible induction of labor with Pitocin (synthetic oxytocin) at the hospital, stimulating massage might be used in conjunction with other methods she may be trying to encourage labor to begin. Massage itself will not induce labor, but will help prepare the mother's mind and body to step into the flow of birth. Acupressure is particularly effective in bringing the body into balance in this way, but detailed technical descriptions are beyond the scope of this book. Some useful points are included in this chapter, however, as they are frequently used by massage therapists and lay people who are not certified acupressurists.

GENERAL TREATMENT

Facilitating relaxation for a mother is one of the most important steps in preparation for labor. Any stress that causes obvious or subliminal tension can impede

Visualization is a practice that can increase relaxation, reduce bodily stress responses and help to manifest desirable situations. For some women, it can be very powerful. Others do not relate to the technique and find it difficult to envision imagery in their mind. Some women visualize easily without guidance, while others want someone speaking to them with a soothing voice and suggesting particular types of imagery. Include visualizations in your sessions when you want to help your client increase relaxation, or revision fearful or negative thoughts. But, before incorporating imagery in your sessions, first determine whether your client has interest or experience using visualizations. Then, search for clues as to what type of imagery has power and significance for her, by asking her in what types of environments she feels safe or relaxed. Where is she most at ease? Use these images in your process. Not everyone will relate to the same type of imagery. Let the client be your guide in how to guide *her*.

Affirmations are often used in conjunction with visualization. Affirmations are positive, encouraging words to help shift fear-based or negative thought patterns. A useful way to incorporate affirmations is to notice negative thoughts that your client may have expressed about herself or her pregnancy, labor, baby, partner, etc. When you have identified these issues, seek a reversal of these thoughts. For instance, if she says "I'm afraid I can't handle the pain of labor," identify the positive mirror of this thought, such as: "Moment by moment, one contraction at a time, I will find ways to ride the waves of contractions," or, "As I relax, the pain will decrease." Avoid using negatives in an affirmation; rather than saying "I will not feel pain," try something like, "I have the ability to cope with the sensations I feel." She may like to have you repeat the affirmations to her, but generally it is more empowering for her to repeat the affirmations to herself, in her mind or out loud, while envisioning imagery that supports the affirmation.

Affirmations rely on the belief that beneath all of our exterior ego personas, we are pure, good beings, supported by a numinous energy that is larger than our ego-selves; it is *that* truth that we want to nurture. We may suggest to a client who feels inadequate about becoming a mother a short affirmation such as, "I have the capacity to be a good mother," or something more involved such as, "I have within me all the strength and wisdom I need to be a good mother, and I am supported by all energies and guidance to become that."

the commencement of labor. Remember that labor involves not only a physical release, but a spiritual and emotional one as well. Supporting her surrender into safety and trust will aid your client as she embarks on the journey of birth.

Help relieve tension with full-body relaxation massage, but also focus on the areas that will need to expand or release during labor. These include the hip adductors, the lateral hip rotators, the legs, the belly, and the groin area. Use flowing effleurage and petrissage to the upper thighs and long strokes down the entire body from head to toes to help mobilize energy. Thorough massage of the hands and feet will relax the mother and stimulate reflexive zones. More advanced work includes release of the perineal attachments and pelvic floor, some of which can be addressed by the client's partner with perineal massage, as discussed later in the chapter.

SPECIFIC BODYWORK TECHNIQUES

Several bodywork techniques that are effective in helping a mother prepare for labor and birth in her final weeks of pregnancy are presented below. Additionally, the following techniques, which are described in previous chapters, are useful in labor preparations as well:

- Femur traction and mobility (see the section "Sciatica and Sacroiliac Pain" in Chapter 6)
- Sacral compression and unwinding (see the section "General Full-Body Relaxation: Sacral Compression and Unwinding" in Chapter 5)
- All techniques in the section "Back Pain: Low" in Chapter 6

Jaw Release

Benefits

There is a reflexive relationship between the mouth and the perineum, and especially between the jaw and the pelvis and cervix. Releasing tension in the jaw can encourage the pelvic area and cervix to relax as well. This may be useful in preparation for and during labor.

Position: Any that provides access to the jaw.

Technique
1. Ask the client to relax her jaw.
2. Before applying lotion or oil to the face, gently palpate the masseter on one side with 1 or 2 fingers. Jiggle the fingers to provide a vibration into the muscle for several moments.

Case Study 7.1
HELPING A CLIENT PREPARE FOR LABOR

Joni was 40 weeks pregnant and planning on having her third child at home. Her friend, Terri, a massage therapist, came to Joni's home to offer a labor preparatory massage. Joni shared with Terri about her current fears and hopes for this birth. She was anxious for labor to begin, yet hesitant as well, due to a lack of support from her husband. She was aware of tension in her belly and in her mind. She hoped a massage would help her to relax and to invite labor with more confidence.

Terri was aware that nurturing touch can stimulate emotional issues to surface, but she was not trained in somato-emotional work. She was comfortable, however, being present with feelings that might arise during a session without having to analyze them. Terri asked Joni if she would like to try incorporating visualization into the massage session, to help Joni relax further. Joni agreed, and knowing that Terri knew her well, asked her to guide her with the types of positive imagery and affirmations that she related to. Acknowledging Joni's issues, they invited what they envisioned as a "Birthing Goddess" energy to enter into their space to assist Joni to surrender into the birth. They also focused their thoughts on the baby, acknowledging the baby's effect on stimulating labor and affirming to the baby that it was safe to come into the world whenever ready.

With Joni lying on her side, Terri began a full-body massage, using general effleurage and petrissage to the back, neck, shoulders, and gluteals. As she worked, she noticed areas of depleted energy and others with tense or full energy. She placed her hands on the depleted areas and envisioned her breath moving through her hands, filling these areas with qi or life-force. Terri then placed her hands on the areas of tension and encouraged Joni to breathe into each area, relaxing the tension as she exhaled.

Next, Terri placed her palms on either side of Joni's spine at the neck and palmed slowly down toward the sacrum to relax the back and connect the head with the pelvis. This also affected the acupressure Bladder meridian, which influences the flow of labor. On the sacrum, Terri did a friction rub, bringing a flush of circulation to the skin and warmth into the pelvis. She then applied deeper stimulating pressure into the sacral foramen, holding and making circling friction on each spot. Joni said this helped release some of the tension she was holding there and made her pelvic area feel more "alive."

To integrate her work, Terri used long strokes from the head and back, drawing energy down and out the extremities with each exhalation, encouraging Joni to envision energy surging down, like a waterfall through her body. While visualizing, Terri noticed tightness in Joni's right hip and groin area. Terri asked her to tighten and then relax that area, and then worked with isometric stretches to open the hips.

Throughout the session, Terri offered encouraging affirmations, as Joni had asked, reminding Joni that her body knew how to labor, that she had done this successfully twice before, that Joni could always rely on the support of the spiritual energy that she related to, as well as on the support of the millions of women who had birthed before her.

On the hands and feet Terri spoke of imagining opening the channels of energy in the upper and lower body so that the energetic river could flow freely. On the feet, she applied thumb pressure around each heel and ankle, stimulating reflexology areas and pressing into an acupressure point in the center of the sole of the foot, just below the ball of the big toe, bringing a calming, grounding, and energizing flow through the body.

Terri then focused on acupressure points that are prohibited earlier in pregnancy, including Spleen 6, Large Intestine 4, Bladder 60, and Kidney 3. On the shoulders, she applied downward pressure into Gall Bladder 21, while speaking about envisioning a soft beam of light streaming down through Joni's body, imagining it softening everything it touched—including the jaw, the belly, and the perineum.

As Terri worked, Joni sometimes noticed areas that felt tight and unwilling to release. Just by talking about these sensations, she was able to let go more, and the tissues softened under Terri's touch.

With warmed castor oil, mixed with essential oils of Clary Sage, Rose, and Jasmine, Terri did a stimulating belly rub, incorporating Joni's back and belly in the work.

In closing, Terri did face massage and included relaxing work to the jaw. She then placed her hands on Joni's heart and belly, asking Joni to visualize love flowing into her belly. As she did this, Joni's tears began to emerge, and she cried quietly for several moments, releasing more tension.

Two days later, Joni's labor began. Her support team was present, and she gave birth without complications to her baby girl. Later Joni said the massage had helped her feel relaxed and more mindfully prepared for what lay ahead of her. She said she was more balanced and connected to her body and felt that the massage, visualizations, and affirmations helped her have a greater sense of trust that all would resolve in the best timing possible.

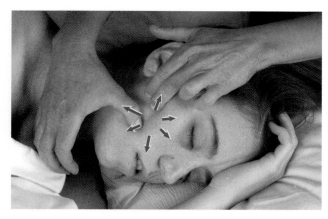

FIGURE 7.1   Slow compression and myofascial release on the masseter.

Apply pressure in opposite directions over the masseter. Gradually, as the tissues and fascia melt away under compression, the fingers will begin to spread apart, sliding through the tissue.

3. Compress into the center of the masseter with two fingertips, allowing them to sink slowly into the muscle as it relaxes under the pressure. Apply a slight traction between the fingers. Gradually, as the tissues and fascia melt away under the compression, the fingers will begin to spread apart, sliding through the tissue. Repeat this compression and stretching in all directions from a central point on the masseter (Figure 7.1).
4. Apply lotion and use a sliding-compression stroke from the insertion of the masseter on the zygomatic arch to the mandible.

Adductor Resistance

Benefits

Some women are uncomfortable thinking about their perineal area being exposed to numerous people who may be present during the birth of the baby. Stretching and relaxing the hip adductors while in the semi-reclining position can offer a chance for her to relax more in preparation for the inevitable exposure that occurs during pushing and birth.

Position: Semi-reclining with knees flexed and soles of feet facing each other, flat together. Let her knees flop down toward the table as far as possible in a relaxed position.

Technique
Note: Be careful to maintain proper draping throughout this work.

1. Place your hands on the inside of the client's knees with light pressure, as she relaxes.

2. As she exhales, ask her to push slightly against your hands isometrically with her knees as you resist against her pressure. Hold for 8 seconds during an exhalation.
3. Have her relax the pushing, then stretch further and repeat.

Sacral Releases

Benefits: In the last weeks of pregnancy, stimulation to the sacral foramen helps release, relax, and prepare the pelvis for birthing. It brings circulation to the area, stimulates nerve function, and helps relieve back pain.

The sacrum has 8 foramen, or openings, through which pass nerves that innervate the pelvic floor. The sacrum shields and protects the uterus and provides stability and somatic grounding. In the late second trimester and throughout the third trimester of pregnancy, many ailments of the low back area can be relieved with careful work to the sacrum.

 CAUTION: Excessive stimulation of the sacral nerves and foramen is contraindicated for those with a history or risk of miscarriage or preterm labor.

Position: Sidelying

Technique
1. Apply slow pressure with fingertips or thumbs into the sacral foramen, one on each side of the sacrum at the same time. The foramen are located about 1 thumb-width out from the center of the sacrum and can be felt as energetic or physical indentations in the sacrum. There are 4 holes on each side of the sacrum. Slide your fingers slowly, with firm pressure, along the sacrum to search for the foramen; sometimes you can see them through the skin as dimples.
2. Communicate with the client about comfortable levels of pressure. Hold each point for several of your breaths or until you feel a softening.
3. Move to the next foramen. Push with your thumbs into each of the sacral foramen, applying even pressure and holding, or making small circles on each hole (Figure 7.3).
4. Perform friction rub on the whole sacrum back and forth, creating heat in the area.

Cupping

Benefits: Increases energy from the pelvis down the legs, opening the circulation and flow of energy.

Position: Sidelying

Self Care Tips FOR MOTHERS:

Squatting Practice

You may want to suggest to your clients to practice squatting during their pregnancy in preparation for birth. Squatting has numerous benefits:

- It helps a woman become familiar with opening her hips as necessary for birth.
- It helps stretch the adductors and perineum, which need to be flexible and expansive for birth.
- It strengthens the legs, feet, and ankles, and reduces leg cramps.
- Encourages evacuation of the bowels, decreasing straining and risk of organ prolapse.
- It increases mobility of the pelvic joints, expanding the pelvic diameter, making space for the baby to descend during birth.
- It lengthens the low back, reducing low back pain.

 CAUTIONS: Squatting should not be painful or stressful. A client with diastasis of the symphysis pubis should not squat.

One method of stabilized squatting practice is to stand with the feet a bit wider than hip width apart and turned out laterally. She can hold onto the back of a stable chair or onto the doorknobs on either side of an open a door. Keeping the elbows straight, she then pulls back and sinks into a squat as in Figure 7.2. She pulls up to return to standing. If it is too difficult to squat, a modified squat can be done by sitting on a small stool, with the hips abducted and the heels on the floor.

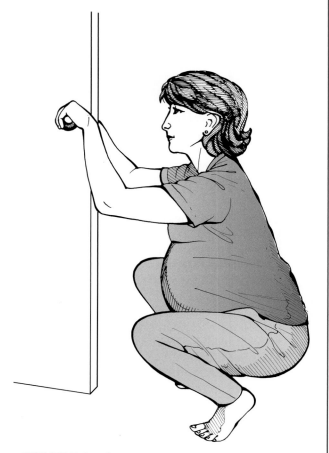

FIGURE 7.2   Squatting with support of the door.

Technique
Stimulate the buttocks and legs with percussive strokes, holding your hands in a cup like shape and patting or hitting lightly from the buttocks down the quadriceps and lateral side of the leg to the foot.

Belly Rub

Benefits: Belly rubs are very helpful at the end of pregnancy to help relieve pressure from the abdomen on the groin and to potentially increase preparedness for labor. If labor is late and contractions are desired, use warm castor oil as an added stimulant, and massage longer, with more stimulating energy than used in a standard belly rub. The addition of essential oils for a belly rub is helpful at this stage of a normal pregnancy. Use these oils only at the end of pregnancy, when labor is due, in the following dilutions: 3 drops of rose (*Rosa damascena; Rosa centifolia*) or lavender (*Lavandula officinalis; L. angustifolia*), 2 drops of jasmine (*Jasminum grandiflorum*), and 2 drops of clary sage (*Salvia sclarea*) to 2 tablespoons of warmed castor oil. If you wish to use other essential oils or other dilutions, consult aromatherapy texts and obtain aromatherapy training for pregnancy.

Technique: See Chapter 5.

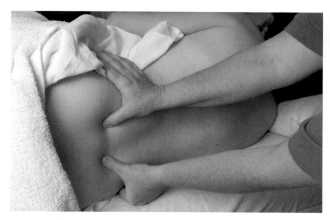

FIGURE 7.3   Circling pressure into the sacral foramen.
Apply slow pressure with fingertips or thumbs into the sacral foramen, one on each side of the sacrum at the same time. The foramen are located about 1 thumb width out from the center of the sacrum and can be felt as energetic or physical indentations in the sacrum. Slide your fingers slowly, with firm pressure, along the sacrum to search for the foramen; sometimes you can see them through the skin as dimples.

DISPELLING MYTHS:
Using Massage as a Quick Route to Labor

When a woman's due date has come and gone, she may develop anxiety about whether labor will ever start. Usually after 41 weeks' gestation, doctors and midwives begin to consider options for inducing labor in an effort to avoid the baby getting too large or the placenta deteriorating. Some women who believe that receiving an "induction" massage might stimulate their labor ask their massage therapist for such help.

Massage does not trigger labor to begin. What massage can do is to help the mother relax. Relaxation helps diminish adrenalin and catecholamine production, allowing hormones, endorphins, and prostaglandins that prepare the body for labor, to function more optimally. Massage can be very beneficial at this late stage of pregnancy, and if a woman's labor does begin after receiving a massage, she may believe it was the touch that stimulated it. However, it is much more likely that it was due to her ability to relax under the touch and be offered reminders of her body's inherent wisdom regarding birth, which allowed the natural development of contractions to occur. In this way, massage was a complementary support, rather than the cause of labor beginning. For many women, labor still does not begin until other elements are in place—physically, psychologically, or spiritually—even after receiving a thorough and focused massage with the intent of supporting labor.

Complementary Modalities:
Acupressure for Labor

The acupressure points that are forbidden during pregnancy are helpful at the end of pregnancy to support the body's preparations for labor. They can be taught to a woman and her partner for use before and during labor. Acupressure is an in-depth study and practice of energy; the following are tips for a generalized approach that can still be effective when combined with a focused intention of support. As long as your client's PCP has affirmed that labor is due, these points can be incorporated into a therapeutic massage and used with any healthy pregnancy after 38 weeks. Gentle pressure to the points is not dangerous and will not cause harm or trigger labor to start suddenly; instead it will support the body to do what it naturally wants to do.

The most common points to support contractions and birth, and to decrease pain, are Large Intestine 4, Gall Bladder 21, Spleen 6, Bladder 60, and the Bladder 31 and 32 in the sacral foramen. These are pictured in Figure 4.3. Touch on these points gently but firmly every half hour when your client is preparing for labor, working both sides of the body simultaneously if possible. Hold each point for at least 5 minutes, encouraging the client to envision the cervix softening and dilating, imagining hormones coming into full strength to promote labor, envisioning energy flowing without blockage throughout her body. Acupressure points are not magic buttons that will cause a change immediately; they need thorough and consistent attention over a period of hours or days to be effective.

When searching for a point, ask how it feels; the woman may notice a special sensitivity when you touch the point, a discomfort, a zing of energy, or a pulsing. Or she may not feel much at all. Maintain open lines of communication; ask her to let you know what a comfortable pressure is for her. Think of the body as a temple in which it is appropriate to enter quietly and respectfully; use that same respect and caution when touching a point. Apply pressure gradually, with attention and intention, as she exhales. Release the pressure with the same attention.

Always initiate pressure from your belly rather than from just your hands or arms, using perpendicular pressure (90 degrees) into the points.

How the Partner Can Help
Perineal Massage

Many women giving birth experience some sort of trauma to their perineal tissues. This is not surprising, considering that a 6- to 10-pound little person has spent minutes or hours pushing her or his way against a woman's delicate innermost mucus membranes. If the baby descends too quickly or if the mother pushes too forcefully, it is possible that these tissues will not stretch adequately and they may tear. Studies are inconclusive as to whether prenatal perineal massage helps decrease perineal tears at birth. However, birth is a process that progresses more smoothly when a woman has familiarity and ease with her perineal area, and perineal massage can facilitate this when initiated up to 6 weeks before the expected delivery time. Many PCPs suggest that their clients practice perineal massage, but few women are given specific instructions for a gentle approach to this work.

Although scope of practice regulations and the sensitive nature of this work prevent a massage therapist from performing it, a client's partner can be taught to do general perineal massage for weeks ahead of the delivery to help prepare, soften, and stretch the tissues and help the mother become accustomed to the sensations of stretching.

The following description of benefits, contraindications, and techniques can be given to your client and her partner.

Benefits

Daily prenatal perineal massage of 5 to 10 minutes, beginning around 35 weeks of gestation, can provide the following benefits:

- Accustom a client to stretching and pressure sensations, enabling her to relax more easily when stretching during delivery.
- Release constricted perineal musculature.
- Allow a partner to be intimately involved with birth preparations.
- Create a pre-birth opportunity to work with possible emotional issues related to perineal trauma or abuse.
- Possibly decrease duration of the pushing stage of birth if emotional issues were addressed during prenatal perineal massage.

Precautions and Contraindications

Perineal massage should not be performed if any of the following situations exist:

- The woman has vulvar varicosities, active genital herpes lesions, yeast infection, or any active vaginal trauma, infection, or sexually transmitted disease.
- The woman does not wish to have the massage.
- The partner is uncomfortable with the procedure and unable to stay present with the woman's sensations, requests, or responses.
- The woman is experiencing preterm labor. If she is, avoid perineal massage until she is at 38 weeks' gestation.
- The woman is on bed-rest for any high-risk condition.

Observe the following precautions when doing perineal massage:

- Avoid rubbing on the urinary tract opening to prevent inflammation or introduction of infection-causing bacteria to the urinary tract.
- Use excellent communication with women who have a history of sexual abuse, as emotions or memories could be triggered during some perineal massage.
- Always clean the hands and fingernails well before and after the massage. Keep fingernails cut short to avoid injuring the perineal tissue.

Guidelines on Performing Perineal Massage

Preparations: While the woman gets comfortable in a well-supported semi-reclining position, warm a few tablespoons of nourishing sweet almond, vitamin E, or avocado seed oil. Do not use mineral oil or Vaseline, which leave a water-repellent residue and may ultimately dry out the tissues. Place a towel under her bottom, to absorb dripping oils. She may wish to take a warm bath or put warm moist washcloths on her perineum to help relax more fully before starting bodywork.

1. *Attunement:* When you are both comfortable, place your hands on your partner's perineum, allowing the palm of your hand to press gently against her outer labia and your fingers to rest on her mons and pubic bone. This gives her a chance to breathe and relax, getting accustomed to being touched in this way.
2. *Lubrication:* Dip your fingers into the warm oils, and gently lubricate the outside of her perineum. When she says she is ready, re-lubricate your fingers and slowly and gently slide one and then two fingers about 1/2 to 1 inch into the bottom of her vagina. Lubricate inside with the oil.

How the Partner Can Help
Perineal Massage (Continued)

3. *Kegels:* Ask her to squeeze her muscles, like a Kegel exercise. If you cannot feel her tightening, she may want to practice strengthening and toning these muscles for birth. Work together for a few moments tightening and relaxing these muscles, having her practice and focus on relaxing them completely in-between squeezes.

4. *Exploring:* Press down slowly in the bottom of the vagina, and then work your way up, pressing on the sides until about half way up toward the top. If you find tight areas, help them relax by using gentle pressure and rubbing. Press into the tissue and slide out, holding the pressure and encouraging opening. Communicate regularly with her to ensure comfortable pressure, speed, and amount of lubricant.

 CAUTION: Avoid rubbing at the top under the pubic bone where the urinary opening is.

5. *Stretching:* Begin again at the bottom of the perineum. Press slowly down with the flats of your fingers, increasing pressure until she feels a burning or tingling or tightness and tells you to stop. Hold the pressure there where she feels the burning for 1 minute as she breathes and practices relaxing her perineal muscles. This should not be painful, but she should feel the stretch. This is a good time for her to practice breathing into her abdomen and relaxing fully with each exhalation. Visualization may help her relax. Verbally affirm her beauty and power and remind her to breathe slowly as she relaxes all of her muscles. Eventually the sensations in her perineum should be numbed or reduced. Repeat this stretching, moving up the walls of the vagina.

6. *Completing:* When completed, place your palm over the outside of her perineum, fingers resting over her pubic bone. Acknowledge and appreciate the work she has done relaxing and opening, and remind her that during birth, she will have the skills to again relax like this to allow the baby to come easily through her.

EMOTIONAL SPACE: LETTING IT FLOW, LETTING IT GO

During a massage, your client may naturally experience a release of deep emotion. There is no need to analyze her feelings or provoke emotional reactions; your role is a massage therapist or birth supporter, not a psychologist, and you must work within the scope of your field of practice. On the other hand, emotions often arise, unsolicited, just because a client feels your nurturing support. The most essential gift the massage therapist can offer is to maintain a supportive space . . . listening, continuing your nurturing touch, allowing her emotions to flow, encouraging her with verbal reassurance, letting her know that you are with her as a witness to her feelings. As emotions are released, blood flow increases throughout her body. Muscular tension along with the emotions that have been stored and held in the restricted muscle tissue are freed.

Crying, laughing, or deep breathing can all be signs of emotions rising to the surface. If these develop during a massage session and you are uncertain about how to help support your client, consider using the following tools:

- Notice your own breath. Maintain grounded, relaxed breathing that can serve as an anchor or grounding cord for your client. Stay calm and connected with breath. Keep your feet solidly on the ground.
- Maintain your touch, but slow it down to holding, rocking, or focused pressure in one particular area.
- If she is extremely agitated, you may consider calling on a higher dimension of support, if you relate to that. Spirit guides, plant spirits, or other spiritual allies can help to ground both of you. This can be done silently or out loud as seems appropriate and relevant for each client.
- Crush a healing herb, such as motherwort, mugwort, mint, or chamomile and have her hold and smell it. The scent and plant presence can be calming.
- Allow time for her to share whatever she would like about the experience afterward,

and leave time for grounding, assimilation, and re-entry into the world.

- Listen rather than judge or give advice. Acknowledge what she is saying, and perhaps repeat it to assure her that you have heard her correctly. Acknowledge that her feelings are valid, while remembering that feelings are transient.
- Affirm the importance and value of her emotional clearing at this time.
- To help your client return to the present moment after an emotional release, you might hold her feet or place a hand on her belly or head, reminding her to breathe into her belly. Help her notice her surroundings, the flowers outside the window, the picture on the wall, the feeling in her feet; this will help her to assimilate and return to the present from her emotional world.

CHAPTER SUMMARY

Any bodywork can help a woman in her preparations for birth; there is not a specific type of work that is necessarily better than another. However, the techniques discussed in this chapter can be useful for a variety of women, and do lend themselves to a focus on birth preparations. Perhaps more important than the type of bodywork done, is the incorporation of emotional safety and support with the touch. Using affirmations, creating a safe environment, encouraging full relaxation, and incorporating visualizations of positive processes and outcomes for birth, along with supporting the release of emotional restrictions—these are the keys for offering the most beneficial pre-birth massage.

CHAPTER REVIEW QUESTIONS

1. Describe a primary focus of bodywork when helping a woman prepare for labor.
2. Explain why releasing the jaw can support labor preparation.
3. Discuss why relaxation is a critical ingredient for labor to begin.
4. Explain how the use of visualization and affirmations can be supportive prior to and during labor.
5. Describe the important application methods involved in utilizing acupressure for labor support.
6. Discuss issues surrounding the practice of perineal massage. Examine what would be necessary dynamics within a couple before beginning perineal massage.
7. Name three contraindications to perineal massage. Name four benefits of prenatal perineal massage.
8. Discuss methods of and tools for supporting a client if strong emotions arise during a massage session.
9. At what point during a pregnancy could you suggest working with labor preparations?
10. Describe the benefits of massage for labor preparation as you would to a client who wants you to work with this focus.

PART II

BIRTH

There is hardly a people, ancient or modern, that do not in some way resort to massage and expression in labor, even if it be a natural and easy one.

GEORGE ENGELMANN, 1884

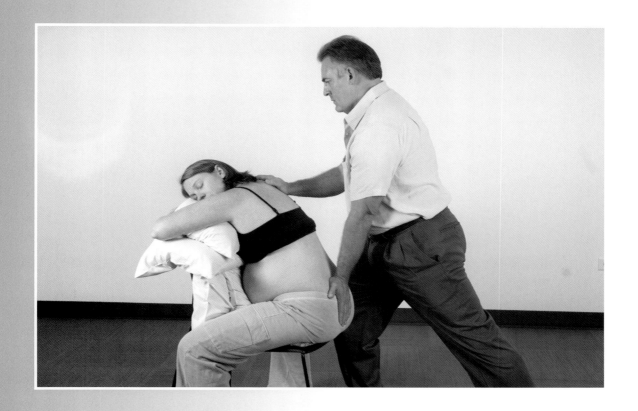

CHAPTER 8

SUPPORTING WOMEN DURING LABOR AND BIRTH

LEARNING OBJECTIVES

After reading this chapter, you should be able to:

- Describe the role of the massage therapist when working with women in labor.

- The physiological and emotional benefits of touch for women in labor.

- Describe bodywork techniques that can facilitate an easier birth.

- Identify the ways in which a massage therapist must have skills of flexibility and creativity to adequately work with women in labor.

- Identify the ways subtle energies or emotions can affect labor progress.

- Explain the relationship between stress and impeded labor progress and describe ways for the massage therapist to help women decrease stress during labor.

- Give an elementary explanation of the Gate Control Theory of pain and how it applies to touch during birth.

*W*e call giving birth "labor," meaning work, travail—the monumental effort involved in bearing new life. In Spanish, to give birth is *dar a luz* or, literally, "to give to light," reminding us that birth is a unique and powerful journey during which women are deeply transformed as they bring this new life and new light into the world.

After 9 months of harboring and nurturing a human being within her body, a woman undergoes this rite of passage in physical and emotional dimensions, as well as for many, a deeply spiritual one. One new mother relayed to her massage therapist that, "The moment my child was born was the most intensely spiritual moment of my entire life!" In many cultures, this spiritual quality of birth is honored as the laboring woman is considered to be in the closest contact possible with a divine energy. Massage therapists touching a woman during her birth may feel this contact themselves as they witness her transformation into the mother of a new child.

As the mother-to-be enters this pulsing dimension of birth potential, she must be able to open herself to an intensity of energy, pain, bliss, and surrender. For this to happen easily, she must be in a safe environment and must *feel* and trust in that safety. For many women, surrendering into this trust involves being strongly supported in the dimensions in which birth occurs, and being reminded of her innate wisdom, which can guide her on this path.

A massage therapist may be at a birth primarily as a physical supporter, but more often than not, she or he will be drawn into the role of emotional supporter as well. Whether or not the mother and the massage therapist have gone through birth themselves or have witnessed another's birth before this one, they may both be inspired knowing that millions of women have journeyed down this well-traveled path. There are ages of birth wisdom to draw on—either resting in the collective unconscious or still practiced in many cultures. Each woman's mother, grandmother, and great-grandmother gave birth in a direct line to

*A*round the world, for generations, touch has been the time-tested practice used to improve a woman's experience of labor (Figure 8.1). Imagine these scenarios of touch around the world. In India, elder women or experienced mothers may surround a woman in labor, anointing and massaging her body, pressing into potent energetic pressure points (marma chikitsa) and massaging her perineal area to help promote birth and relieve pain.[2,3]

In Jamaica, midwives would incorporate touch and massage frequently during birth, massaging the woman's belly to encourage the baby to move into an optimum birthing position and using warm cloths to pull and rub behind the back and create a soothing friction.[4]

Efe midwives of the Congo might support a laboring woman with the touch of breath, song, and hands, encouraging her to be like the river as she pushes her baby into the world.[5]

At a homebirth in the United States, a woman breathes deeply as her friend sits with her, massaging her hand and encouraging her with quiet songs. The baby's father rubs her forehead and softens her jaw with his touch. Candles flicker in the dawn light; the midwives sit in a corner, watching and waiting.

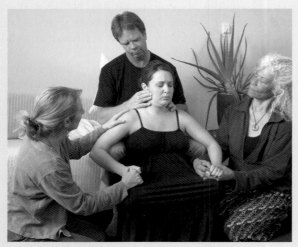

FIGURE 8.1 **Friends and partners have been supporting women through birth for thousands of years with touch, verbal reassurance, and encouragement.**

herself, and their presence, subconsciously or in person, may provide this woman with support as *she* now becomes mother.

A well-known traditional midwife, Ina Mae Gaskin, has said, "Motherwit, or mother wisdom, includes knowing that every woman has the knowledge within her about how to give birth, and that for her to have access to this knowledge, she must be protected from fear, distraction, and abusive treatment."[1] A massage therapist can join in supporting a woman to discover this motherwit and help create the optimum safe environment for birthing.

Meaningful touch and attentive encouragement are often a significant part of creating this safe and precious birth environment. Massage has been repeatedly demonstrated to help a mother have a safer, more relaxing birth, as touch stimulates the parasympathetic nervous system, helping a woman to relax while simultaneously increasing attentiveness. In this chapter, we will explore the role of the massage therapist in supporting a woman during birth, and the benefits of massage during this time.

THE MASSAGE THERAPIST SUPPORTING BIRTH

Intuition, trust, and deep relaxation — these qualities, cultivated throughout a pregnancy and labor, promote a healthy environment for a baby to develop in and be birthed into. A massage therapist can help to nurture these qualities through touch. However, isolated massage techniques will not ease a woman's labor. They must be combined with grounding emotional support and applied in an ever-changing situation.

Massaging during labor is unlike any other massage. Rarely is the client lying still, as on a massage table. The type of touch that is helpful may change with every contraction, demanding that the one touching rely constantly on intuition and creativity and be willing at any moment to stop touching all together if it has become an undesirable mode of support. Those who support the laboring woman are embarking together with her on perhaps the most intense experience of her life, journeying into deeply personal and intimate spaces.

Touch therapists must be grounded in an appreciation for and understanding of this transformative energy of birth. Touch that is disconnected from the unique needs of the woman in labor can cause irritation or distraction rather than ease or relaxation. The most effective touch for a woman in labor is touch that offers not only physical nurturing, but emotional as well. To provide optimum bodywork services, one must attune not only to where tension may be developing in a woman's muscles, but also to subtler influential forces, such as how her energy may be blocked due to fears or unexpressed emotions. Often, through the use of nurturing touch, these emotions are freed, allowing labor to progress more fluently. With subtle influences in mind, pay attention to your own thoughts and energy as you enter a woman's birthing domain. Attempt to become fully present to each moment and to leave behind your personal daily concerns. If you have underlying tension, this may impact how well a woman will relax during labor.

Understanding the importance of creating a safe environment during birth, recognizing how fear affects labor, and learning ways to offer nurturing touch during birth will help you become an ideal support person. The following chapters will give you tools and ideas that can be implemented during labor. The words and pictures in the chapters will help you cognitively understand how to support a laboring woman, but the true instruction will be the actual practice of opening your heart to each individual birth as a woman "brings to the light" a new life.

BENEFITS OF MASSAGE DURING LABOR

Touch can affect how a woman experiences labor and influence the progression of labor. The benefits of sensitive and nurturing touch during labor are numerous. These are discussed below:

- *Improves Physiological Functioning:* Nurturing touch and emotional support increases oxytocin levels; oxytocin helps decrease anxiety, blood pressure, and cortisol levels, and can have a sedative effect, helping women manage contractions more easily.[6-9]
- *Speeds Labor:* Nurturing touch helps speed labor and decreases the need for augmentation of contractions with synthetic oxytocin,[10-12] and possibly, when using effective stimulating abdominal massage, may increase the strength and/or frequency of contractions.
- *Relieves Muscular Discomfort:* Massage is commonly used to reduce muscular aching and cramps. During labor this is especially helpful with common leg cramps or low back aches.
- *Decreases Use of Pain Medications:* Touch can increase a woman's pain perception and threshold therefore decreasing the use of pain medications.[6,11-15]
- *Relieves Muscular Discomfort:* Massage is commonly used to reduce muscular aching and cramps. During labor this is especially helpful with common leg cramps or low back pain.

- *Improves Back Pain:* Touch techniques to the low back can relieve "back labor" and general low back pain.[16,17]
- *Increases Dilation:* Many midwives and massage therapists find that massage to the jaw, or the "upper mouth" can help to relax the "lower mouth," or the vagina and cervix, promoting dilation and birth.
- *Helps the Baby Reposition Appropriately:* Belly rubs, used in conjunction with other techniques and supervised by the client's PCP, might be helpful for encouraging babies to move from posterior positioning to anterior, optimizing delivery.
- *Renews Energy:* During a long labor, the use of invigorating strokes or acupressure can help increase energy.
- *Increases Satisfaction:* Quality support, as well as nurturing touch, improves a woman's ability to cope with contractions and increases her level of satisfaction with her birth.[11,13,18]
- *Offers Birth Companions Effective Support Tools:* Gives the labor support team specific ways to feel useful and improve a woman's experience.
- *Decreases Anxiety:* Touch provides emotional support and reassurance and decreases anxiety and fear, helping a woman to relax and have increased confidence in herself and her process, thereby improving the progression of birth.[12,14,18,19]
- *Reduces Medical Interventions:* Continuous emotional and touch support during labor reduces the incidence of medical interventions such as cesarean birth, forceps, and the use of synthetic oxytocin hormone—pitocin.[10,11]
- *Reduces Depression:* Touch during birth has been shown to decrease the incidence of postpartum depression.[9,12]
- *Increases Maternal Attention Toward Infant:* Studies have shown that women who receive loving support and nurturing touch during labor, touch and interact with their infants more than those who do not receive that support.[20-22]

EFFECTS OF STRESS ON LABOR

Paramount to a satisfying birth experience for many women is having the support of a massage therapist or **doula**—a caregiver specialized in offering laboring women emotional encouragement and physical touch. More than the relief of pain, it is the emotional support and safety that develops between these types of birth companions and the laboring woman that helps her to feel empowered to cope with her contractions and which leads her to a sense of satisfaction about her birth.[18, 23] If women have an unsafe environment with no solid emotional support during birth, fear and accompanying stress increase. When people experience stress, hormones called **catecholamines**, such as adrenaline, are released into the bloodstream.[24,25] Catecholamines cause an increase in heart rate, blood pressure, and respirations and divert blood away from digestion.[24,25] They also relax smooth muscle. Fearful thoughts during labor, such as the fear of pain, fear of the unknown, fear of the coming contraction—are stressful, causing an increase in circulating catecholamines which can relax the uterine smooth muscle and result in slowed or stalled contractions. Fear is also often accompanied by shallow breathing, muscular tension, and vasoconstriction,[24,25] responses which further diminish effective uterine contractility. Essentially, if the laboring woman subconsciously or consciously suspects her environment is not safe for any reason, labor will often stop, and for good reason—who wants to birth a baby into a dangerous situation? Inadequate support or distracting touch can add to a woman's disease and fear.

One way to create a safe birthing environment and reduce the mother's stress is to have a support team or individual with her during birth. Over the past two decades, studies representing over 12,700 women have demonstrated that positive support and nurturing touch creates more personally satisfactory birth experiences for women, decreases medical interventions, and speeds labor.[11,26-29] The compiled results of some of these studies can be seen in Table 8.1.

Because of the obvious benefits of this assistance during labor, more professional massage therapists specialized in the perinatal cycle are finding a niche in supporting women during labor, and hospitals are beginning to recognize a need for their services. Oregon Health Sciences University Hospital in Portland has collaborated at times with local massage schools, allowing student therapists to offer massage to women in the labor and postpartum units. Mid-Columbia Medical Center in The Dalles, Oregon, has hired massage therapists to provide services to all patients, including women in labor and postpartum. In recognition of the benefits of emotional and nurturing touch support, the Hearts and Hands Volunteer Doula Program was started at San Diego University Hospital in 1999. It offers doula training and free doula services to all women in labor. Part of their training includes hands-on touch, massage, and acupressure support.

TOUCH INCREASES PAIN THRESHOLD

Simply the *presence* of a supportive person has been found to help ease labor, but by adding the element of *touch,* the body's natural ability to relax is increased dramatically. Touch has been shown to stimulate the production of oxytocin—the hormone commonly associated with stimulating contractions. Current research on oxytocin indicates that the hormone also increases pain thresholds, has anti-anxiety effects, and increases social and emotional connectivity and compatibility in mammals, including humans.[6-8]

In evidence of this, women who participated in studies in Turkey, Taiwan, England, and the United States in which they received massage or acupressure during labor described their experience of labor pain as significantly less than those who received none.[6,13-15, 29] Those who received touch daily for 2 weeks prior to labor and then during labor were found to have an increased pain threshold, so that the same level of stimulation felt less painful than it did prior to massage, even though cortisol, a hormone produced in stressful situations, remained the same for those who received the touch as for those who did not.[6,15]

Table 8.1	Laboring With and Without Continuous Nurturing Support	
Birth Experience	**Without Support**	**With Support**
Duration of labor	9.4—19 hours	7.4—9 hours
% of labors resulting in natural birth	12%	55%
% of labors resulting in cesarean sections	18%	8%
% of labors resulting in use of epidurals	55%	8%
% of labors resulting in use of pitocin	13%—44%	2%—17%
% of labors resulting in use of forceps	26%	8%

Statistics for table gathered from analysis of studies described in Klaus MH, Kennell JH, Klaus, PH. Mothering the Mother. Reading, MA: Addison-Wesley, 1993.

As women labor, just as for those who run a marathon, the body will naturally release **endorphins** due to physical exertion and regular breathing.[31,32] Endorphins are hormones that decrease pain and give us sensations of relaxation, ease, relief, ecstasy, and pleasure. These molecules of sedating, pain-relieving hormones link to opiate receptor sites in the brain, the same receptor sites that cause pain medications such as morphine to be effective.

The presence of endorphins does not mean birth will not be painful or difficult, but a woman may find herself entering what some consider an altered, trance-like state and lose focused awareness of her surroundings. For some women, their experience may be somewhat euphoric, despite what may appear to onlookers as suffering. She may at times sound and look as though she is in agony, yet many women, when asked later, will say their contractions were a "bearable" pain or that they were in another dimension, without awareness of how they appeared to others. For many of these women, the element of *touch* helped them relax enough to enter this altered, endorphin-flowing state of mind.

Along with being a source of comfort and helping increase pain thresholds, touch also reduces transmission of painful sensations by affecting the amount and type of nerve impulse transmission to the central nervous system. The gate control theory explains how this happens.

APPLICATIONS OF THE GATE CONTROL THEORY FOR MASSAGE DURING BIRTH

In the 1960s, Dr. Ronald Melzack and Patrick Wall at McGill University developed theories about people's perceptions and experiences of pain, based on emotional as well as physical considerations. The essence of these theories is still widely accepted. One aspect of the Gate Control Theory, explained here very simply, is that there is only a certain amount of stimuli that the central nervous system (CNS) can handle at once. If too much stimulus tries to enter the CNS, its sensors will essentially short circuit—blocking or inhibiting some nerve transmissions. This is known as the "gate control" theory and may explain why victims of serious accidents initially feel less pain than one would expect.

Melzack and Wall also found that different nerve pathways were stimulated by different types of sensations and that the nerve stimuli moved at different speeds toward the CNS. Testing different stimuli, they found that sharp and sudden pain signals traveled on narrow and slower moving nerve fibers. Dull, lingering, and aching sensations traveled on larger and faster pathways. These faster moving nerve fibers could also be stimulated tactilely with vibration, scratching, and cold, as well as pressure. These sensations seemed to inhibit or bypass the painful sensations moving along the slower fibers. Because the faster moving impulses arrive more quickly to the gateway, they overwhelm and fill it, preventing or reducing the access of the slower moving painful stimulation. These fast-moving nerve pathways are stimulated by special tactile receptors, called **corpuscles**, found in different layers of the skin. Different types of corpuscles are sensitive to specific types of touch.

Meissner's corpuscles, which respond to pressure, are located in the superficial skin layers in hairless areas of the body—especially in the face, lips, fingertips, palms of hands, and soles of feet. They can be stimulated by squeezing hands or by acupressure or massage of the feet, rubbing the lips, kissing, or touching soft things with one's fingertips. Pacinian corpuscles are in the subcutaneous tissue and respond to deep pressure and vibration. Tension, pressure, or continuous deep touch, such as cuddling or being held firmly, stimulate the Merkel's disks, located in the superficial layers of skin, in both hairy and hairless areas of the body.

Melzack and Wall also studied the emotional and psychological elements of pain and found that pain increases with attention: the more one fights against or gives attention to pain, the stronger it becomes. *Thoughts* of pain breed fear and tension, raising blood pressure and increasing pain perception. The pain perception increases fear about the pain, and thus the cycle becomes self-perpetuating. Meanwhile, positive thinking and visualization has the effect of decreasing pain, thereby decreasing stress.[33]

A study comparing American and Dutch women with regard to their expectations of birth pain found that American women expected labor to be very painful and that they would need medications.[34] Few Dutch women expected this much pain. The results of their thoughts were manifested in the following results: 5 in 6 of the American women were medicated for pain in birth, whereas only 1 in 3 of the Dutch women used pain medications.

With these understandings in mind, the massage therapist can offer touch during labor that, at times, focuses on stimulation of the touch receptors that speed pleasurable sensations to the central nervous system, and can also include positive verbal encouragement to help diminish a woman's stress-producing thoughts.

PAIN DURING LABOR

While some women may experience birth as a highly sensually pleasurable experience,[35,36] many women

MASSAGE THERAPIST TIP — Labor Without Touch

*W*hile comforting touch soothes and relieves discomforts for many women during labor, there are also women who find that any sort of touch is a distraction. Their ability to tune inward and focus on contractions and the energies of birth is optimized by support from a distance, or with touch in-between contractions. Be prepared to moderate your assumptions about how to support or touch your client in labor, if you find that she does not want touch-contact for much of the labor. As labor progresses, her needs and desires may change, and touch may at some point again become desirable. Perhaps only one specific *area* will feel good to be touched, or only one *type* of touch will be comfortable. Explore, try different techniques, and respect the desire of your client as you find what works and what doesn't work for her in each moment.

describe it as painful. Pain is a subjective experience, but it is not uncommon for women to claim that birth was the most painful experience they have ever endured. Carol Burnett is often quoted for her description of childbirth: "Having a baby is like taking your bottom lip and pulling it up over your head."

Many women have developed fear about the sensations of giving birth and, in the United States, make plans well-ahead of labor, to have epidural anesthesia in hopes of numbing all birthing sensations. However, epidurals and pain medication are not always available when a woman wishes for it. A woman who hoped for an epidural may learn that she still must labor for some time before it can be initiated. Most women must experience the sensations of birth for a certain period of time, whether they choose pain medications or not. This is an important reason to provide your client with reassurance, respect, and grounding tactile stimulation. The use of complementary nonpharmacological modalities such as touch, warm water, and emotional encouragement can become vital tools for many women through at least part of their labor.

In American culture, pain is generally associated with something "wrong" that needs to be "fixed." But pain does not always indicate a problem, nor does it have to indicate suffering. Imagine pain as existing in three categories: functional, emotional, or dysfunctional. Dysfunctional pain indicates something *is* "wrong." For instance, in labor, the baby's position may be creating relentless painful pressure on a woman's sacrum or ribs. Or pain may be due to more serious problems or be representing danger, such as with a complicated or high-risk situation. An extreme example would be a woman with abdominal pain due to a uterine rupture or placental abruption—a life-threatening situation. In general, dysfunctional pain may need to be managed medically to minimize its sensations and/or dangers. Massage often cannot offer primary relief for this type of pain, and anxiety will frequently be a normal component of it.

Functional pain is a "normal" sensation during birth due to the normal processes of cervical dilation and opening. Each woman will relate to and interpret these sensations differently. With a history of stress

Traditional Birth Practices: Traditional Cultures and Pain

*H*ere is an Ainu birthing chant: "Wherever you may be, my little grandmothers, please help today a suffering woman!"[4(p88)]

For some traditional cultures, pain is considered a normal part of labor and therefore not something special to talk about. As compared with many industrialized cultures, these societies sometimes have a higher tolerance for and/or greater stoicism toward and less expression of pain. One source states that the Yucatan Mayans have seen pain as "the very hallmark of labor progress rather than as a symptom to be treated or an evil to escape."[38] Since pain is often related to fear, these cultures focus more on *alleviating that fear* than on the actual pain itself. Emotional support, encouragement, and reassurance, as well as reminding a laboring woman that this process is normal, that the pain is normal, and that there is nothing "wrong" with her body, are all part of relieving the tension that can surround a painful experience.

In Malaysian and Indonesian homebirths, midwives use massage throughout pregnancy and then rely on that touch as the primary tool to alleviate pain during labor.[39] In old Hawaiian culture, the healers or priests had ways of helping women relieve their discomfort by transferring the painful sensations to others in the community who might have been more "deserving of the pain" and who would suffer during the labor, while the woman experienced an easier birth.[40]

> ## MASSAGE THERAPIST TIP
> ### Reminders About Birth
>
> - A nurturing, protective environment is critical to healthy birthing. If a woman feels stress, fear, or anxiety, the catecholamine release will interfere with labor. Use massage as well as verbal and emotional support to help cultivate a safe environment.
> - Recognize that for some women, birth can be an experience of empowerment, a sexual experience, or a spiritual experience. For some, it may be an experience of unbearable pain and uncertainty. Your role is to support each woman and accept what is her experience; to listen, watch and feel how she meets her labor; and to offer nurturing touch to help her ground and focus on creating a calm and trusting relaxation response to contractions.
> - Remember to touch the hands and feet, which are especially responsive to pressure and vibration. This touch can decrease experiences of pain in labor. Simple holding and pressing techniques for the hands and feet can be taught to willing labor companions who want to share effective touch as part of their support.

Case Study 8.1
SUPPORTIVE TOUCH TO ENCOURAGE CONTRACTIONS

Katie's bag of waters broke at first light on Sunday, but contractions were few and far between, despite hours of brisk walking, herbal concoctions, and emotional processing. By Monday morning, her cervix was 5 cm dilated. She was exhausted, and the midwives were questioning whether the potentially large size of this baby was the cause of the slow progress. While the midwives conferred, they requested that the massage therapist rub her belly and help motivate contractions with the use of touch.

The massage therapist entered the bedroom where Katie labored with her husband Aaron. Katie was curled on her left side on the bed, breathing and trying to relax with contractions. Aaron sat at her feet, holding and rubbing them. Sitting behind Katie's back, the massage therapist warmed oil in her hands, and began to rub Katie's sacrum and belly simultaneously. She massaged in large circles around the belly, around the back, and down the thighs and buttocks. Understanding that the emotional, spiritual, and physical realms are intertwined and influential on one another, the therapist offered verbal encouragement for Katie and her husband.

Aaron continued holding and rubbing Katie's feet, stimulating reflexology areas and acupressure points that he had been shown, while the therapist continued a rhythmic touch, imagining energy moving through her hands to help Katie's cervix relax and open and applying finger pressure on the sacral foramen to stimulate opening and releasing in the pelvic area. She made long, firm strokes down Katie's back, drawing the energy down from her shoulders to her sacrum, uniting the strokes with full circles with her flat palm around Katie's belly and back.

During the massage, with Katie and Aaron's agreement, she encouraged them to visualize energy flowing through Katie's body like a river. Within 10 minutes of rubbing, Katie said she was feeling strong pressure, like she wanted to push. As she spoke, she began to grunt, uncontrollably pushing with the urge that moved through her body. "It hurts, it feels different . . ." she said.

The midwives were called up to the room to check Katie's cervix. It was completely dilated. Katie pushed for an hour to deliver her baby boy, who was much smaller than anticipated. The reason why became evident within the hour, when, as another contraction arrived, the head of an unexpected twin emerged!

Later, when asked about the effect of massage on her labor, Katie verbalized that because she trusted the massage therapist implicitly, she relaxed completely whenever she laid her hands on her body. She found herself able to attune to whatever part of the body the therapist touched, focusing there and letting go of tension in that particular area. She felt as if the therapist was pulling, pushing, or drawing energy through her body, clearing out tense areas, regenerating tired areas, and opening a movement of energy in areas of resistance. Under the hands of the therapist, Katie felt utterly supported, safe, and cared for, and felt that it significantly increased her endurance and fortitude for such a long labor.

and anxiety related to psychological trauma or unpleasant memories, the functional pain can become more intense and more difficult to manage, as it becomes complicated by *emotional* pain. Unprocessed emotions tend to intensify a woman's relation to pain and decrease her pain threshold.[37] Nurturing touch can be a potent form of support to help mediate both functional and emotional pain.

Women who do not think of labor as painful may describe contractions as "squeezes" or "sensations." Contractions, they say, feel like a tightening that can *become* painful, although they note that it was generally their *fear* that increased the sensations of pain. They also describe that with massage, emotional support, and the maintenance of a safe and nurturing environment, their birth was a moment-to-moment journey—each moment unique, each moment a chance to breathe, to feel the waves of power moving through them, to open again and again into the energy spiraling through their body.

However a woman experiences her birth, touch can often be integral to improving her response to it. Even if you are not invited to your client's birth, you can have an influence on the ease with which she meets her labor, by sharing with her partner or support companions, if they desire, simple touch techniques that they can use during labor. Having a nurturing touch-supporter through labor can help the mother-to-be create the type of birth she would most like to have.

CHAPTER SUMMARY

For many women, the essential ingredients for a safe and satisfying birth include a sense of empowerment and success in coping with or transcending the experience, in addition to having solid, positive encouragement from a support companion. The massage practitioner can enhance these ingredients by adding knowledgeable, caring touch which can decrease pain, increase relaxation, speed labor, and reduce medical interventions. Serving women in labor, witnessing a baby's birth, and positively influencing a mother's responsiveness to her infant are unique and powerful opportunities. Being invited to serve in this capacity indicates that you have skill in helping a woman feel at ease. Keep in mind that your presence and loving touch may have a deeper impact on your client than you even realize, as your presence will forever be a part of her and her child's birth story.

CHAPTER REVIEW QUESTIONS

1. Explore and discuss how a massage therapist might offer her or his services to women in labor

and options for charging for your services. Some choose to do an hourly rate with a limit to the number of hours. Others choose a flat rate for an entire birth, and others work for free. What might be appropriate for you within your community?

2. Name three effects of oxytocin on a woman during labor.
3. Name five benefits of touch during labor.
4. Describe three ways that touch can influence the progress of labor.
5. Explain how nurturing touch might decrease the need for pain medications or pitocin induction or augmentation.
6. Describe how the birth and environment, as well as thoughts, have the power to affect the progress of labor.
7. Describe why a woman who feels unsafe and unsupported in her birth environment may have difficulties or lack progress in her labor.
8. Discuss three measures you might take to help relax a woman who is developing tension in response to contraction sensations and expresses fear about "making it" through labor.
9. Describe the roles of oxytocin, endorphins, and cortisol in the birth process and their relation to touch.
10. Explain the relevance of the Gate Control Theory to labor. How can the massage therapist use this information?

REFERENCES

1. Gaskin IM. Midwifery and women's power. Woman of Power. Summer 1989;28(14):27–29.
2. J Chawla. Rites of Passage. Life Positive: Your Complete Guide to Holistic Living. July 1997. Last accessed online July 2007 at: http://www.lifepositive.com/spirit/death/deathrites.asp.
3. Mira S. In: Mira S, ed. Her Healing Heritage: Local Beliefs and Practices Concerning the Health of Women and Children: A Multi-State Study In India. Compiled by Vd. Mita Bajpai. India: Chetna Publication, 1996; March (25):216.
4. Dunham C. Mamatoto: A Celebration of Birth. New York: Penguin Books, 1991.
5. Jackson D. With Child: Wisdom and Traditions for Pregnancy, Birth and Motherhood. San Francisco: Chronicle Books, 1999.
6. Lund I, Yu L-C, Uvnas-Moberg K, et al. Repeated massage-like stimulation induces long-term effects on nociception: contribution of oxytocinergic mechanisms. Eur J Neurosci 2002;16(2):330–338.
7. Uvnas-Moberg K, Petersson M. [Oxytocin, a mediator of anti-stress, well-being, social interaction, growth and healing] [Article in German] Z Psychosom Med Psychother 2005;51(1):57–80.

8. Uvnäs-Moberg K. Oxytocin may mediate the benefits of positive social interaction and emotions. Psychoneuroendocrinology 1998;23(8):819–835.

9. Field T, Hernandez-Reif M, Diego M, et al. Cortisol decreases and serotonin and dopamine increase following massage therapy. J Neurosci 2005;115(10): 1397–1413.

10. Scott KD, Klaus PH, Klaus MH. The obstetrical and postpartum benefits of continuous support during childbirth. J Womens Health Gend Based Med 1999;8(10):1257–1264.

11. Hodnett ED, Gates S, Hofmeyr GJ, Sakala C. Continuous support for women during childbirth. Cochrane Database Syst Rev 2003;3:CD003766. DOI: 10.1002/14651858.CD003766.pub2.

12. Field T, Hernandez-Reif M, Taylor S, et al. Labor pain is reduced by massage therapy. J Psychosom Obstet Gynaecol 1997;18(4):286–291.

13. Yildirim G, Sahin NH. The effect of breathing and skin stimulation techniques on labour pain perception of Turkish women. Pain Res Manag 2004;9(4):181–182.

14. Chang MY, Wang SY, Chen CH. Effects of massage on pain and anxiety during labour: a randomized controlled trial in Taiwan. J Adv Nurs 2002;38(1):68–73.

15. Nabb MT, Kimber L, Haines A, et al. Does regular massage from late pregnancy to birth decrease maternal pain perception during labour and birth?—A feasibility study to investigate a programme of massage, controlled breathing and visualization, from 36 weeks of pregnancy until birth. Complement Ther Clin Pract 2006;12(3):222–231.

16. Guthrie RA, Martin RH. Effect of pressure applied to the upper thoracic (placebo) versus lumbar areas (osteopathic manipulative treatment) for inhibition of lumbar myalgia during labor. J Am Osteopath Assoc 1982; 82(4):247–251.

17. Simkin P, Ancheta R. The Labor Progress Handbook. Malden, MA: Blackwell Publishing, 2000.

18. Leeman L, Fontaine P, King V, et al. The nature and management of labor pain: part i. nonpharmacologic pain relief. Am Fam Physician 2003;68(6):1109–1112.

19. Sommer P. Obstetrical patients' anxiety during transition of labor and the nursing intervention of touch [doctoral dissertation]. Dallas: Texas Women's University, 1979.

20. Klaus MH, Kennell JH, Klaus PH. Mothering the Mother. Reading, MA: Addison-Wesley, 1993.

21. Hofmeyr GJ, Nikodem VC, Wolman WL. Companionship to modify the clinical birth environment: effects on progress and perceptions of labour and breast feeding. Br J Obstet Gynaecol 1991;98:756–764.

22. Wolman WL. Social support during childbirth: psychological and physiological outcomes. Masters' thesis. University of Witwatersrand, Johannesburg; 1991.

23. Lowe N. The nature of labor pain. Am J Obstet Gynecol 2002;186(Suppl 5):S16–24.

24. Lundberg U. Catecholamines and Environmental Stress. Stockholm University Department of Psychology for the Allostatic Load notebook. John D and Catherine T. MacArthur Research Network on Socioeconomic Status and Health. Last revised September, 2003. Last accessed online July 2007 at http://www.macses.ucsf.edu/Research/Allostatic/notebook/catecholamine.html#Health.

25. McRee LD, Noble S, Pasvogel A. Using massage and music therapy to improve postoperative outcomes. AORN J 2003;78(3):433–442, 445–447.

26. Kennell J, Klaus M, McGrath S, Robertson S, Hinkley C. Continuous emotional support during labor in a US hospital. A randomized controlled trial. JAMA 1991;265(17):2197–2201.

27. Campero L, Garcia C, Diaz C, et al. Alone, I wouldn't have known what to do: a qualitative study on social support during labor and delivery in Mexico. Soc Sci Med 1998;47(3):395–403.

28. Rosen P. Supporting women in labor: analysis of different types of caregivers. J Midwifery Womens Health 2004;49(1):24–31.

29. Madi B. Effects of female relative support in labor: a randomized controlled trial. Birth 1999; 26 4–8.

30. Chung UL, Hung LC, Kuo SC, Huang CL. Effects of LI4 and BL 67 acupressure on labor pain and uterine contractions in the first stage of labor. J Nurs Res 2003;11(4):251–260.

31. Arsenijević L, Kojiç Z, Popoviç N. [Plasma levels of cortisol and opioid peptide beta-endorphin during spontaneous vaginal delivery] Srp Arh Celok Lek 2006;134 (3-4):95–99.

32. Fettes I, Fox J, Kuzniak S, et al. Plasma levels of immunoreactive beta-endorphin and adrenocorticotropic hormone during labor and delivery. Obstet Gynecol 1984;64(3):359–362.

33. Adams B, Bromley B. Psychology for Health Care: key terms and concepts. New York: Macmillan Press, 1998.

34. Senden IP, van du Wetering MD, Eskes TK, et al. Labor pain: a comparison of parturients in a Dutch and an American teaching hospital. Obstet Gynecol 1988;71(4):541–544.

35. Harper B. Gentle Birth Choices. Rochester, VT: Healing Arts Press, 1994.

36. Tonetti-Vladimirova E. Birth as We Know It: The Transformative Power of Birth [DVD]. 2006.

37. Simkin P, Klaus P. When Survivors Give Birth: Understanding and Healing The Effects of Early Sexual Abuse on Childbearing Women. Seattle: Classic Day Publishing, 2004.

38. Lieberman AB. Easing Labor Pain. Boston: Harvard Common Press, 1992:33.

39. Kanagaratnam T. Coconut Belly Rubs: Traditional Midwifery Care in Malaysia and Indonesia. Int Midwife1995;1(3).

40. Pukui MK. Hawaiian beliefs and customs during birth, infancy, and childhood. In: Meltzer D, ed. Birth: an anthology of ancient texts, songs, prayers, and stories. New York: North Point Press, 1981]:132 [originally from Occasional papers of the Bernice P. Bishop Museum. Vol 16, No 17 (March 20, 1942). Honolulu: Bishop Museum Press].

CHAPTER 9

MASSAGE FOR THE STAGES OF LABOR

LEARNING OBJECTIVES

After reading this chapter, you should be able to:

- Identify the different stages and phases of labor, the mother's experience, and general bodywork techniques and comfort measures appropriate for each stage and phase.

- List topics that should be clarified with a client before joining her as a support person in labor, and explain why this is important.

- Describe specific ways to help establish a comfortable and nurturing birth environment.

- Describe methods of incorporating breathing and visualizations into a birth.

- Describe 5 different positions that may be comfortable for a client during labor. Describe the types of bodywork techniques that can be helpful in those positions.

- Identify ways the massage therapist can care for her or his body and reduce the risk of injury during a woman's labor.

*I*f you are invited to support and massage a woman through her labor, it will be useful to understand what you might expect regarding the physical and emotional changes occurring during the actual process of birth. This chapter will review the basics of what occurs at the end of pregnancy and the beginning of labor, the various stages of birth, and comfort measures to help you support your client.

OVERVIEW OF LABOR

Labor is a nonlinear journey that is unique to each woman and child who undergoes it. It is a mix of hormones that physically induce uterine contractions in labor, but also suppress the rational mind, inviting the mother into altered levels of consciousness where a natural process of opening and releasing can occur. As discussed in the previous chapter, this usually occurs best when a mother is well supported in a safe, nurturing environment. Oxytocin, prolactin, endorphins, and catecholamines all play a role in the labor dance. Below is a simplified overview of labor, including its beginnings and its three primary phases.

Length of Pregnancy

A normal gestation is between 38 and 42 weeks. At this point a fetus' lungs have fully matured and the baby will be strong enough to breathe well at birth. If born before 37 weeks, a baby is considered premature, and depending on its gestational age, could have difficulty adapting to life outside the womb. After 42 weeks' gestation, the baby in utero will be very mature and growing larger. The placenta begins to degrade, and gradually the amniotic fluid decreases, but the baby is usually born before serious problems develop.

Due Date

Your client may tell you her **due date**, also known as the EDC, or "expected date of confinement." This date is an *average* based on a woman's last known menstrual period. The name is a relic of days when women were kept separated from family or community during birth. Only 10% of women actually deliver on this date, with a majority delivering within 2 weeks on either side of the EDC.[1] However, many women become attached to the actual *day* they are told, and when the due date is passed, anxiety may develop about whether labor is ever going to begin. This anxiety and anticipation could actually delay the onset of labor. Massage can alleviate some of this anxiety and remind a mother of the need for patience and trust.

When Labor Begins

For a baby to be born, the maternal uterine **cervix**—or bottom neck of the uterus—must **dilate,** opening to its maximum capacity, measured as 10 centimeters (cm). The cervix must also **efface**—thinning or shortening—from its normal 3 to 5 cm length to being as thin as a flannel sheet. The rhythmic uterine contractions of labor have the express purpose of opening the cervix and pushing the baby out. It is not clear what initiates labor, but current theories indicate that chemicals from the baby's adrenal glands stimulate a release of maternal birth-inducing hormones.[2,3]

As the uterus contracts, the upper fibers of the **uterine fundus** (the top of the uterus) pull up the lower fibers, shortening the uterus. In general, when uterine contractions are lasting 60 to 90 seconds from the start to the end of one contraction, have been occurring consistently every 2 to 3 minutes for at least 2 hours (contraction frequency is measured from the beginning of one contraction to the beginning of the next), and are also causing cervical changes, a woman is considered to be in active **labor**. In the process of labor, the uterus gradually contracts into itself, while pushing down so that the baby's head is pressing against the cervix, helping it to dilate.

If you put a hand on top of a woman's belly during a strong contraction, you may feel it getting hard and then softening again as the contraction subsides. The woman may feel the contraction as pressure in her cervix, a tightening in her lower belly, or as a pain in her low back, sacrum, or legs. Sometimes it will radiate around from her belly to her back or settle into her hips.

Length of Labor

How long labor lasts is variable. The child influences the progress and outcome of the birth by its position in utero. The mother can influence it due to her emotional and physical states, as well as her birth history. Typically, first-time mothers or those with many years between children have longer labors (12 to 30 hours), whereas those having their third or more child often have relatively fast labors (2 to 8 hours). Yet one mother having her third child could struggle with immense discomfort and exhaustion for 16 hours, while another has a first birth that lasts for 2 hours, with little pain. No two women have the same experience, and no two births are the same even for the same woman!

Descent and Position of the Baby

Usually, before birth, the baby descends from higher in the mother's abdomen into the pelvis. At some point before or during labor, its head will normally become **engaged**, with the widest diameter of its head settling down behind the mother's pubic bone, readying for birth. When this occurs the mother will feel a sense of relief as the pressure against her diaphragm is decreased and she can breathe more easily. This is known as lightening. You might notice a distinct change in how she is carrying the baby if you see her several times at the end of pregnancy.

To help facilitate the baby's passage, not only do the maternal pelvic joints loosen so as to open wider, but the baby's skull bones are movable so that they can mold together to fit better through the pelvis. Vaginally-born babies often have a somewhat cock-eyed or conical shaped head from this molding. This will resolve over the first few days after birth. Craniosacral bodywork is quite beneficial in realigning the skull bones of a newborn.

By the time labor begins, the majority of babies will be in the vertex or head-down presentation. Optimally, they will also be facing toward the mother's sacrum with the occiput at the mother's anterior side (Figure 9.1A). A vertex baby is sometimes positioned **posterior**, with its occiput aimed toward its mother's sacrum and its face looking toward the mother's abdomen (Figure 9.1B). This posterior position is often associated with unrelenting pain in the low back and sacrum for some women, known as **back labor**. There are a number of bodywork techniques that can significantly improve back labor discomfort or eradicate it all together, at least temporarily. Other techniques might help the baby to rotate anteriorly, allowing for an easier delivery and less painful labor.

Babies sometimes position themselves in other ways. Breech presentation, with the head up and bottom down, is one of the most common malpresentation (Figure 9.1C). Attempts may be made with manual external manipulations to make the baby move to vertex, as there are increased risks with breech position during a vaginal birth. Some babies, on rare occasions, are positioned sideways, or in a

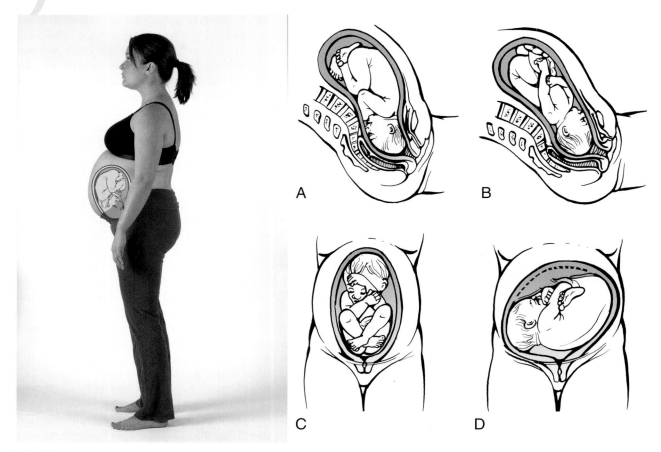

FIGURE 9.1   Presentations of the baby.

(A) Vertex (Anterior): the most common position for the baby to be in and the easiest for a vaginal delivery. The baby's head is down, with the occiput facing the mother's anterior. (B) Vertex (Posterior): the baby will be head down, but with the occiput toward the mother's sacrum or posterior torso. This can lead to slower, more difficult, and more painful births. (C) Breech: the most common malpresentation, with the buttocks down instead of the head down. (D) Transverse lie: the baby is sometimes positioned with its spine sideways to the mother's spine. This type of presentation does not allow for a vaginal birth.

transverse lie, to the pelvic opening (Figure 9.1D). These babies, if not able to be moved to vertex, must be born via cesarean section.

Signs of Impending Labor

Some clues indicating that labor is impending may include the baby dropping into the pelvis, and increasing frequency or awareness of Braxton-Hicks—or "practice" contractions. These tightenings of the uterine muscle do not cause cervical dilation, but are considered to be a warm-up for labor. Sometime before labor commences (or sometimes in the midst of labor), a woman may notice the loss of her **mucous plug**—thick mucous, sometimes streaked with old blood, that has prevented bacteria from entering the uterus. There may also be some **bloody**

show—a brownish, reddish discharge as the cervix begins to dilate. These signs could happen anytime in the weeks prior to labor as well as up to the day of labor.

Amniotic Fluid

Also called the bag of waters, the **amniotic sac** is a membranous container inside the uterus that holds the baby and amniotic fluid safely intact. The membranes must rupture at some point for the baby to be delivered, though on rare occasions, a baby is born still inside the sac. Normally, the sac breaks spontaneously during, or sometimes before, labor. Often a doctor will intentionally break it during labor, thinking it may speed labor and also to be able to assess the quality of the amniotic fluid.

Traditional Birth Practices:
Recognizing Labor

*E*very culture has its clues for recognizing impending labor. We pay attention to the due date, lightening, or the loss of the mucous plug. Malaysians recognize labor as commencing when the feet or big toe is cold. They claim that the heat of the body is moving away from the extremities and being directed toward the womb.[4]

Ancient Hawaiians determined the time of impending labor by observing the linea negra, or "alawela," developing on the midabdomen. Labor was known to be imminent when a line commencing from the top of the belly met the one commencing from the pubic area.[5]

If the bag of water should spontaneously break before labor, contractions are usually not far behind. Normally the amniotic fluid is clear with either a slightly sweet odor or none perceptible. Sometimes the baby has had a bowel movement, known as **meconium,** inside the uterus, making the fluid a greenish color. If this has occurred, it is assumed the baby was or may be stressed in some way in utero, and the baby's heart rate will be watched more closely through labor.

Phases of Labor

The journey of birth can take anywhere from 1 hour to days, depending on how many babies a mother has had previously, how big this fetus is, how psychologically and physically ready a mother is for the birthing, and how effective the contractions are. If you are to attend a birth and expect to be present from beginning to end and into early postpartum period, make time to be available for several hours to several days.

Labor is often described as having several phases and stages. The **first stage of labor** involves the dilation of the cervix and includes several phases. **Prelabor** is the very earliest phase in the first stage of labor. In this phase, a mother may be having contractions, but they are gentle, irregular, and having little effect on dilating her cervix.

When the cervix does finally begin to dilate, it is considered to be the phase of **early labor**. As the contractions grow closer together and more intensive, **active labor** is said to be underway. The final phase of

the first stage is **transition**, when the last of cervical dilation is occurring and the mother is preparing for the **second stage of labor**: pushing. After birth, the delivery of the placenta is considered the **third stage of labor**. These phases and stages are discussed in more detail later in this chapter.

ROLE OF THE MASSAGE THERAPIST DURING BIRTH

When giving birth, a woman may look into the face of both life and of death. Nothing is more real than each moment that she feels the force of life bearing down through her pelvis and reaching its way through her body. She may wonder at times if she can survive such a force, which seemingly pushes her with its own will, beyond what she has known before. She herself is being born in a new way, to a new self as she births her child.

As a massage therapist participating in birth, your role is to be supportive, to offer methods for a woman (or her birth companions) to relax and feel refreshed, and to help her remember, in the toughest moments, why she is laboring. Sometimes your role is to simply watch and wait for a time when your services are desired or appropriate.

 CAUTION: You should not perform any techniques for inducing or speeding up labor unless you have clearance for this from the doctor (if in a clinical setting), the midwife, or the doula responsible.

There is no special massage routine for labor, since every birth is different. If you understand the stages of labor and possibilities of what you might encounter and have some experience with comfort measures that may help her through the particular stages, you will be better prepared to meet the needs of women in varying situations. You must be flexible—willing to follow the laboring woman from place to place if she is walking, from one position to another as her needs change, and through all emotions, from outbursts of frustration to inward spaces of peace and meditative calm. You will become embedded in the story of her birth, and in some ways, the journey will change who you are, as it is rare to share in the experience of birth and not be profoundly affected by its power.

There are many methods to deal with the intensities of labor. Epidurals, medications, TENS (transcutaneous electrical nerve stimulator) units, and sometimes baths and showers are tools used in hospitals.

Case Study 9.1:
A CASE OF RUPTURED AMNIOTIC SAC DURING MASSAGE

Jenna was 39 weeks pregnant with her first baby when she came to Carol for a massage. She had been coming each month during her low-risk pregnancy, enjoying how massage helped relieve her backaches. Her pregnancy was still progressing normally, but as she moved to change positions from one side to the other, she felt a sudden gush of water running down her legs. Carol noticed the immediate pooling of water over the massage table and down to the floor, and both of them were surprised and nervous. Obviously, Jenna's bag of water had just broken. Carol collected towels to soak up the fluids, while Jenna called her PCP. The clinic nurse asked her several questions: Is there any sign of an umbilical cord? (no) Is the fluid clear? (yes) Have contractions started? (no) Has she felt the baby moving? (yes). The nurse told Jenna to go to the hospital where she planned to labor to confirm that the baby was fine and to assess for contractions. She said that Jenna did not need emergency transport.

Carol later discussed the situation with another skilled pregnancy massage therapist and decided on several new protocols for working with her pregnant clients:

1. Carol decided to put a waterproof protective cover on her massage table under her sheets. While she realized it is a rare occurrence for a client's bag of waters to break during a massage, it is an unpredictable one, and since she regularly saw pregnant clients, she felt better having extra table protection just in case it should happen again. Additionally, she ensured that she had a few emergency menstrual pads stocked in the office bathroom, recognizing that in a situation such as this, as well as during the postpartum period, women may be leaking fluids vaginally and may be in need of an absorbent pad.

2. The situation made her aware that at any time during pregnancy and postpartum, linens and covers may get wet from leaking body fluids, such as amniotic fluid, breast milk, or vaginal secretions. She ensured that she had rubber gloves available in case they were needed for changing soiled sheets, as a universal precaution against skin contact with clients' body fluids.

3. She learned from the client's nurse more about amniotic fluid: A client should always call her prenatal care provider when her bag of water breaks. As long as the fluid is clear and she is not having an urge to push, it is not an emergency situation, unless she is less than 37 weeks' gestation. Other concerning situations are the appearance of green meconium-stained fluid, which would indicate that baby had a bowel movement and could be stressed. Immediate emergency transport is necessary for red or port wine-colored fluid or if part of the umbilical cord appears with the leaking amniotic fluid.

Breathing, relaxation, and visualization are tools taught by childbirth educators. Different types of massage and touch, including acupressure, reflexology, hydrotherapy, Reiki, and aromatherapy may be used by bodyworkers. Each situation demands accessing something slightly different to help each woman find her strength and focus to make it through labor. You will not know ahead of time which method will work for which woman, though you may have some ideas.

Your ability to support a woman in labor can be strengthened by understanding some of the issues that may be entertaining her psyche as she approaches birth. Before you join a woman at the time of birth, meet with her and the other supporters if possible, to establish a common understanding about expectations. Clarifications *before* labor begins will help alleviate confusion and uncertainty during the birth, when she may be too distracted to talk about details.

To help create the environment she envisions for her labor, explore her ideas about birth, her desires regarding emotional and physical support, and clarify your specific role. The questions that follow may help you with this discussion:

- What is the mother's ideal vision of her birth?
- What type of touch, words, or actions make her feel supported?
- Who does she want as her primary caregivers and supporters?
- Does she want the massage therapist there for just a few hours or for the entire labor and for the actual birth?

Respecting the Role of the Client's Partner

*A*void interfering with the natural bonding that can occur between partners during this important episode in their lives. It is a rite of passage for the partner or father as well as for the mother and child. Teach and encourage the partner, if necessary, to also touch the woman, unless she has specified desires for the massage therapist to be the primary touch support. See Case Study 9.2 regarding this issue. Note that although the story in this case study is about a woman's two friends who attend the birth, the same role and boundary issues need to be addressed with a professional massage therapist.

- What arrangement for payment (if any) will be made if the therapist is to be there for the entire birth of an unknown duration?
- If during the labor, the mother wants the therapist or another person to leave, how and with whom will it be easy for her to share that request?
- What is the best way for the massage therapist to support the mother and her partner or team, during labor? For example, the client may want the massage therapist to support and teach the partner while the partner mostly massages the mother.

Reminders for Supporting Birth

Keep in mind some essential tips that establish a comforting, nurturing environment for all involved in the birth.

- *Share with the Support Team*: In addition to doing massage at a birth, take the time to offer to teach the support team touch techniques that are useful during labor. Share basics of touch that will not overwhelm a lay person. For instance, open palms and smoothing stokes, moving consistently in one direction, are more effective and soothing than erratic strokes. Pick some tools that you have found to be the most consistently helpful during births and share a few of the best with the support team.
- *Birth Environment*: As a massage therapist, your role is to support whatever environment the mother desires for her birth. While it is

generally found that low lighting and relative quiet will help women relax more easily, some personalities may choose environments with bright lights and a variety of friends or family to be present. If you are noticing that your client is having a difficult time relaxing in the environment that has developed around her, you might ask whether she would like you to do some focused bodywork in a quiet space to help her relax. During this time, she may become aware of changes she can ask for to make her environment more supportive for relaxation. As discussed in Chapter 8, a woman who cannot relax in her environment will labor less efficiently and effectively; hence, cultivating and maintaining a relaxing "womb room," space is critical.

- *Visualization*: Remember to encourage the client to visualize images she finds empowering if this method is effective in helping her relax or stay grounded.
- *Things Change*: Even if you have practiced various massage techniques before labor, *during* labor, a woman may not want to be touched at all or may need an entirely different type of touch than you have used during pregnancy. Be open and creative. Do not take it personally if she does not want to be touched. For some women, touch may become too distracting.
- *Consistent Strokes and Pressure*: When massaging, move the energy all the way to the end of each extremity, working with gravity and the direction of baby's descent with long, slow, firm and consistent strokes. Help her stay focused with your touch by using deliberate strokes. Energy often collects in the abdominal-pelvic region, the jaw, shoulders, and inner thighs. Help this energy to move down and out of the body; keep it flowing like a river. Maintain skin contact as much as possible, rather than picking up your hands at the end of every stroke.
- *Practice Ahead:* If you have not worked with this client before, offer to massage her a couple weeks before labor is expected, if possible. This will accustom you and your client to working together so that during labor there is already a familiarity between you and she knows that she can trust you with your touch. She may also develop an automatic relaxation response when you are near, if she is comfortable with how you have touched her before.
- *Remember Calm*: A woman in labor absorbs subtle energies like a sponge. Each individual

Case Study 9.2:
A LACK OF PRE-BIRTH COMMUNICATION

Meredith planned to birth her twins at home. Her friends, Sue and Erin, planned to arrive at Meredith's home across the country two weeks ahead of the due date to connect with Meredith and clarify her needs during their stay. Erin was a massage therapist and new labor and delivery nurse who had been to a number of births. This was the first birth for Meredith and Sue, but not for Meredith's husband, Roy, who had two other children. Erin and Sue did not know Roy well nor feel connected with him, but they hoped relations would become more comfortable once they had a chance to visit and talk before labor.

That chance never came; Meredith's labor began earlier than expected. Sue and Erin arrived just after Meredith had been transferred to the hospital due to some unexpected complications with the twins. When the women arrived, Sue set herself up at Meredith's bedside, breathing with, massaging, and encouraging her. Erin assumed what she believed to be "her position" at the other side of the bed and began to massage Meredith's hand and shoulder. Variations of this support continued for 20 hours while Roy sat quietly in a corner. It was the three friends who talked, made decisions, and finally agreed to a cesarean section after it was clear labor was not progressing.

Throughout the labor, Sue and Erin felt annoyed with Roy, who seemed nervous and was not getting involved as a coach, as they thought he should. Yet they also did not encourage or invite him to join in, ask if he wanted time alone with Meredith, or offer to show him ways they thought he could be supportive. Instead, they judged him for his lack of participation, while increasing their own supportive efforts. They never knew if perhaps this was the role Meredith had asked of him—to be present, but not in Meredith's face—yet still they felt it was his duty to offer her more obvious support.

When the four of them reviewed the birth together later, Erin and Sue came to understand that, while Meredith had indeed *wanted* Roy to be more of a support, he had felt overwhelmed by the friends who had easily stepped into the role of doula and massage therapist for Meredith. They had not made space for Roy, and he was intimidated and uneasy about his role in the midst of women who acted as though they "knew exactly what they were doing."

Erin later became a doula specialized in massage during labor. Upon reflection of this earlier labor, she realized her opinions and judgments had interfered with Meredith and Roy's ability to connect during the birth of their first children. She determined to make it a priority as a doula to establish the following protocol: If she could not meet together with a client and her labor supporters one month or so prior to the due date (and a bit earlier than that for twins, who often come early), she would set up a phone conference. During that conference, she would clarify needs and boundaries, and would explore the hopes and expectations of both the mother and partner with regards to Erin as the massage therapist/doula, as well as expectations for the partner or other birth companions who might be present. She found this to be a very helpful practice that ensured she was the kind of support team member her clients hoped for.

---

energy in her environment can benefit or impede the progress of her birthing. If you, as a support person, have fears or anxiety during a birth, it could have a negative impact on the laboring woman. Enter the birth room with clarity and grounding, and if, during the birth, you notice that you are having difficulty staying present, leave the room, take a break, practice your own methods of relaxation, and return when clear.

• *Remember Reassurance*: Regular positive, convincing, verbal encouragement can help a woman relax with each contraction. When possible, maintain eye contact with your client while touching during active labor contractions. Focus on what is working and how well she is doing.

• *Remember Breath*: Pay attention to your breath and to your client's breathing patterns. Help her to maintain relaxed or focused breathing throughout labor. Breath-holding increases anxiety and tension.

• *Remember Self-Renewal*: Nurture yourself regularly. Hours spent bending over a bed or applying counterpressure to a sacrum can leave you with a strained back and make you ineffectual as a continuing support. Check in with yourself every hour. Do you need food or drink? Do you need to raise the bed up so you are not hunched over?

- *Remember Relaxation*: Note where your client may be holding tension. Where is she clenching, resisting, or feeling pain? Touch those specific areas, as well as the areas that mirror this original tension at the opposite side of the body. For instance, when the cervical area is tight, massage to the feet or sacrum may help relax the neck. When the jaw or throat is tight, the pelvic area or abdomen may also be constricted and need attention. Massage to the hands can help relax the shoulders.
- *Remember Intuition*: If images or thoughts arise in your mind about techniques, or activities that might offer safety, relaxation, and pain relief for the mother, explore them. Birth is an intuitive experience and supporting birth is a creative, variable, and fluid job. If a situation arises where you simply have no idea how to help, consider the options listed in Box 9.1.

PRECAUTIONS AND CONTRAINDICATIONS FOR MASSAGE DURING LABOR

For the safety and comfort of your client during labor and birth, it is important to remember a few precautions and contraindications, discussed below.

Precautions

Here are two primary precautions for the massage therapist to keep in mind during labor. These are addressed below.

Watch the Client, Not the Monitor

In the hospital, the condition of the baby and the frequency of a mother's contractions are monitored electronically. Watching the fetal heart rate and uterine contraction monitor can become a focal point for a woman and those supporting her. There have been instances when a support person has begun to encourage the woman to breathe and relax because she or he saw a contraction being recorded by the

---

BOX 9.1 | Support Tools for Labor

Below is a reminder list of general actions you can take to support a laboring client when you are not sure what else to do.

- Encourage slow abdominal breathing into the abdomen
- Apply cold or warm packs to the sacrum or neck
- Help her change positions
- Take a break
- Change the music in the room
- Hold her hand
- Remind her of why she is doing this
- Offer her a cool drink
- Knead her buttocks or apply pressure to her sacrum
- Stroke down her thighs to her feet
- Massage her hands and feet
- Apply warm cloths to her perineum
- Hold onto her toes
- Make long, firm strokes down her whole body
- Give other supporters a shoulder rub

The birthing toolbag: Be prepared for a birth with special massage tools and self-care items. Put these in your car a few weeks before the expected birth so that you do not forget them! Support tools might include the following:

- Massage tools: rollers, rocks, tennis balls, or a rolling pin (for rolling over fleshy areas to give your hands a break).
- Hairbrush: brushing hair can be an easy distracting sensate experience for a mother. You can also use the brush against her skin if that feels good to her.
- Acupressure and reflexology charts, if needed for reminders.
- Massage lotion/oil.
- Hydrotherapy tools: ice packs, hot water bottle, bags for ice, small towel.
- Essential oils and an aromatherapy diffuser.
- Music and a CD player.
- Snacks.
- Visualization ideas to help the mother focus during contractions.
- Self-care items such as toothbrush, snacks, and water and other hydration, hair ties, medications, glasses, clean clothes.

monitor, and yet it was not something that the woman was actually feeling. On the other hand, a woman may be feeling a great deal that is not recorded by the monitor, and supporters have nearly ignored her because they could not see on the monitor what she was reacting to. Watch and listen to the birthing woman. Let her be your focus and avoid the seduction of constant monitor watching!

Epidurals

Epidural anesthesia—the use of numbing medication placed in the epidural space of the lower spine—is often chosen in American hospitals to numb the sensation of contractions. Massage does not have to stop just because a woman has an epidural. Now is a good time to massage the neck, shoulders, jaw, back, arms, and hands.

Contraindications

There are no reasons why absolutely all touch would be contraindicated in labor. At the very minimum,

---

DISPELLING MYTHS:

Epidurals Alleviate the Need for Nurturing Touch

Many women choose to receive an epidural as a means of managing their discomfort. Once it has become effective and the woman is comfortable, it is not uncommon for everyone in the room to breathe a sigh of relief, and step back into a more relaxed posture. The continuous and focused support that may have been offered while the woman was feeling her contractions, no longer seems necessary. This distancing from the demands of contractions can lead to what some midwives call, "epidural abandonment." Suddenly leaving a laboring woman without the close emotional and physical contact she had just moments ago can lead to an emotional let-down that may not be recognized immediately, but which may later lead to feelings of disappointment. She is still in labor, but only the electronic monitors and the baby can tell. The adrenaline and endorphins that powered her experience earlier, diminish. While a woman is numb from the waist down with an epidural, there is no reason that massage cannot or should not continue on other parts of her body. In fact, at this point, it may still be quite valuable for helping the mother recover from the stresses she has just endured with the first part of her labor. Focus on her head, face, shoulders, arms and upper back.

---

there is always room for holding a hand or for energy work such as indicated under Type II bodywork in Chapter 4. Even this simple contact can have a major impact on the well-being of a birthing woman by significantly reducing anxiety. There are a few times when certain *types* of touch or massage to certain *areas* may be contraindicated. In addition to these listed below, the standard massage precautions listed in Table 4.1 also apply during labor.

1. *Abdominal massage is contraindicated for the following:*
   - If there is a known dangerous condition or strong potential for one with the baby or placenta and the PCP determines that abdominal massage is inappropriate
   - If the mother refuses it or if it makes her more uncomfortable
   - If it interferes with external fetal monitoring that is particularly critical at that time

Note: If there are known problems with the placenta or baby, nonstimulating, relaxing massage to *other* parts of the body may be very helpful to ease a mother's anxiety. If there are any concerns for the safety of the mother or baby, obtain permission from the prenatal care provider before continuing with massage.

2. *General Type I massage is contraindicated for the following:*
   - If the mother refuses it
   - If the PCP determines it could endanger the health of the mother or baby or would otherwise be inappropriate

BODYWORK MODALITIES HELPFUL DURING LABOR

Numerous complementary bodywork modalities are especially valuable during labor. These are sometimes more appropriate or easier to use than massage. This section addresses tools such as breathing, visualization, and hydrotherapy. It also covers some useful reflexology zones and some acupressure points specifically helpful during labor. These latter techniques are intended for therapists who have experience and training in their use. If you do not, it is recommended that you seek such training before performing the techniques with clients.

Breathing

Stress during labor causes women to hold their breath, which increases tension and slows labor. During labor, a woman's breath can be a comforting and stable focal point to reduce anxiety, improve her coping abilities, and increase her ability to relax with contractions. On a physiological level, conscious breathing can reduce lactic acid buildup and increase oxygen flow to the mother and baby, improving outcomes for both. Breathing also helps a woman stay present in each moment, rather than focus on concerns about what the next contraction will bring. On a spiritual level, breath is the most fundamental connection with life energy, a continuous reminder that we are alive. When we make breathing conscious, this innate connection to a life force becomes more potent.

Using Breathing

There are innumerable ways to use breath during birth. Incorporating attention to breathing during prenatal massage sessions can increase a woman's potential for utilizing this tool during labor. Generally, inhaling through the nose and exhaling through the mouth helps to circulate a flow of renewing energy through the body. Some women find certain patterns of breathing useful for relaxation and concentration, whereas others find that normal, slow, but conscious breathing throughout labor is helpful for them. Some women, often along with their partners, will want to use specific breathing exercises learned in childbirth education classes. Work with the approach she has learned and that is working for her, while suggesting additional techniques that may complement it.

Here are some general suggestions for working with breath.

- *Cleansing breaths:* Encourage a relaxed jaw and a full refreshing breath at the start and end of each contraction to cleanse away tension.
- *Intuitive breath patterns:* A woman who is listening to and trusting the inner and intuitive needs of her body will often be guided in the type of breathing most appropriate for each moment.
- *Ineffective breathing patterns:* Breathing too quickly often leads to hyperventilation, dizziness, and exhaustion, while breathing too shallowly or slowly may not bring enough oxygen to nourish her cells and baby.
- *Sipping breaths:* A woman who becomes frightened and anxious will commonly hyperventilate. Encourage her to take short sips of air, gradually allowing the breath to become deeper and fuller. Often it is helpful to maintain eye contact, guide her breath with yours, and hold firmly to her feet, hands, or shoulders to help ground her and diminish fear.
- *Observing breath:* Counting each breath helps some women focus, while just observing the natural breath coming in and out without shifting it helps others.

Specific Breathing Practices

The following breathing practices can be encouraged and taught to a mother while she is being massaged. Practice these techniques yourself to ensure that you can teach them adequately and can utilize them yourself to help you stay calm and centered during a woman's labor.

Abdominal Breathing   To help relax and surrender, use abdominal breathing. Inhale through the nose, allowing the breath to slowly fill the belly and be released in a gentle slow exhalation through an open mouth or pursed lips. The in-breath and out-breath should have the same duration.

Whale Breathing   To help release frustrated energy, inhale fully through the nose and exhale with a puff through the mouth, like a whale or dolphin blowing as it comes to the ocean's surface to clear its blowhole.

Ujjayi Victorious Breathing   This is a yogic breath that, when done for at least 3 minutes, can strengthen the nervous system and energy movement through the spine, while also expanding consciousness. It calls on one's inner strength, the victorious one who can withstand hardship and stay calm and centered during difficulty. It is useful anytime there is pain or discomfort.

Instruct the woman to breathe in through the nose, but to feel the breath in the back of the throat. There may almost be a sense of strain with the breath, and there will be a louder sound than is present with normal, slow nostril breathing. Bringing the chin forward and down very slightly will increase the ease and effectiveness of the breath. The breath massages the back of the throat. Imagine breathing on glasses to fog them before cleaning them; this breath has a similar guttural action, though the mouth is closed or only slightly parted and the breath comes through the nose. Imagine the sound of ocean waves in the distance; that is how the breath will sound. Let the breath begin in the abdomen, filling up the chest from there with full, deep breaths. Pause for as long as comfortable at the top of the inhalation before doing a controlled exhalation.

Visualizations and Affirmations

Positive imagery and words are often used during pregnancy to help establish a woman's readiness for labor and prepare her body and mind for what is to come. During labor, their use may continue to be beneficial for recalling her inner strength and funding more energy, relaxation, and trust throughout the process. Combining breath with affirmations such as "I am safe," "I can do this," "All is well," "Everything is flowing smoothly. My body knows how to do this," will increase the power of each breath. Incorporating specific relaxing or empowering imagery with affirmations and breath increases the effectiveness of both.

Use inventive but simple imagery that your client relates to and finds easy to envision in conjunction with your touch. For instance, when needing to increase energy or trust, she might visualize generations of women in a direct line to herself, giving birth successfully, standing and cheering her along, passing along their wisdom to her. Or she may imagine as a contraction begins, a warmth building up like a fire to heat her belly. She can watch the heat spread through her whole body, melting and relaxing all it touches. As it subsides, the firelight lessens, the flames die down to coals. The following is a more detailed example of dilation imagery. If your client relates to this type of imagery, you can share this with her between contractions, guiding her into a sensory scene that she can continue to envision during a contraction.

Contraction/Dilation Imagery

Imagine a still pool of water in a peaceful forest glade. The pool is lined with pink, yellow, and purple water lilies floating on its surface. Imagine soft, gentle clouds above dropping small raindrops into this still pool. See each raindrop land on the water, merge with it, and radiate out perfect, small circular waves from the center where it made contact, spreading across the entire pool. Feel the movement of that circular wave, expanding, opening simply and smoothly across the pool, growing ever wider. Sense your perineum and cervix relaxing and opening just like these water rings, as they soften and stretch. Roll your tongue around in your mouth and feel the softness of the cheek walls. This is how soft your cervix is. Let your mouth relax; let the mouth open from pursed lips to an ever growing circle. Open your mouth and breathe out, imagining your cervix opening in the same way, with the same ease.

Contraction–Relaxation

During labor, tension often develops in the jaw or shoulders, possibly causing simultaneous restriction in the pelvis or cervix. Muscle resistance work, combined with visualizations and breath, can be beneficial to help relieve this type of tension. Below is an example of this:

1. Notice where the client is holding muscular tension during contractions; it may be in her shoulders, in her solar plexus, in her pelvis and inner thighs, or in her hands.
2. Between contractions, have her exaggerate that tension. For instance, if her shoulders are tense, have her shrug her shoulders up even tighter toward her ears, as far as she can while inhaling and holding her breath.
3. On an exhalation, instruct her to completely relax her shoulders, allowing them to fall into their natural resting position.
4. Place your hands flat on the top of her relaxed shoulders and push down to stretch them slightly. Ask her to shrug her shoulders up while exhaling, pushing against your resistance, increasing her tension. Give resistance, but let her "win" so that her shoulders end in a shrug. Then have her inhale and relax the shoulders entirely again.
5. Ask her to relax completely as she feels the warmth of your hands on her shoulders.
6. As the next contraction begins, notice the tension developing again in her shoulders, and immediately place your hands on them, reminding her of that sensation of relaxing under your hands that she just felt moments ago. She can practice relaxing again now, while envisioning the warmth of your hands spreading down to her belly, back, pelvis, and legs.
7. During this resistance work, encourage the mother to visualize softening, opening, releasing, and letting go.

Hydrotherapy: Hot and Cold Applications

The use of water during pregnancy can amplify healing for many women. As a woman enters water during labor, she enters another dimension unlike her life on land (Figure 9.2). She is weightless and floating, just as her baby has been. Many of her aches and pains are relieved with this immersion and so some women choose to labor in and birth their babies into water. Many women who immerse in water during active labor find it easier to relax with contractions. They often have shorter, easier labors, a reduced use of medications, and they report a less painful and more satisfying birth experience.[6-9] Massage can often be continued when the client is immersed in water. Hands, head, feet, shoulders and back can still be touched if the client is in a birthing tub.

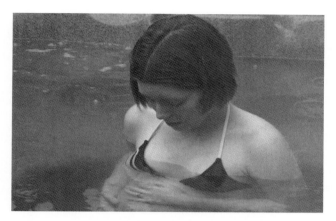

FIGURE 9.2 **Immersion in water can be very soothing for some women, and has the capacity to slow or speed labor.**

Hydrotherapy can also be effective when applied as moist hot and cold compresses or water sprays from a shower. For any applications of hot or cold water, always test the temperature on your own skin before applying to the client. Place 1 to 2 layers of protective cloth between her skin and the warm or cold pack.

 CAUTION: Avoid heat or ice applications to numbed areas on women with epidurals.

There are numerous methods of using water in labor. See Box 9.2 for a few examples.

Reflexology

Massage to the feet is grounding and comforting for many women during labor. Reflexology, however, is much more exacting in its approach than massage, applying direct pressure into areas that reflexively relate to specific parts of the body. Reflexology studies done with laboring women in England and Denmark have shown it to be effective for relief of contraction pain and for shortening labors.[10,11]

See Figure 9.3 for a diagram of reflexology zones located on the soles and tops of the feet. Reflexology on the uterus, ovary, pituitary, hip, spine, and sacral areas of the feet can help ease labor discomforts, encourage contractions, and renew the body. If you have studied reflexology techniques, work on the following areas during labor.

- The solar plexus/diaphragm area can influence breathing and increase relaxation.
- The hips and pelvic area can help reduce low back pain.
- The breast and pituitary area can influence hormonal releases that support labor.
- The head area can influence the mind, relaxation, anxiety, and shoulder tension.

Acupressure

Acupressure is practical and valuable during labor, as sometimes it is easier to hold 1 or 2 acupoints than to start and stop massaging every time the woman moves or changes position. If you are familiar with and trained in the use of acupressure, you can use these simple techniques of holding points as well as instruct interested birth companions in their use as well.

The acupressure points discussed in Chapter 4 that were contraindicated during pregnancy are now important points used to relieve pain, stimulate contractions, and help the baby to move downward.

BOX 9.2 | Hydrotherapy Tools for Labor

- Rub ice on acupressure point Large Intestine 4 to relieve pain. (See Chapter 10.)
- Apply cool cloths to the forehead, back of the neck, wrists, and low back.
- Apply friction massage using cold moist washcloths wrapped around your hands.
- Use frozen juice cans or a frozen rolling pin to roll over soft tissue of the body.
- Stimulate energy and lagging contractions with short cold bath immersions.
- Spray water on the back or belly with a hand-held shower.

- Support immersion in a warm tub or birthing pool.
- Offer water massage or Watsu® during early labor.
- Apply warm, moist compresses to the low back, across the belly, in the groin, just above the pubic bone, or on the perineum.
- In early labor, if she is comfortable in a sitting position, she can immerse her feet in cool or warm water followed by foot massage.
- Massage the jaw, head, and neck while she sits in a warm hip bath, with water only up to groin to help relax the perineum.

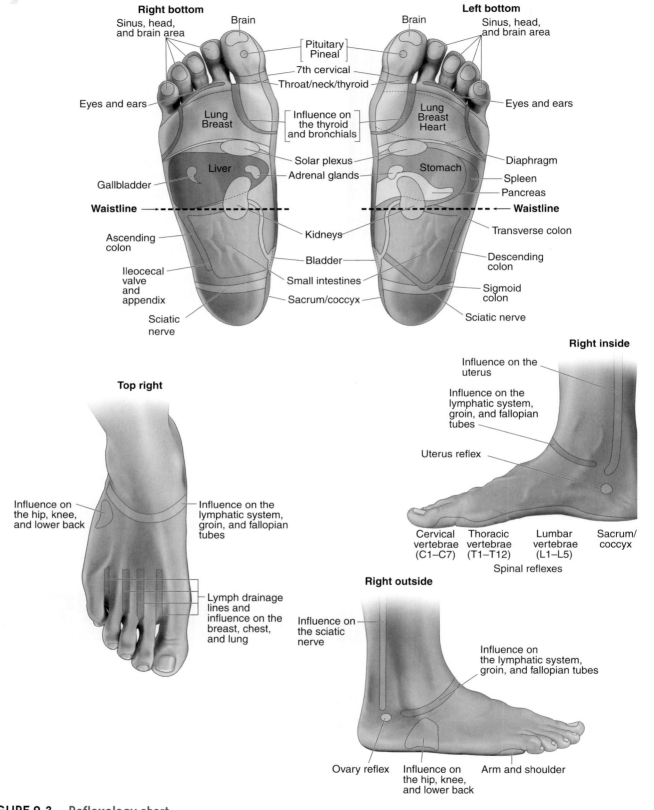

Right bottom
Sinus, head, and brain area
Brain
Pituitary / Pineal
7th cervical
Throat/neck/thyroid
Eyes and ears
Lung
Breast
Influence on the thyroid and bronchials
Liver
Gallbladder
Solar plexus
Adrenal glands
Waistline →
Ascending colon
Kidneys
Ileocecal valve and appendix
Bladder
Small intestines
Sacrum/coccyx
Sciatic nerve

Left bottom
Brain
Sinus, head, and brain area
Eyes and ears
Lung
Breast
Heart
Diaphragm
Stomach
Spleen
Pancreas
← **Waistline**
Transverse colon
Descending colon
Sigmoid colon
Sciatic nerve

Top right
Influence on the hip, knee, and lower back
Influence on the lymphatic system, groin, and fallopian tubes
Lymph drainage lines and influence on the breast, chest, and lung

Right inside
Influence on the uterus
Influence on the lymphatic system, groin, and fallopian tubes
Uterus reflex
Cervical vertebrae (C1–C7)
Thoracic vertebrae (T1–T12)
Lumbar vertebrae (L1–L5)
Sacrum/coccyx
Spinal reflexes

Right outside
Influence on the sciatic nerve
Influence on the lymphatic system, groin, and fallopian tubes
Ovary reflex
Influence on the hip, knee, and lower back
Arm and shoulder

FIGURE 9.3   Reflexology chart.

The entire body is reflected in the feet, as illustrated in this chart. Reflexology has been shown to be very useful during pregnancy and labor for relieving pain and encouraging the birth process. (Adapted from Williams A. Spa Bodywork: A Guide for Massage Therapists. Philadelphia: Lippincott Williams & Wilkins, 2007.)

There are other points used by advanced practitioners, but we will look only at the common points, which are easy to locate. Numerous studies have investigated the benefits of acupressure for labor and found particular points to be especially effective in reducing pain, starting or speeding labor, and reducing cesarean section rates.[12-15] The points most commonly researched in these studies were Large Intestine 4 and Spleen 6—the two most strongly prohibited points during pregnancy.

Using Acupressure During Labor

Acupressure points can be used throughout labor. Press in slowly to a point, compressing with a light or firm pressure, depending on how it feels for the mother. During contractions, pressure may be fairly firm on points. They should not feel *painful* to the mother, though some points are quite sensitive.

In early labor, stimulate the points for 5 to 10 minutes at least every 2 hours. As labor progresses, these points can be held either during every contraction or in between contractions. If that is not possible, stimulate the points at least every 30 minutes in the following manner: press and hold the points for 10 to 15 seconds, then release for one to two long breaths. Repeat 3 to 5 times.

If neither the mother nor you are noticing any difference within 10 minutes using a pressure point, try a different one. There are times when a woman may not be noticing a difference with a point, but her supporters may notice that her coping abilities have increased significantly. The pain is not gone, but her ability to relax with it may have improved. In this case, continue using the point if she agrees.

Intersperse massage techniques with the holding of acupressure points to help the client relax even more.

Common Points

The following points (shown in Figure 4.3) are the most commonly used:

- Large Intestine 4: This point helps release stuck energy, stimulate stronger contractions, relieve pain, and open gateways of energy in the upper body. It is especially useful when the bag of water has already broken but contractions have not yet begun or are weak. Spleen 6: Helps increase contractions, dilate the cervix, regulate hormones, and is excellent for pain relief. Studies have also documented reduced cesarean rates in labors where this point is used.[12]

- Gall Bladder 21: Moves energy downward, helping to bring the baby down into the pelvis. Relieves pain and eases difficult labors.
- Bladder 60: Draws energy down the body and the baby into the pelvis. It clears excess energy, especially from the head, supports contractions, helps reduce pain, and alleviates pain. It is also useful for difficult labor.
- Bladder 31 and 32: These sacral points are helpful for stimulating contractions, relieving back pain, and encouraging dilation of the cervix.
- Kidney 3: Helpful especially for back and contraction pain and increasing stamina. Hold together with Bladder 60.

GENERAL MASSAGE FOR BIRTH

Some massage techniques are useful at any stage of labor and are simple enough to learn and use throughout labor. They can be quite effective for pain relief and for emotional support. Long strokes, petrissage, and work on the hands and feet are nearly always effective. The use of a long piece of fabric (rebozo) to provide friction and hip movement, the use of a "birthing" ball as a means for a client to rock the hips while contracting and being massaged, and the inclusion of other massage tools such as handheld or electronic massagers may prove advantageous in some situations.

Techniques from other chapters that are useful at any time during birth include "Sacral Compression and Unwinding" in Chapter 5 and all techniques in Chapter 7 for labor preparation.

Petrissage

Use slow, relaxing petrissage to any areas of obvious tension.

Hand and Foot Massage

Massage to the hands and feet has a greater benefit for women in labor than simply alleviating muscular tension in the extremity itself. It influences the entire body at once—decreasing sensations of pain by affecting the transmission of nerve impulses to the central nervous system, and stimulating reflexology areas and acupressure meridians.

The following work to the hands can be repeated on the feet.

1. Hold the client's hand (or foot) with her palm (or sole) resting on the upward turned fingertips of both your hands, and your palms

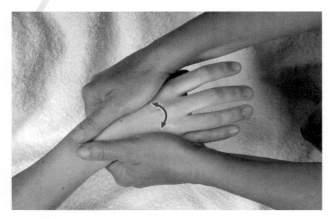

FIGURE 9.4   Hand massage.
Massage of the hands offers a mother a relaxing and beneficial experience. Press your palms and the fleshy base of your thumbs into the tops of her hands as you press up into her palm with your fingertips.

wrapped around the dorsal side of the extremity.

2. Press your palms and the fleshy base of your thumbs into the top of her hand (foot) as you press up into her palm (sole) with your fingertips.
3. Squeeze out to the side, sliding your palms off her hands. Repeat, working your fingertips into the palms of her hands (Figure 9.4).

4. Work from the tip of each finger down to its base, pushing excess fluid back into her circulation, spiraling down the finger.
5. Rotate each finger in small movements to help loosen and relax.
6. Turn her hand over, so the back of her hand rests in your palms. Work with your thumbs into the fleshy parts of her palms, making circles and fanning out from the base up toward the fingers and sides of the hand.
7. Make long strokes down her arms and all the way out her hands and fingertips, imagining drawing all excess energy from her upper body down and out.

Long Strokes

No matter what position the mother is in, you can always make long, slow, firm-pressured strokes with the palms of your hands, moving down her body from head to toe, on the front or back, or just fully down the arms or legs. Two people can work together do this with a full-body grounding stroke as follows.

Two-Person Grounding Stroke

With the mother standing, leaning forward onto a bed or table with pillows, two people can stand on either side of her and make long strokes down her back to her feet (Figure 9.5A). Work together with firm, slow

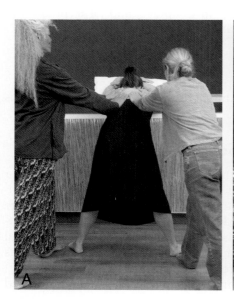
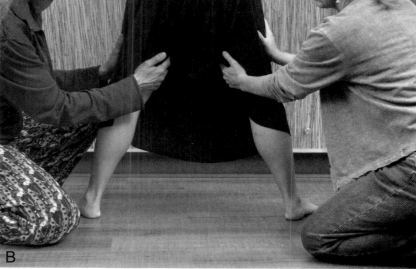

FIGURE 9.5   Two-person grounding stroke.
(A) To help ground a laboring woman, move energy downward, open the cervix, and relieve back discomfort, two people can stand on either side of her and make long strokes down her back to her feet. Work together with firm slow strokes. (B) Squeeze into either side of the ankle or Achilles tendon or into the arch of the foot at the end of each long stroke to help ground and stimulate acupressure points.

strokes. Squeeze into either side of the ankle or Achilles tendon or into the arch of the foot at the end of each stroke to help ground and stimulate acupressure points (Figure 9.5B).

Sacral Counterpressure

With the client on hands and knees, leaning over a bed or table or straddling a chair, or in any position where you can access her sacrum, place your open palm with fingers pointing toward her feet on the center of her sacrum. Apply pressure directly on her sacrum during contractions. Use as much force as you can that is comfortable for her, pushing in and down caudally toward the coccyx (Figure 9.6). Gently release when the contraction is over. She can increase the pressure by pushing her hips toward your hand. Often you will need to use a significant level of pressure, especially if the mother is experiencing back labor; ensure that you are using proper body mechanics to avoid causing yourself strain.

> *Case Study 9.3:*
> DRAWING ENERGY DOWN
>
> Rosa was having a difficult time sitting still during her labor, and chose to walk around her birth room at the hospital as much as possible. When the nurse, Sally came in, she found Rosa leaning over the raised hospital bed during contractions. Her husband stood by her, uncertain what to do. This was their second child.
>
> Sally had checked Rosa's cervix 30 minutes earlier when she had been 6 cm dilated. Sally suggested that Rosa's husband, Jorge, and she work together to do some long grounding strokes down Rosa's back and legs. They both placed their hands at her shoulders, and stroked down Rosa's back, squeezing her thighs as they stroked down to her feet. There, they squeezed on either side of the ankles and the soles of the feet. They repeated this with each contraction for about 15 minutes, as Rosa said it felt good; she could feel her perineum relaxing with each stroke. Rosa would squat or sink down into her knees slightly with each stroke down her back until the contraction passed. After this period of time, Rosa's legs began to tremble, and Sally found suddenly with the next contraction, the baby's head hanging between Rosa's legs. Rosa had relaxed and opened so fully that the baby had just slipped out without effort. The doctor happened to be close at hand and helped catch the baby just as the rest of his body emerged.

 CAUTION: Always be sure that pressure is centered on the sacrum and not on the lumbar spine or to one side of the sacrum, which can move the sacrum out of alignment.

Rebozo Massage

Throughout pregnancy and labor, many Mexican and Central American midwives use a long shawl or "rebozo" to massage the mother, to help the baby move, to provide comfort, and to relieve pain. Numerous methods can be implemented at any time during labor, using a sheet, long scarf, or other cloth. Two methods, rebozo friction and rebozo hip jiggle, are presented below.

Rebozo Friction

1. Have the client relax in a chair.
2. Place a long, smooth cotton or silk shawl or cloth behind the small of the back.
3. Stand or kneel in front of her, holding the cloth on either end and sliding it back and forth across her low back, creating a warming friction against her low back. (Figure 9.7A). This can also be done with oil lubricating the back, sometimes allowing the cloth to slip across the skin more easily.

Rebozo Hip Jiggle

1. The mother has her knees on a blanket or other padding as she rests forward onto her forearms with her buttocks in the air.
2. Place the rebozo around her buttocks, with your hands holding the scarf close to each hip. Jiggle and rotate the hips (Figure 9.7B). The rebozo does not slide across the skin, but stays put on the buttocks and hips. The therapist's movements help to rock and jiggle the hips.
3. For some women this can help relieve back ache, bring energy to the pelvis, and help the baby move from posterior to anterior.

FIRST STAGE OF LABOR: CONTRACTIONS AND CERVICAL CHANGES

Labor has been described as having three stages. In the first stage, the contractions normally become regular and strong, causing the cervix to dilate from 0 to

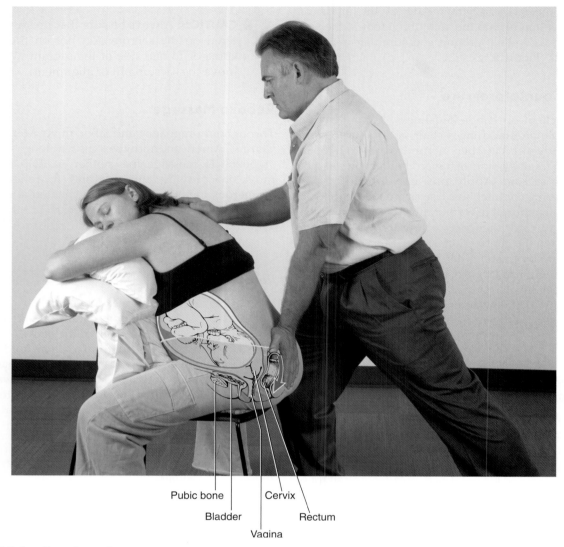

Pubic bone   Cervix

Bladder   Rectum

Vagina

FIGURE 9.6   Sacral counterpressure.

The client can be in any position that gives access to the sacrum. Direct pressure toward the coccyx. The mother can push up into the hand to increase force of pressure if desired and able.

10 cm. This section examines each phase of this stage of labor, how the woman may experience it, and what types of support measures may be most appropriate.

Pre-Labor

At the start of the labor journey, a woman might have ongoing, mild contractions for days and yet have no cervical dilation. This occurs more frequently with a first pregnancy. If your client is seen by her PCP during this time, she will probably be told she is not in labor yet. Discouragement and disappointment are common along with questions about whether she is doing something "wrong" to cause

her to suffer these seemingly useless contractions. By the time she begins active cervical dilation, she could be thoroughly exhausted from days of little sleep or rest.

This **pre-labor**, also called *prodromal* or *latent* labor, is not useless; the body is readying itself for labor. The cervix may be softening and effacing, or thinning out and the baby's head may be starting to settle into the pelvis. Frequently, there is an emotional component to pre-labor. Be aware that your client may be experiencing some type of ambivalence or emotional discomfort about beginning labor, or entering into motherhood, and she may verbalize some of this during a massage.

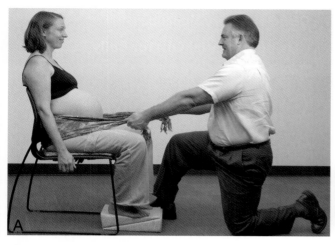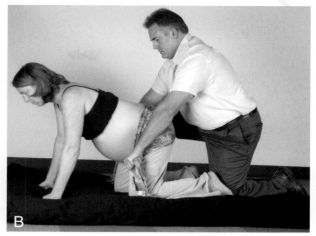

FIGURE 9.7   Types of rebozo massage.
(A) Rebozo friction: Hold the cloth on either end, sliding it back and forth across her skin, creating a warming friction against her low back. (B) Rebozo hip jiggle: With the client on her hands and knees, wrap a rebozo over her buttocks, holding the cloth close to the hip, and jiggle the hips, rotating and wiggling, to help relieve back ache and move the baby, if necessary.

In ancient Hawaiian culture, pre-labor contractions were viewed as "sympathetic pains" for other women in labor. A woman with ineffective contractions was made to rest and eat nourishing warm food as a means to reduce or relieve her of her discomfort.[5]

Characteristics of the pre-labor phase are the following: ***

- Contraction frequency: irregular. The uterus is warming up with mild contractions.
- Dilation: The cervix may be thinning and softening, but not dilating. The baby may be moving into the pelvis more securely.
- Duration: Hours to days.
- Mother's Experience: A woman may experience some, all, or none of the following:
  - Contractions are usually mild, but some women experience them as strong, until they begin to compare them with more active contractions.
  - Frustration, anxiety, discouragement, excitement, and jubilance are common feelings.
  - A "nesting" urge is felt, and the mother is preoccupied with final preparations for the baby's arrival.

General Supportive Measures

Laboring and birthing in water is becoming popular around the world. In early labor it can slow down labor. This may be helpful for a prolonged pre-labor when the woman just needs to sleep. Encourage her to take a bath and relax.

A mother can walk, exercise, and continue life as usual to avoid focusing on these early contractions.

Massage for Pre-Labor

A full body massage can promote relaxation and possibly sleep, perhaps allowing the body to have time to gather its resources to set in motion a more active labor. Techniques from Chapter 7 are appropriate if stimulation rather than relaxation is important.

Early Labor

Eventually, contractions begin to come more regularly. The woman pays attention to them, but usually she can talk and continue with other activities without having to stop or give all her attention to them.

Characteristics of the early labor phase are the following:

- Contraction frequency: 15 to 20 minutes apart, increasing gradually to 5 to 10 minutes apart; lasting 40 to 60 seconds.
- Dilation: 0 to 4 cm.
- Duration: 3 to 20 hours or more.
- Mother's Experience: A woman may experience some, all, or none of the following:
  - Mild to moderate contractions.
  - Possible bloody show.
  - Contractions gradually becoming longer, stronger, and closer.
  - Possible backache, exhaustion, exhilaration, and excitement.

How the Partner Can Help
Belly Rubs for Contractions

*D*uring labor some women do not want their bellies touched at all, while others find it relieving to be massaged between or during contractions. Learn more belly rub techniques in Chapter 5. The following is a useful technique to teach a willing partner if the client is enjoying her belly touched. It can provide some pain relief for the mother as well as offer an intimate touching time between them both.

Have the client sit and recline against the partner who is in a comfortable chair or bed with the head up. Alternatively, have the client stand in front of the standing partner. To lift away the pain during or between contractions, the partner can begin with hands resting low on the mother's belly, fingertips pointing toward the pubic bone. Draw the hands up along the groin and out toward the hips and repeat, hand over hand (Figure 9.8). Stroke up from the pubic bone to the umbilicus area as well. Make all strokes move in one direction, up and out. Create a steady, smooth rhythm from the beginning to the end of the contraction.

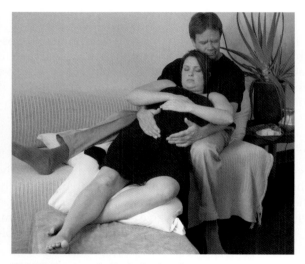

FIGURE 9.8   Belly Rubs for Contractions.
Client can be semi-reclining or standing while you lift away pain during or between contractions. Begin with the hands resting low on the belly, fingertips pointing toward the pubic bone. Draw the hands up along the groin and out toward the hips and repeat, hand over hand. Stroke up from the pubic bone to the umbilicus area.

- Contractions that are felt in the abdomen generally are felt higher in the uterus initially, rather than lower in cervix.
- Bag of water may break.

Complementary Modalities:
Using Essential Oils for Belly Rubs

*F*or labor, certain essential oils can have an influence on stimulating contractions or helping a mother relax. You might choose to make ahead of time the following safe oil to use on the belly during labor. If you want to use different oils than those described here, refer to a prenatal aromatherapy text as listed in Appendix B. To 2 ounces of warmed castor oil add 8 drops of clary sage (*Salvia Sclarea*), 5 drops of rose (*Rosa damascena; Rosa centifolia*), and 4 drops of jasmine (*Jasminum grandiflorum*). Shake it well before using. Massage with the intent to relax, renew, and help the mother connect gracefully to her contracting belly.

 CAUTION: Jasmine and clary sage have strong scents that some might find offensive during labor. Always get approval from the mother before using a scent.

- Frustration if it is going on for a long time or if she is told labor is not progressing.

General Supportive Measures

- It is usually more helpful for a woman to stay busy for as long as possible with normal activities until the contractions begin to *demand* attention; otherwise, she may grow weary before the hardest work has begun. At the same time, relaxation is the key to allowing labor to flow and keeping a reserve of energy; alternating activity and rest will preserve a mother's energy for more active labor.

A bath or shower can help to relax or sometimes stimulate contractions.

- Once the client is no longer able to talk through contractions, slow, focused breathing may be appropriate.

When resting, help her practice relaxing visualizations, such as imagining being in a peaceful setting where she feels totally safe. She may wish to play music that she associates with relaxation or good feelings.

Massage for Early Labor

- All techniques in Chapter 7 are beneficial in early labor.

- All techniques under the sections "Bodywork Modalities Helpful During Labor" and "General Massage for Birth," above.
- Full-body massage.

Active Labor

As labor progresses, the contractions grow closer and stronger, effacing and dilating the cervix. The woman gradually becomes less interested in outside distractions and more focused on her inner process. If she has had children before, this phase is likely to be shorter than the first time she labored. Her bag of water may rupture, causing her to leak fluids continuously or with each contraction. Linear thinking is gone; the woman is entering a watery dimension where she is responding bodily, psychically, and emotionally to all the energies around her; any type of provocations can influence her and her labor.

Characteristics of active labor are the following:

- Contraction Frequency: 2 to 5 minutes apart; lasting 60 to 90 seconds
- Dilation: 4 to 7 cm
- Duration: 1 to 8 hours, or more
- Mother's Experience: A woman may experience some, all, or none of the following:
  - Contractions feel moderate to strong.
  - She may be more uncomfortable and introspective.
  - She may be very tired, sleeping in the moments between contractions.
  - She may be leaking fluids and having bloody show.
  - She may have backache, groin pressure, or back labor.

General Supportive Measures

- Help her remember to drink plenty of fluids.
- Help her remember to urinate every hour (a full bladder can diminish the effectiveness of contractions).
- Labor tends to flow more effectively if the mother changes positions regularly.
- If she is becoming anxious, remind her of why she is doing this and use visualization that help her meet one contraction at a time, without thinking ahead to the next one.
- Encourage opening, surrendering, and focusing.
- Immersion in warm water now can be a helpful way for her to relax and promote the progress of birth.
- If she has back pain, she may need to change positions, especially using positions that let the belly fall forward, such as on her hands and knees with pillows supporting the belly.

Massage for Active Labor

- All techniques under the sections "Bodywork Modalities Helpful During Labor" and "General Massage for Birth," above.
- With the client standing or in sidelying position, stroke up the inner leg with one hand and simultaneously stroke down the outer leg. This stimulates the yin and yang meridians of energy and brings balance to the body.
- Effleurage the abdomen and upper legs. Petrissage and knead the buttocks.
- Long strokes down the inner legs help to relieve shaky legs and groin tension and relax the cervix and perineum.
- Two-person grounding stroke as described above.
- Knead the buttocks and apply pressure to the sacrum.
- Walk down the sacrum with the palm of your hand, thrusting in slightly to stimulate nerves that help release the pelvis for delivery.

Varying Positions

Most women feel more comfortable and are able to tolerate the sensations of contractions if they can move regularly. Sometimes, in hospitals, this can be difficult to do if the woman is continuously electronically monitored. However, if there are no risks to the mother or baby, she should be allowed or encouraged to walk frequently, to use the shower, or to change positions. Frequent and regular changes of position during labor assist cervical dilation, rotation of the baby, enhancement of contractions, circulation of blood, relief of aches and pains, and improvement of a fatigued mind. Sometimes a woman will not feel like moving at all, but despite her resistance, she may find relief when she moves into another position. If you are massaging a woman who has just moved into a new position, suggest she try this position for several contractions before she decides that it is not beneficial. Standing or walking is often more comfortable than lying down. The massage therapist must be prepared to work in a variety of positions that the mother finds comfortable. The following section describes common positions and some techniques to use in each. See Table 9.1 for a summary of positions and their benefits during labor.

Straddling a Chair This position affords access for massage to the back, head, jaw, shoulders, hips, and hands and is usually quite comfortable. The woman

Table 9.1 Labor Positions and Benefits

Benefits

Position	Helpful for back labor	Easy access for long strokes and sacral pressure	Restful for support companion	Restful for mother	Good for pushing	May encourage contractions	Widens pelvic outlet	May help baby descend in pelvis
Semi-reclining With hips flexed			✓	✓	✓		✓	✓
Straddling chair leaning forward	✓	✓		✓			✓	
Supported squatting with companion in chair			✓	✓	✓	✓	✓	✓
Kneeling leaning forward	✓	✓*	✓**		✓			
Standing leaning forward	✓	✓				✓		
Hands and knees	✓	✓			✓			✓
Walking		✓			✓	✓		✓
Sidelying				✓				✓
Water immersion				✓		✓***		

* Companion standing behind woman.
** Companion seated in chair before woman.
*** Only in active labor.

sits straddling a chair (or toilet) facing backwards and leaning into pillows.

- Make thumb circles or press points down either side of the spine from the neck to the sacrum.
- Press into the sacrum, and rub in the sacral foramen.
- Make long strokes down the back from the neck and squeeze into the hips from both sides.
- Stand in front of her and lean into her shoulders with your forearms (Figure 9.9).
- Make long strokes from her head down to her sacrum or all the way down to her feet.
- Place the palm of one of your hands on your client's forehead and the other supporting her head from behind. Squeeze gently, holding, supporting, and being still for a moment—as if your hands are a container for her mind.

Supported Squatting in Front of a Chair   In this position, you get a little break by being seated in the chair, while the mother squats in front between your knees. This gives you access to her shoulders, head, and jaw (Figure 9.10).

- Massage, tap on, and stroke her shoulders, head, neck, and jaw.
- Apply traction to her neck.

Sitting in a Chair   The laboring mother is not often sitting in this position, but a technique can be used to alleviate some pressure in her pelvis and low back, help open the sacroiliac joint, and sometimes realign the pelvis. With the woman sitting normally in a chair, push against her knees, moving her femur back into

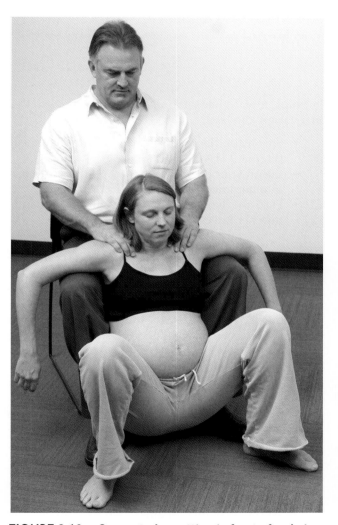

FIGURE 9.10   Supported squatting in front of a chair.
A good position to share with support companions or partners who can get a little break seated in the chair, while the mother squats in front, between the knees. This allows access to the shoulders, head, and jaw.

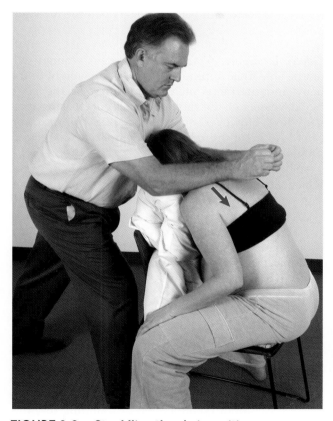

FIGURE 9.9   Straddling the chair position.
This position offers good access into the shoulders. Save your hands by using the forearms to lean into the shoulders.

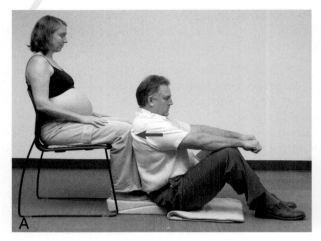 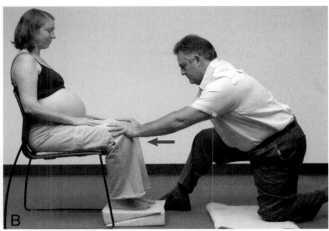

FIGURE 9.11   Sitting in a chair.

*This allows two ways to push against her knees. This pushes the femur toward her sacrum, alleviating some pressure in the pelvis and low back, opening the sacro-iliac joint, and sometimes realigning the pelvis. **(A)** Sit on the floor and lean back into her knees. **(B)** Or simply face the woman and push with your hands into her knees.*

her hips, toward her sacrum. You can accomplish this in a variety of ways:

- Sit on the floor and lean back into her knees (Figure 9.11A).
- Lie on your back at the mother's feet and push into her knees with your feet.
- Face the woman and push with your hands into her knees (Figure 9.11B).

Hands and Knees, Kneeling Leaning Forward, or Leaning Over a Counter or Chair   Leaning forward helps relieve pressure on the low back and can be a nice change from other upright positions. This position affords you access to the client's back and sacrum and ease with making long strokes down her body.

The client can be on her hands and knees or leaning forward over a table or counter, or against a wall.

She can also kneel and face you, resting her arms and head in your lap, as you rub her head and shoulders. A second person can rub or press into her back in this position.

- Long strokes and the two-person grounding stroke can be used in this position.
- Apply pressure against her sacrum as she pushes back into your hand.
- Forearms and elbows can be used on the gluteal and sacral areas.
- Sacroiliac relief: see Chapter 10.

Birth Ball   Some women find sitting and swaying their hips and pelvis on a large ball very relaxing. Kneeling and leaning forward over the ball while rocking forward and back can also open the hips and pelvis.

Sidelying, Supine, or Semi-Reclining   A woman will not be able to lie supine for long, as the weight of the baby and uterine contents can compress the large blood vessels of the mother's back, decreasing oxygen flow. However, she may choose this position briefly to have the rebozo work done, as described previously.

She may also choose to use the sidelying position, which can be very restful and which gives the massage therapist good access to the whole body for all types of massage.

The semi-reclining position is another reclining choice that opens the pelvis if the hips are flexed. This position also gives the therapist access to the head, neck, shoulders, arms, hands, belly, and legs.

Transition

Transition can be like walking across the coals of a fire; it can require intense focus. If fear is going to arise in a labor, this is the most likely time it will appear. If the woman is going to state that she absolutely cannot go on longer, proclaiming that this is the last time she will ever get pregnant, this is the likely time for that to occur! If she is going to be nauseated, vomit, or have uncontrollable shaking, it normally happens now. All physical energy is preparing for completion of dilation of the cervix. Once this occurs, the energy shifts and the mother can focus on pushing the baby out.

Your support is critical at this time. For many, this is usually the shortest phase of labor, but may be the most challenging time for a woman to stay present. Transition is a good sign; it is heralding the second stage and the end of labor. Remind her of this and that the baby will soon be in her arms.

Characteristics of the transition phase are the following:

- Contraction Frequency: Usually 2 to 4 minutes apart; lasting 60 to 90 seconds
- Dilation: 8 to 10 cm
- Duration: Anywhere from several contractions to several hours, or more
- Mother's Experience: A woman may experience some, all, or none of the following:
  - Moderate to strong contractions
  - Possible spontaneous rupture of the bag of waters
  - Pressure in the vagina, pubic bone, and rectum
  - Nausea, vomiting
  - Leg cramps
  - Uncontrollable shaking of the legs, arms, and jaw
  - Sensitivity to touch
  - Drowsiness
  - Cold feet and a flushed face
  - Restlessness, fear, irritability, sense of being overwhelmed, as if she cannot go on
  - Desire to escape
  - Desire to push before fully dilated

General Supportive Measures

- Support her in maintaining focused breathing and relaxation.
- Support her in position changes as needed.
- Encourage her and reassure her that this is the shortest stage. This is the beginning of the end. Stay with her and maintain eye contact if that helps her stay grounded.

Massage for Transition

- For some women touch will feel uncomfortable during transition and hands-off support may be more appropriate.
- Apply long, grounding massage strokes, using firm pressure or holding of the hands, feet, or sacrum, as in the two-person grounding stroke, discussed above.
- Petrissage to the buttocks will help them relax as tension develops with increasing perineal pressure.
- With the client on hands and knees or in the sidelying position, hold warm compresses to the inner legs and perineum. The woman's partner can place a gloved hand and warm cloth over the woman's tailbone and anus, fingers pointing up toward her sacrum. This firm pressure can help her relax her perineum, ease pressure sensations, and prevent her from pushing until the cervix is fully dilated.
- Apply light strokes down inner legs with warm oil.
- Hold her great toe and next two toes on both feet with both hands to help relieve pain and relax the perineum.

The Lull

Sometimes between transition and pushing there can be a lull in contractions. This is normal and need not be hurried. It is the body and nature's way of giving the woman a break and letting her collect her resources for the pushing effort. The uterus, too, is gathering its energies, revitalizing itself so that it can most effectively do the next work. The uterus is a muscle (the strongest muscle in a woman's body), which tires and may need a break before it can work efficiently again.

Characteristics of the lull are the following:

- Contraction Frequency: None
- Dilation: 10 cm
- Duration: 10 minutes to 1 hour
- Mother's Experience: A woman may experience some, all, or none of the following:
  - Cessation of contractions
  - Rest

General Supportive Measures

- Offer fluids to drink.
- This is an appropriate time for the mother as well as support people to sleep briefly, rest, and recover.
- Focus on relaxing areas of tension.

Massage for the Lull

- Perform general relaxation massage.

- Hold and compress the occiput and forehead between two hands, to rest her mind.
- Massage neck, jaw, and shoulder.
- Apply slow fingertip circles on the temples.
- Perform hand and foot massage as described in the section, "General Massage for Birth," above.

SECOND STAGE OF LABOR: PUSHING AND BIRTH

After the dilation of the cervix is complete and transition is over, the second stage of labor begins: pushing the baby. Birth is imminent, and often the mother and support companions may feel some renewed energy.

Pushing

When the cervix is completely dilated to 10 cm and contractions are continuing or have resumed, the mother will begin pushing. Normally the woman will have an urge to bear down that occurs spontaneously and involuntarily. For some, there can be what Michel Odent describes as the fetal ejection reflex,[16,17] where, if left undisturbed, the mother will have a quick and natural delivery of the baby without having to actually work at the pushing. Since most women in the United States deliver in hospitals, it is rare for this undisturbed ejection reflex of the baby to occur. Instead, their experience may be that pushing is a relief, relative to the rest of labor. Finally, she has a chance to do something active, rather than just face the challenge of surrendering to contractions over and over. For other women, pushing may feel overwhelming, exhausting, or more painful than active labor. Pushing can last from just one push to 3 hours or more depending on the size of the baby relative to a woman's pelvis, the number of previous deliveries, the position of the mother and baby, and the effectiveness of the contractions and of the woman's efforts.

The mother must move into an appropriate position that opens the pelvis. In a home birth, this might include squatting, being on hands and knees, or in sidelying position with the top leg flexed to the side) to push effectively. In the hospital, the most likely position, used for doctor convenience, is the semireclining position, with the woman pulling her knees up to her sides or resting them in stirrups, while the support team assists by pushing against her feet and flexing her hips, opening her pelvis further.

As the baby descends through the pelvis and onto the perineum, the perineal musculature will begin to stretch, thin, and expand. Soon, the baby's head fills the vaginal opening—this is known as **crowning.** The mother may feel sensations of burning or tearing—this is often called the **ring of fire**. You can imagine a little how this might feel, by sticking a finger in either side of your mouth and pulling out to the side until you feel a burning. If you did this very suddenly and very forcefully, the pain sensations would be much stronger and more difficult to tolerate than if you did it gradually and slowly with some control. Either way, it will not be a comfortable feeling.

This is similar to perineal stretching. If the tissues are allowed to stretch gradually, often with the woman placing her hand on her perineum and the baby's head to facilitate control, she can adapt to the sensations, greatly reducing the chance of tearing or cutting. Teaching and encouraging the practice of perineal massage in the last 4 to 6 weeks of pregnancy will aid in this birth process, and skin tears that sometimes occur at birth can be avoided.

It is possible that a doctor or midwife will cut the tissue to help the baby be born faster — this is called an **episiotomy**. This procedure is generally a practitioner preference and is rarely necessary unless there is an emergency situation requiring rapid delivery.

Characteristics of the pushing phase are the following:

- Contraction Frequency: Usually 2 to 4 minutes apart; lasting 60 seconds
- Dilation: 10 cm to birth
- Duration: 1 push to 5 hours, or more.
- Mother's Experience: A woman may experience some, all, or none of the following:
  - Moderate to strong contractions.
  - Grunting deep and low or holding the breath with contractions.
  - Urge to push becomes stronger as the baby descends.
  - Pressure on the stretching perineum and widening hips.
  - May feel pressure in the rectum and the need for bowel movement.
  - Crowning "ring of fire."
  - Amazement, relief, and a sense of satisfaction.
  - Exhaustion, feeling like it is too much work or more pain.
  - Leg cramps due to positioning and the strain of pushing.
  - Shakiness between contractions — the whole body may shake uncontrollably or just the legs.
  - Whole body tension after each contraction.

General Supportive Measures

- Provide verbal encouragement to support her pushing.

- Applying continuous warm moist cloths to the perineum is very effective to reduce ring of fire pain.
- Apply a cold cloth as needed to the head and neck.
- Remind her of how she relaxed with prenatal perineal massage sessions.
- Offer her sips of water between pushes.

Massage for Pushing

- Reflexology and acupressure techniques as discussed in the section, "Bodywork Modalities Helpful During Labor," above.
- Touch to her feet, shoulders, jaw, or hands, reminding her to relax completely until the next urge to push.
- Extend and stretch the legs, arms, and hands and massage between contractions. Perform calf massage between contractions to prevent leg cramps. To address cramps further, see the section "Leg Cramps" in Chapter 6.
- Hand-holding: Acupressure point Large Intestine 4 increases the effectiveness of pushing and movement toward releasing the baby and, especially if the mother is getting tired. Hold during contractions if the mother is not using her hands; otherwise, squeeze between contractions along with performing hand massage.
- Foot massage: Pressing into the bottom of the foot can help the perineum to relax and open.
- Pressing into the top of the shoulders on acupressure point Gall Bladder 21 (Figure 4.3) can help the baby to descend and move the birth energy downward.
- If the mother is in the sidelying or hands and knees position, place your palms on her upper back and walk them, hand over hand, down either side of the spine.
- Stroke down the inner thighs over and over with long strokes to help relax the perineum between contractions.
- Massage the jaw muscles to reflexively release the perineum (see "Jaw Release" in Chapter 7).

Birth—Emergence

A final push, and the baby's whole head finally emerges from the vagina. As soon as the baby's head is out and before the first breath, many doctors and midwives will suction the mouth and nose to remove fluids, particularly if the baby had meconium in the fluid. Each shoulder and the rest of the body then comes slipping out, and the baby is on her or his own. Soon the lungs begin inflating with air for the first

Traditional Birth Practices: Softening the Perineum

Many women know the benefits of applying lubrication, warmth, and water to the perineum to help it relax during labor. In Uganda, Bugandan women use herbal sitz baths. Women in Sudan may squat over a pot of steaming infusions. Moroccan women use hot salt water and steam to keep the perineum soft, clean, and healthy during pregnancy and labor. [18]

There is record of a 17th century English midwife using a special mixture of olive, linseed, and hollyhock oils and bird fat to soften the perineum and "Sople the privie place."[19] Midwives today may use vitamin E oil to do perineal massage before and during labor to help the mother feel more at ease with the sensations of stretching to the area and to attempt to help the tissues stretch further.

Traditional Birth Practices: Power of the Placenta

Around the world, people have tended to the placenta carefully. The Jicarilla Apache Indians put the placenta in the top of a spruce tree, connecting the child's health to that of the long-living tree. The mother would keep a part of the baby's dried umbilical cord; without this protection, it was thought that the child would die. When the mother died, the cord, which may have been kept for years, would then be placed on a spruce tree, as had the placenta.[20]

The umbilical cord was also dried in some African cultures and in Haiti and Japan and often saved for a lifetime to ensure the owner's safety. It was sometimes boiled in hot water as a tea when needed for special healing. Some people were known to keep the cord of their dead mother for a lifetime or for generations. In Haiti, to prevent evil spirits from taking a placenta and using it in curses against the child, a hole might be dug in the birth room and the placenta buried there.[21]

Each island in ancient Hawaii once had a specially designated site for placing the umbilical cord.[5]

In the United States, many hospitals freeze the placenta after delivery to be sold to cosmetic companies for use in their products, as it is believed to have beneficial components for skin.

The ancient Egyptian pharaoh's placenta was especially important, exhibited for others to see in temples and in processions.[4]

time. Once the baby is born, what happens next varies depending on whether one is in a hospital, home, or birthing center. Eventually the umbilical cord, attaching the baby to the placenta, will be clamped off and the cord cut.

THIRD STAGE OF LABOR: BIRTH OF THE PLACENTA

The final stage of labor involves the delivery of the placenta, after which the real labor begins: the next hours, weeks, and years may be the most challenging work of a woman's life—being a parent!

Placental Delivery

After the baby is born, the placenta—the organ that nourished the baby in utero—must also be delivered. This is the third stage of labor, which normally occurs within 5 to 30 minutes after the baby's birth. Usually, the woman will feel a strong cramping as the placenta detaches itself from the uterine wall and emerges at the vaginal opening. The side that was attached to the uterine wall is raw and meaty looking, while the other side is smooth with large blood vessels on its surface like tree branches spreading out across it; some call this the Tree of Life.

The placenta tells us many stories about the health and intrauterine life of the baby. The doctor or

---

Case Study 9.4:
MASSAGE CLIENT UNKNOWINGLY IN ACTIVE LABOR

Martha was 40 and having her first child. She was 39 weeks pregnant and came for her weekly massage. When she arrived at the therapist's office, she told Sara, the therapist, that she had been having contractions all day, but that they were mild. She said she believed that this was still very early labor.

Martha situated herself on the massage table for her session, but quickly found that she was uncomfortable lying on her side; she felt better standing. The therapist continued with the massage, with Martha leaning forward over the massage table, rocking her hips and saying that she was worried that if things were this intense during early labor, she couldn't imagine what active labor would be like.

Sara was a labor and delivery nurse, as well as massage therapist, and had worked with hundreds of women in labor. She could see that Martha was acting more like a woman in active labor, but Martha was so convinced that she was going to have a long labor that she initially convinced Sara as well that this was so. Soon, however, Martha began to feel nauseated and vomited into the nearest waste basket. At that point, Sara expressed her concerns more strongly that this was active labor and asked Martha when she had had her last exam with her PCP. Martha then admitted that yesterday at her prenatal appointment she had already been 3 cm dilated! Sara insisted that Martha call her husband for a ride and leave now for the hospital where she planned to deliver her baby. Martha left with her husband soon after that and delivered her baby 1-1/2 hours later, 30 minutes after arriving at the hospital.

The cardinal signs of active labor and transition that Sara recognized during Martha's massage were the following:

- Inability to lie still comfortably
- Focused breathing and difficulty talking as she was having contractions
- Contractions every 3 to 5 minutes
- Nausea and vomiting (a common symptom at transition)

If Martha had been in early labor, it would have been an excellent time to get a massage. In active labor, Martha also appreciated the massage; however, her birthing center was a 1-hour drive from the therapist's office. With no previous birth history, there was no way to gauge her proclivity toward a long or very short labor. It is not possible to predict the course of labor, but if she had had previous births that were very fast, or had had even one birth before, chances were good that she could have a relatively quick labor this time. Since she had been having contractions all day and because she was 3 cm dilated the day before *without* having had many contractions, and was having difficulty relaxing with them, there was clear indication that she was in active labor and likely progressing. When Martha said she was having contractions, Sara should have asked right away when her last cervical exam was and how far dilated she had been; the information, in this case, may have given her quicker clue to what was happening in her massage office on this day.

midwife examines the placenta after birth to be certain that it is intact and to look for any abnormalities that might indicate problems for the baby.

Once the placenta is delivered, many women experience a profound state of bliss or excitement. The endorphins are circulating through her body, she has just finished what could be likened to a marathon with regard to her physical and psychic workout, and she may have a great sense of accomplishment as well as overwhelming emotion at meeting her baby for the first time. Some women may also feel ambivalence, exhaustion, or distance from the newborn and herself.

If the woman had any perineal tears or cutting at delivery, she will need to have stitches, which will be done now.

Characteristics of the placental delivery are the following:

- Contraction Frequency: Usually one big contraction to release the placenta
- Duration: Normally occurs 5 to 30 minutes after delivery of the baby and takes 1 to 2 contractions to deliver
- Mother's Experience: a woman will experience any or all of the following:
  - Moderate to strong cramping
  - Mixture of feelings of pride, exhaustion, exhilaration, hunger, and thirst
  - Sometimes heavy bleeding or cramping during or after delivery of the placenta

Massage for Placental Delivery

- The mother is usually, at this point, engaged with the baby and not paying much attention to the placental delivery. Avoid touch that is distracting to her at this time.
- There are many complementary bodywork modalities that are beyond the scope of this book but that are useful for helping the placenta to detach if it is stuck or to help stop bleeding.
- Massage of the uterus is used by the doctor or midwife after placental delivery to stimulate the uterus to contract, expel clots, and stop bleeding.
- Gentle touch to the mother's head may be appropriate.
- Perform a neck and shoulder rub if the mother is without the baby and feeling tense.

CHAPTER SUMMARY

It is an exciting opportunity to share in the labor and birth journey of your client. Key elements for providing optimum attention to your client during labor include using long, slow strokes that flow out from the center of the body to the extremities. Focus on areas that can relieve muscular stress, and when appropriate, encourage relaxation through breathing, visualization, and affirmations incorporated with your touch. The simplest touch—holding a hand, squeezing the toes, pressing onto the sacrum—can profoundly and beneficially impact a woman's ability to relax. Stay focused and grounded and take regular breaks to refresh yourself and provide the most renewing and beneficial touch. If you are present throughout labor, your attentive energy will be rewarded by sharing in this most intimate and profound experience as a new life emerges into the world and takes her or his first breath.

CHAPTER REVIEW QUESTIONS

1. Define the phases and stages of labor.
2. Describe three labor support tips that can enhance the cultivation of an environment of safety and relaxation. Explain why this is important.
3. A woman with an epidural will be monitored continuously and should not be feeling any or many sensations related to her contractions. What should the massage therapist pay attention to at this time? Explain why massage after epidural anesthesia may still be very valuable for a woman in labor. What contraindications apply to bodywork and epidurals?
4. Read the breathing and visualization practice. Try each one. How do they make you feel? Can you relate to the imagery? What would work better for you? Practice guiding someone through a visualization after identifying imagery that they specifically relate to.
5. Discuss the use of two different complementary modalities useful for supporting a woman during labor. Describe the benefits of each.
6. Describe a labor situation for which the following techniques may be especially beneficial:
   a. Foot massage or reflexology
   b. Drawing energy down the body
   c. Abdominal massage
7. Describe general bodywork techniques you might use with a woman who is in transition and having fear and resistance to the experience.
8. A client has been laboring in her bed for 3 hours. Her cervix has been at 5 cm dilation without change for that time and the contractions seem to be less strong than before she got in bed. What might she try doing to stimulate labor? What type of bodywork might you suggest that could be helpful?

9. Explain why a massage therapist might be at increased risk for injury during labor massage. Name three ways you could avoid strain to your body when working with laboring women. Identify three tools you could use to preserve your hands when offering touch for hours on end during labor.

10. Consider and describe what bodywork techniques could easily be taught to the partner or labor companions if they wish to support the laboring woman with more touch.

REFERENCES

1. Beers M, Berkow R, eds. Merck Manuals Online Medical Library. Home Edition for Patients and Caregivers. Merck & Co. 1999–2007. Available online at http://www.merck.com/mmhe/sec22/ch261/ch261b.html.

2. Nathanielsz PW. Comparative studies on the initiation of labor. Eur J Obstet Gynecol Reprod Biol 1998; 78(2):127–132.

3. Beshay VE, Carr BR, Rainey WE. The human fetal adrenal gland, corticotropin-releasing hormone, and parturition. Semin Reprod Med 2007;25(1):14–20.

4. Jackson D. With Child: Wisdom and Traditions for Pregnancy, Birth and Motherhood. San Francisco: Chronicle Books, 1999.

5. Pukui MK. Hawaiian beliefs and customs during birth, infancy, and childhood. In: Meltzer D, ed. Birth: An Anthology of Ancient Texts, Songs, Prayers, and Stories. New York: North Point Press, 1981:129-136. [originally from Occasional papers of the Bernice P. Bishop Museum. Vol 16, No 17 (March 20, 1942). Honolulu: Bishop Museum Press].

6. Cammu H, Clasen K, Van Wettere L, et al. To bathe or not to bathe during the first stage of labor. Acta Obstetricia et Gynecologica Scandinavica 1994;73(6): 468–472.

7. Grodzka M, Makowska P, WielgoÊ M, et al. [Water birth in the parturients' estimation] [Article in Polish]. Ginekol Pol 2001;72(12):1025–1030.

8. Cluett ER, Nikodem VC, McCandlish RE, et al. Immersion in water in pregnancy, labour and birth. Cochrane Database Syst Rev 2004;(2):CD000111. Update of: Cochrane Database Syst Rev. 2000;(2):CD000111.

9. Geissbühler V, Eberhard J. Waterbirths: A comparative study: a prospective study on more than 2,000 waterbirths. Fetal Diagn Ther 2000;15(5):291–300.

10. Motha G, McGrath J. The effects of reflexology on labour outcome. Nursing Times, Oct. 11, 1989 C, Forest Gate, London, England.

11. Liisberg, GB. Easier births using reflexology. Tidsskrift for Jordemodre, No. 3, 1989.

12. Ingram J, Domagala C, Yates S. The effects of shiatsu on post-term pregnancy. Complement Ther Med 2005;13(1):11–15.

13. Chung UL, Hung LC, Kuo SC, et al. J. Effects of LI 4 and BL 67 acupressure on labor pain and uterine contractions in the first stage of labor. J Nurs Res 2003;11(4): 251–260.

14. Lee MK, Chang SB, Kang DH. Effects of SP6 acupressure on labor pain and length of delivery time in women during labor. J Altern Complement Med 2004;10(6):959–965.

15. Chang SB, Park YW, Cho JS, et al. 30 minutes of pressure on SP 6 reduces C-section rate: Taehan Kanho Hakhoe Chi 2004;34(2):324–332.

16. Odent M. The fetus ejection reflex. Birth 1987; 14(2):104–105.

17. Lothian J. Do not disturb: the importance of privacy in labor. J Perinat Educ 1004;12(3): 4–6.

18. Goldsmith J. Childbirth Wisdom From the World's Oldest Societies. Brookline, MA: East West Health Books, 1990.

19. Dunham C. Mamatoto: A Celebration of Birth. New York: Penguin Books, 1991:52.

20. Opler ME. Myths and tales of the Jicarilla Apache Indians. In: Meltzer D, ed. Birth: An Anthology of Ancient Texts, Songs, Prayers, and Stories. New York: North Point Press, 1981:103–107. [Originally from Childhood and Youth in Jicarilla Apache Society. In Publications of the Frederic Webb Hodge Society Publication Fund. Vol.5. Los Angeles: The Southwest Museum/Administrator of the Fund, 1946.]

21. Herskovits MJ. Haitian birth customs. In Meltzer D, ed. Birth: An Anthology of Ancient Texts, Songs, Prayers, and Stories. New York: North Point Press, 1981: 108–114. [Originally from Life in a Haitian Valley. NY: Alfred A. Knopf, 1937.]

CHAPTER 10

COMMON COMPLAINTS DURING LABOR

LEARNING OBJECTIVES

After reading this chapter, you should be able to:

- Describe six complaints or conditions of labor for which bodywork can be helpful.

- Describe bodywork techniques that can be applied in a variety of maternal positions.

- Explain reasons why labor may slow or stall and describe how touch can help improve the situation.

- Describe the use of visualization or verbalizing feelings to benefit a stalled or slowed labor.

- Explain one common reason for a woman to experience "back labor" and describe ways of using bodywork and positioning to address the discomfort associated with it.

- Describe four common reasons for experiencing back pain during labor.

One cannot predict exactly what a woman will encounter as she steps onto the path of labor. However, there are some common conditions that many women experience at some point in the process. This chapter examines a few of these conditions and describes bodywork techniques that may be helpful for each. These techniques or approaches may or may not work; offering touch during labor requires flexibility and creativity. If one type of touch is not working, try another approach. Even if it worked fabulously for the last contraction, it may not work for the next. The massage therapist must learn the rhythm of each woman's dance in labor and the energy that best matches it and then be prepared for it all to change with the next contraction.

ANXIETY/FEAR

For a variety of reasons, anxiety and fear, sometimes progressing to panic, may arise during labor. A woman might begin to doubt that she has the strength or fortitude to make it through labor and begin to feel afraid, or the pain or sensations of her contractions may cause her anxiety. Sometimes memories of former sexual abuse are stimulated during labor by the sexual nature of birth, and suddenly a mother may have to confront feelings she has been keeping at bay. Sometimes there are concerns about the baby's well-being during labor, or there may be questions about the need for a cesarean section or other medical interventions, any of which can stimulate anxious thoughts and a stress response in the body. Hyperventilation may occur if a woman is feeling panicked and/or using inappropriate breathing techniques, leading to dizziness and increased anxiety that something is wrong.

General Treatment for Anxiety

Helping a woman to "ground" herself can allay anxious thoughts. "Grounding" is a term used to refer to making electrical wiring shockproof. In emotional grounding, the desired outcome is the same—we want to ground the mind and emotions in a safe container that can help prevent a client from experiencing an overload of energy or emotional shock, and yet still allow the natural flow of energy to move through her. Sometimes having the client inhale the scent of fresh, crushed pungent herbs, such as rosemary, sage, motherwort, or any green aromatic plants, can help ground her by connecting her to the support of the Earth.

Stay grounded yourself. If you are getting scared, your fear can be transmitted to her. This may mean that you must leave the room, take a walk, lie down for some time, or speak with someone who understands what is happening to help reassure you.

If she is hyperventilating or using erratic breathing, use nurturing touch while reminding her to slow her breathing, which will not only decrease hyperventilation dizziness, but also decrease anxiety as well. Make eye contact and tell her to breathe *with* you if she is having difficulty focusing. Remind her to breathe slowly into her belly, into her feet, and into her perineum. Sometimes fears can be released simply by having the woman acknowledge the fears verbally. If she can name the fear, the naming may break its chains or diminish how big it feels in her mind and she may perceive more clearly how to let go of it.

Do your own grounding techniques first if necessary before working with your client.

Specific Techniques for Anxiety

If you encounter a client who is struggling with anxiety during labor, try using the following touch techniques with her.

Hand Pressure

Hold her hand and press into the center of the palm (Figure 10.1). Firm hand-holding is reassuring and an acupressure point in the center of the palm supports calming energy. Firm pressure to the hand also stimulates neuropathways that can transmit pleasurable sensations faster than pain transmissions, reducing pain and helping ease anxiety.

Grounding the Feet

Hold onto her feet, pressing into the soles of her feet—the place of grounding earth energy—while making eye contact and speaking in reassuring tones and words to help soothe anxious thoughts (Figure 10.2). Squeeze and hold several of her toes together while encouraging her to breathe slowly into her belly.

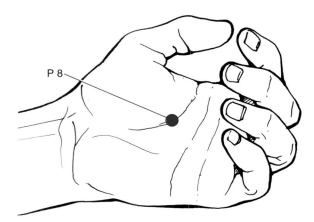

FIGURE 10.1   Hand pressure.
Hold her hand and press into the center of the palm. Firm hand-holding is reassuring, and an acupressure point in the center of the palm (P 8) supports calming energy.

Drawing Energy Down

Press on either side of her spine, from the neck to the sacrum, with both hands, applying pressure into her back as she exhales, releasing pressure and moving down the spine 1 hand-width on the inhalation. Alternatively, use long strokes or the two-person grounding stroke, as described in Chapter 9. Any of these will help draw her energy down and out of her head.

Circular Massage

Massage the temples, chest, and solar plexus with slow circles and gentle effleurage while encouraging her to breathe slowly. To enhance the work, massage with the following mixture of essential oils added to 2

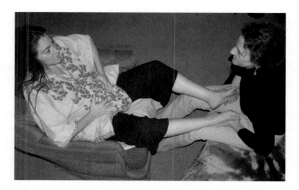

FIGURE 10.2   Grounding the feet.
Hold onto her feet, pressing into the soles while making eye contact and speaking with reassuring words that soothe anxious thoughts.

tablespoons of carrier oil: 2 drops of neroli and 4 drops of lavender.

Chakra Massage

Emotional or spiritual issues, whether obvious or subtle, can cause anxiety and can be addressed with touch and attention to the centers of energy in the body—the **chakras**. A Chakra is a Sanskrit word referring to a spinning vortex of energy located in specific areas of the body. Seven primary chakras are spaced between the crown of the head and the base of the spine and deal particularly with emotional and spiritual energy. The chakras are open funnels of energy, on the front and the back of the body, with the top and bottom chakras open toward the sky and earth. Incorporating awareness of the emotional aspects of the chakras can deepen the quality and enhance the effectiveness of body-mind bodywork.

- *Solar plexus:* This is a place often associated with power and self-assurance. If she is holding her breath, hyperventilating, or seems tight in her solar plexus/diaphragmatic area, place your palms gently over the solar plexus. Breathe with her and remind her that she has all the resources she needs within her to move through this birth. Slide your hands down to her belly, helping to root energy in the center of her body.
- *Third eye:* If she seems to lack trust in the birth process, hold her head in your palms and touch on her "third eye," between and slightly above the eyebrows on the forehead. Hold there while the two of you breathe together and envision awareness of and connection to the things that can give her emotional and spiritual strength.
- *Heart and womb:* If she seems concerned about her or the baby's well-being or difficulties with her support team, place one hand on her heart and one on her womb or sacrum. Make a connection between the two energetically, having her imagine bringing love to her womb from her heart. Encourage her to slow her breathing, to feel your hands on her body, and to let her breath fill up the spaces beneath your hands.

Breathing

Breathing is grounding. Intentional breathing reorients a woman's focus to a calmer place inside.

- Encourage her to bring her breath into her abdomen, making low, guttural sounds. Help her to avoid breathing high in the chest or making high-pitched throat sounds that lead to energy exiting through the head.
- Have her practice Ujjayi breathing (see Chapter 9).

Revisioning

What is the fear? What images does she associate with her fear? How does she verbalize her anxiety? Explore ways of revisioning these images with words and visualizations that are more positively reinforcing. For instance, Penny Simkin, a renowned physical therapist, doula, and childbirth educator, describes a woman who fears her baby will not fit through her "tiny tight opening." This imagery must be adjusted positively. Simkin suggests talking about the "little baby nuzzling its head down in that soft, stretchy place."[1]

If the mother expresses the belief that she will not be able to continue any longer or that the contractions are getting too strong for her to cope with, encourage her by helping her to visualize the rising and falling of the ocean tides and waves, imagining how well she is able to relax and ride those waves into a shore over and over again.

Positioning

The client might change positions if necessary, to ones that are more grounding and that help her feel the strength of her body:

- Walking brings attention to the feet.
- Squatting plants the feet on the floor.
- Sidelying is relaxing and may feel safe.
- Kneeling and resting forward on a partner's lap can feel supportive.

EXHAUSTION

In a long labor, energy reserves can become especially drained. Depending on each situation, a woman may need to either cultivate more energy in the moment (if it is time to push or there is no break in strong contractions) or find ways to relax and regenerate through rest. Below are suggestions for both relaxing and renewing energy and for stimulating energy.

Relaxing and Renewing Energy

- Apply warm compresses to the low back, low belly, and perineum.
- Suggest that the client might wish to immerse herself in warm water immersion in a pool, tub, or shower.

- Perform relaxing full-body massage with slow, soothing strokes to help her nap in between contractions and renew her energy. Rub her temples and jaw in slow, small circles. Massage her feet and slowly rotate her ankles and toes in circles.
- Suggest restful positions including sidelying and draping over a ball, rocking back and forth, and sitting in a rocking chair.

Stimulating Energy

- Press into the soles of the feet with your thumbs just below the ball of the foot in the center of the sole; this opens the doorway for her energetic grounding roots to draw in qi.
- Perform stimulating full-body massage.
- Perform friction rubbing to the sacrum and low back. This is enhanced by adding essential oils to the massage lotion: 3 drops each of clary sage and lavender, and 2 drops of peppermint to 2 tablespoons of carrier oil.
- Apply cool hydrotherapy cloths to the forehead, chest, wrists, and feet or have her take a cool shower.
- Suggest she practice whale or Ujjayi breathing (see Chapter 9).
- Use stimulating massage strokes to renew energy: tapotement to the shoulders and down either side of the spine.
- If she changes position, it may help change her view of the environment around her and shift her exhausted energy. Walking if she has been sitting for some time, or lying down or rocking on a ball if she has been walking may help her adjust her energy.

STALLED OR SLOW LABOR

Sometimes labor slows or stops altogether for a while. This could be due to a dysfunctional problem with the pregnancy and labor or, more often, could reflect emotional or physical blocks. It could also be that the uterus, baby, and mother's body are simply regenerating energy for a new round of contractions. If so, it can be a perfect time to have the client rest, take a bath, or sleep if possible, and allow things to take their own time. Even without regular contractions, the cervix could still be softening and effacing and the baby could be moving into a better position. The mother and supporters may take this time to be in a space of "no time, no mind."

It is also possible, however, that the stalled labor is due to problems such as cephalic-pelvic disproportion (the baby's head is larger than the pelvic outlet) or a malpresentation (such as a transverse lie or the head angled strangely transverse or another difficult position). In most of these conditions, waiting or doing bodywork techniques will not change the situation at hand and medical intervention may be needed.

In the hospital, when a labor slows, stalls, or has difficulty starting, Pitocin is used to help stimulate or augment contractions and encourage the labor along. Bodywork can help stimulate labor also, but for it to be really effective, one must additionally consider the multiple layers of a woman's personal life story. Many life issues affect birth. As you make choices about what type of bodywork to use in any particular situation, take a few moments to consider what may be transpiring on emotional or spiritual levels. Remember that the progress of labor often reflects the personality of the mother and/or her baby.

Many types of bodywork explore the mind-body connection; stay within your scope of practice while maintaining an awareness of the effect of emotions and psyche on birth. If the client's PCP determines that labor must be stimulated and approves of you using bodywork to assist in this effort, there are a number of techniques you can use.

Traditional Birth Practices:
Touch for Labor

Around the world, touch is not only a natural response in an effort to help a woman in labor, but it is also used to stimulate contractions and to ease labor pains.[2] In Jaipur, India, a midwife kneels over a laboring woman, massaging her abdomen and thighs to encourage contractions, before having her get up and walk again.[3] During pushing, a traditional midwife may use her foot or toe to apply supportive pressure to the mother's perineum to prevent tearing. In Yemen, a mother's community of women support her with touch, hugs, kisses, and holding continuously throughout labor.[4] An anthropologist describes women assisting at a birth in Mexico as hugging and holding the mother who was "surrounded by intense urging in the touch, sound, and sight of those close to her."[5] In a Nepali Newar village, a midwife rubs and pushes on the laboring mother's abdomen to encourage the baby to drop down against the cervix.[6]

General Treatment for Slow Labor

To help stimulate a slow or stalled labor, address important concerns in the following order, if appropriate:

1. Physical impediments to labor should be considered by the PCP and birth attendants, such as the baby's position, the mother's position, hydration/dehydration, a full bladder, or lack of movement.

   To address these impediments, the client might try the following: changing position; changing the environment (music, activity); if appropriate and desired, she may want to get into or out of a shower or tub; you might help her and all the labor companions to monitor fluid intake and stay well hydrated. Offer bodywork that can encourage a woman to surrender to the natural process of birth by incorporating visualizations; breathing techniques; and long, slow strokes while also reminding her that her body knows exactly how to do this. Focus on methods to help release the sacrum, pelvis, jaw, and neck. The more relaxed these areas become, the more easily energy will flow. Soothing or familiar music can enhance the mother's and supporters' abilities to relax. Help her to verbalize her feelings about coming to the completion of her pregnancy, and remind her of the joy of seeing her newborn soon.

2. Consider emotional impediments: fear, thoughts about the partner, sexual abuse, unrealistic expectations.

   To address these impediments, try the following: visualization and breath attention, grounding in the feet, and verbalizing fears.

We can also utilize traditional birth wisdom by investigating symbolic and metaphorical conditions of the birth: Look for anything that symbolically represents a freeing of energy and that may encourage the birth energy —untying knots, opening windows, loosening pulled-back hair, etc.

Specific Techniques for Slow Labor

The specific techniques in this section may be useful for stimulating a stalled or slow labor. In addition to the ones discussed in detail below, a number of techniques presented in earlier chapters are also useful, including the following:

- All techniques from the section "Bodywork Modalities Helpful During Labor" in Chapter 9
- The techniques for labor preparation in Chapter 7
- Contraction–relaxation technique in Chapter 9
- Two-person grounding stroke in Chapter 9

Full-Body Massage

Full-body massages allow a woman to relax and let her energy flow. Use long, slow, firm strokes. Effleurage and petrissage to the upper thighs, hips, and gluteals can enhance relaxation in this area.

Stimulating full-body massages help to shift and move "stuck" energy. Use brisk touch with tapotement, rocking, and jiggling.

Hands and Feet

General massage to the hands and feet can open the energetic pathways of the upper and lower body. Acupressure point Large Intestine 4 (see Figure 4.3)

Self Care Tips FOR MOTHERS:

Two Important Reminders

*R*emind your client of the following key self-care tips.

Stay Well-Hydrated

Dehydration leads to ineffective contractions and slow labor. An increase in fluid intake is necessary to keep up with the demands of active labor. Two cups of noncaffeinated drinks should be taken every hour.

Change Positions

If contractions are not strong in one position, use that position for rests, but then reposition again to find one that seems to elicit stronger contractions. Try to change positions at least every hour. Being on hands and knees, leaning over a table, walking, and upright positions often help to strengthen contractions.

also helps promote contractions and ease a difficult labor.[7]

Sacral Palming

With the client on hands and knees or in the sidelying position, place your palm on her sacrum, fingers facing toward feet if possible, and apply pressure. Move the palm incrementally down toward the coccyx with each of the client's inhalations, pressing in during her exhalation, releasing on the inhalation.

Sacral Foramen Stimulation

Use your thumbs, knuckles, elbow (carefully), large round-end eraser, or other implement to push into and make circles on the sacral foramen as shown in Figure 7.3. Pressure to the second foramen is especially effective in helping stimulate contractions. The client can be in any position in which you have access to her back.

Toe Hold

Hold the big toe pads on both feet and squeeze with a solid pressure, asking the client to imagine a stream of energy flowing from her head down through her toes.

Visualization

Offer visualizations that help to clear the spiritual and emotional blocks that may be preventing labor from commencing. Envision surrendering to the flow of great rivers, to the rising and falling of waves and tides. Imagine floating gently down rivers, trusting that its flow will take her ultimately to the great ocean. Envision seeing the baby being born and in her arms.

Jaw Release

A woman may develop frustration in labor when dilation is occurring more slowly than she had hoped.

The jaw is a common place to hold tension that develops from frustration and anger. Due to a "reflexive" relationship between the jaw and the perineum, tightness in the jaw might result in tightness in the cervix or affect the relaxation and dilation of the cervix. Helping to release the jaw tension can help release cervical tension and tension overall. See Figure 7.1 for one method of working with the jaw. The following tools are also helpful if the woman has a cervical "lip," where her cervix is nearly completely dilated, but a small stubborn bit of cervix has not released fully yet.

Changing Positions

For a slow labor, position changes are one of the primary useful tools to stimulate contractions. See Chapter 9 for more details about positioning. Below are two other positioning ideas.

- Hands and knees: This is especially helpful if the woman is in a place where she can go outside. Encourage her to crawl on her hands and knees, moving around making contact with the earth (or imagining earth beneath the floor). Encourage her to feel the touch of earth under her hands and knees and the way it supports her if she lowers onto her forearms and places her forehead to the earth. Suggest that she breathe in the smell of earth, make belly sounds, and release her worries into the earth.
- Squatting OM: The woman might hold onto her partner, the back of a chair, or a rope hanging from above and squat down deeply. As she squats on an exhalation she may want to make low and deep sounds or the sound of OM, breathing in as she stands again. Others may want to join in, together making the OM sound to massage with a sound vibration that can powerfully support and encourage opening. OM is a sound that in India is said to be the sound of the creation of the universe.

MASSAGE THERAPIST TIP   Have the Partner Massage the Client

Sometimes it is the closeness of a dear friend or partner that helps a mother feel safe enough to surrender yet another layer of resistance, expectations, or fear. Teach the woman's partner, if she or he is willing, to massage with warmed massage oils all around the mother's sacrum, low back, inner thighs, belly, and pelvic area. Encourage the use of soothing, sensual, circular, firm touch with repetitive movements to help release the area. Talking can also help release feelings and promote the flow of labor.

BACK PAIN DUE TO A POSTERIOR BABY

"Back labor"—feeling contractions in the back, rather than in the abdomen—may be a normal way for some women to experience contractions. For many, however, it has a basis in the baby being in a "posterior" position, with the baby's face toward the mother's abdomen, instead of toward her back (see Figure 9.2B). This position forces the back of baby's skull to push against the mother's sacrum with each contraction, and this bone-to-bone contact can cause the woman severe pain. Babies are positioned posteriorly in early labor in up to 25% of all labors.[8] These labors are generally longer and more painful and create more difficulty when pushing. For a variety of reasons, for some women and babies, this may be the best position for their birth, however.

When in a posterior presentation, the baby's spine is not always directly lined up with the mother's. More often, the baby is slightly to one side or the other, which gives the care providers a better chance at helping the baby move around to a more anterior position with massage or maternal positioning.

General Treatment for a Posterior Baby

It is possible that the position most commonly assumed by a pregnant woman will affect the baby's position in utero.[9] Many women work at jobs that require sitting at a desk for 8 hours a day, often causing her to collapse in the midback, with shoulders hunched forward and the pelvis tilting posteriorly. This posture confines the baby much more than when the mother is upright, walking, squatting, or repositioning regularly. Posterior-facing may become the baby's most comfortable position in this situation.

Specific maternal positions that can help expand the pelvic outlet or that make use of gravity can help the baby to rotate into a more comfortable or anterior position. Walking upstairs or flexing one hip by placing a foot onto a stepstool or chair can sometimes encourage repositioning. There are also massage techniques that can encourage the baby to move or help a mother cope with the discomfort of back labor. The mother, midwife, or attending care providers may be aware of positions that can be helpful for moving the baby. Techniques used for moving a posterior baby can be read about in midwifery journals and in many of the writings of Penny Simkin. (See Appendix B.)

One optimal position to help the baby move from posterior to anterior is with the mother on hands and knees or standing and leaning forward. This creates more space in the pelvis and allows gravity to help the baby to rotate. Other methods are recommended below. To be successful at all, the baby must be awake and active; if the baby is sleeping, she or he will not move just because the woman has moved.

Unless you are trained as a doula or skilled in labor support, follow the lead of the woman and birth companions. Massage her in the positions she chooses as opposed to directing her into different positions you think she should be in. As much as possible, the mother needs to choose positions that allow movement and expansion of the pelvis. You can massage her as follows:

- *Straddling a chair leaning forward on cushions.* This position gives good access to the back as you can see in Figure 9.11.
    - While the client is in this position, apply pressure to the sacrum and press with thumbs or fingers into the sacral foramen. If you can comfortably work on her feet, as well, stimulate the ovarian and uterine reflexology areas just below and around the ankles. Squeeze the outside edge of the little toe (Figure 6.13) to stimulate the acupressure point Bladder 67 that helps the baby to move.
- *Knee raise/lunge: standing with one leg up on a chair or steps.* The lunge position creates different space in the pelvis by rotating the symphysis pubis and encouraging a posterior baby to reposition. The pelvis opens on the side that the leg is lifted to, so if the baby is more definitively on one side, lift the knee of or lunge to the side where the baby's back is (Figure 10.3).
    - If the client is using this position, the therapist or partner can massage her low back or her shoulders, or apply pressure on acupressure point Gall Bladder 21 (Figure 4.3).
- *Sidelying*: If the PCP determines that the baby's back and occiput are more to one side, have the client lie on that side. For instance, if the baby's back is more to the mother's left side, with feet kicking toward her right, the mother should lie on her left side. If the woman wants to lie on her other side, place a couple of pillows under her abdomen and upper leg and have her lie forward from that side as much as possible, rather than directly perpendicular to the bed. If she lies with her hips straight up to the side, the baby may have a tendency to fall more deeply into a posterior position.
    - During sidelying resting, full-body massage can be done to help the mother relax, as well as belly massage to encourage the baby to move to anterior. (This should be done with the guidance of the PCP as to which direction the baby needs to move.)

avoid rocking backward, increase the pubic separation. If she has carpal tunnel syndrome, the pressure on the wrists when in the hands and knees position could increase pain. Have her fold her fingers under and place pressure on fists rather than on open palms, or have her use alternate forward positions such as leaning forward onto her forearms.

- *Walking/standing/leaning forward*: Gravity and upright positioning along with frequent walking can help the baby to move as well as descend into the pelvis. It can also improve oxygen flow to the baby and make contractions stronger. The client may wish to stand with her arms over her partner, slow dancing and rocking back and forth. She can also stand and lean forward over a counter or against a wall. Consider using music that encourages hip swaying and undulating hula or belly dancing.
  - Long strokes down the back or rubbing on the low back can be used during contractions when the mother has paused in the upright position.
- *Moving in bed*: Sometimes midwives will encourage their clients to move every 15 minutes, or every 3 to 4 contractions, from left sidelying, to sitting up, to right sidelying, to hands and knees. This can be exhausting for an actively laboring woman, but may help the baby to move.
  - Use massage techniques that are appropriate for each short-term position. This may include foot massage and acupressure, hand massage, head and neck massage, and relaxing strokes to the inner thighs and belly.

Other Techniques to Move a Posterior Baby

The following tools may help a baby to reposition from posterior to anterior.

Hot and Cold Therapy

Applying a cold pack on the client's abdomen, in the area of the baby's back, and a warm pack in the area you want the baby to move to may encourage the baby to move toward the warmth (Figure 10.4).

Belly Rubs

During labor, belly rubs sometimes help the baby to reposition. See the section "Belly Rubs" in Chapter 5. If the PCP has told you the baby's position and

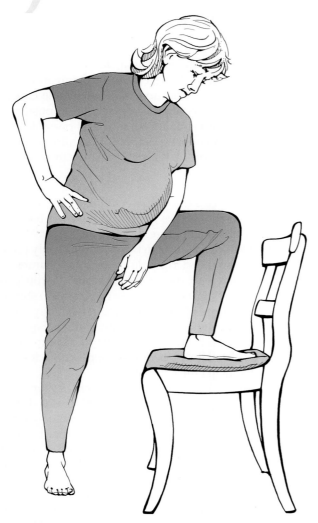

FIGURE 10.3   Knee raise/lunge.
The lunge position creates different space in the pelvis by rotating the symphysis pubis and encouraging a posterior baby to reposition. The pelvis opens on the side that the leg is lifted to, so lift the knee of or lunge to the side where the baby's back is.

- *Hands and knees:* Allow gravity to help the baby rotate. Resting over a birth ball, hanging over the back of a hospital bed with the head raised, or being in the standard hands and knees position and rocking the hips back and forth and side to side, might dislodge the baby so she or he can move into an anterior position.
  - Massage to the back and sacral pressure can be used easily in this position.

 CAUTION: If a woman has a separation of the symphysis pubis, use caution in the hands and knees position. Have her keep her knees closer together, avoid strain with movements, and

*H*ow does one know which way the baby is positioned? An experienced birth attendant will normally feel externally through the abdomen or internally through a dilated cervix which way the baby is facing. For the less experienced, an easy way to determine which position the baby is in is to feel where the most kicking is when the baby is awake. The back may be directly posterior or slightly to one side or another. The back is most likely opposite to where the activity is observed or felt. A mother usually can tell which way the baby is facing.

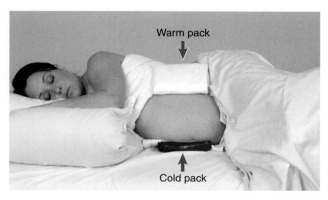

FIGURE 10.4   Hot and cold therapy.
Applying a cold pack on the client's abdomen in the area of the baby's back, and a warm pack in the area you want the baby to move to, may encourage the baby reposition toward the warmth.

direction of desired movement, and has approved abdominal massage, position the mother on the side that the baby is closer to, as explained above under sidelying. When the baby is awake, stand behind the sidelying woman's back, reach over her belly, toward the bed, and under the abdomen. Slide up and across her belly toward her upper side, thus encouraging the movement of baby's back toward the abdomen. Use gentle massage with firm touch to lightly "push" or "pull" her or him over. Do nothing forceful. Envision that the baby wants to move to a more comfortable position for the mother. With subtle touch encouragement, talk to the baby, asking it to rotate so that the back is toward the front of the woman's abdomen.

 CAUTION: Encouraging the baby to move with abdominal massage is appropriate only if you know which way the baby should move and have PCP approval or guidance. Never *force* the baby to move to a new position. The technique

should always be comfortable for the mother and baby. Apply the touch between, not during, contractions.

GENERAL BACK PAIN

At least 30% of women experience back pain at some point in labor.[12] But not all back pain is the continuous unrelenting pain associated with "back labor" and a posterior baby. There are several causes for back pain during labor. It may be due to the following:

- Posterior-positioned baby, as discussed above
- Functional contraction pain from labor that is just felt in the back rather than abdomen
- History of back injury
- Musculoskeletal strain or misalignment from pregnancy

General Treatment for Back Pain During Labor

There are various ways to help decrease back pain sensations in labor:

- General petrissage to the buttocks and hips can ease back pain.
- If within your scope of practice, use any of the complementary modalities and massage techniques mentioned in Chapter 9, including acupressure, hydrotherapy, visualization, reflexology, and changing positions.
- If the mother has been in the same position for some time, she may find that a new position decreases back pain.
- Use deep and continuous pressure and vibration to the hands and feet to close the gateways to the central nervous system through which pain is transmitted (see the discussion of Gate Theory in Chapter 8).

Self Care Tips FOR MOTHERS:

Belly Lifts

*B*elly lifts can alleviate back pain with a posterior baby, as well as speed delivery. With PCP approval, you might teach a woman, or her partner to do this technique. You could do it to her as well.

With the mother in the standing position, she can place her hands under her abdomen, palms against her belly, just above the pubic bone. As a contraction begins, she gently begins to lift the abdomen, as if pulling the baby up and in closer to her spine. This is not a stroking, but a holding, lifting the baby off the pubic bone and directing her or his position more upright for better alignment with her pelvis. Hold for the duration of the contraction. While lifting, the woman may rock her pelvis forward during a contraction and relax it back between contractions, as if doing pelvic tilts with contractions.

The partner or therapist can do this by standing behind the woman, and reaching around and under her belly to lift (Figure 10.5). More can be learned about this technique in JM King's book, *Back Labor No More*.

 CAUTION: Belly lifts are to be done only with birth attendant approval. At times this technique may speed a delivery. Be in a place where the mother is comfortable birthing the baby before attempting this maneuver!

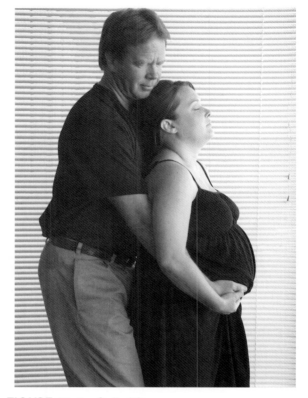

FIGURE 10.5   Belly lift.
Standing behind the client, place your hands below the belly near the pubic bone and lift the baby up and in to align the baby better with the mother's spine. While being done, it may relieve back pain and help a posteriorly positioned baby move down into the pelvis for an easier delivery.

- Distract the client's mind away from the fear of current pain or the expectation of future pain with visualizations and breathing techniques.
- Reduce stress by relaxing the client's body and mind, decreasing catecholamine release and increasing circulating oxytocin and serotonin.
- Encourage the client to focus on the sensations in the body, noticing them come and go, without reacting to them or labeling them as "pain."

In addition, if the baby moves, its position change may decrease back pain.

Specific Techniques for Back Pain During Labor

The specific techniques in this section are useful for back pain. In addition to the ones discussed in detail below, a number of techniques presented in earlier chapters are also useful, including the following:

- Sacral compression and unwinding (Chapter 5)
- Techniques for low back pain (Chapter 6)
- Rebozo massage, Ujjayi breathing, sacral counterpressure, straddling a chair and leaning forward position (Chapter 9)

Complementary Modalities:
Turning a Baby With Acupressure

*B*ladder 67 (seen in Figure 6.13) is a very specific acupuncture point that is often stimulated by acupuncturists with needles or burning moxa (the burning of mugwort plant on the point) to encourage a baby to move from one position to another.[7,10,11] Bladder 67 is the most common point for moving a baby, whether posterior, breech, or acynclitic (when the baby's head is not perfectly lined up with the birth canal). Acupuncture techniques are used after 34 weeks' gestation until a baby moves, though it should be stopped if the baby becomes overly active or has already moved to vertex.

The point can also be stimulated with acupressure by those trained in the modality. Generally it is more effective to use acupuncture or moxa. The use of moxa is not within the realm of massage therapy practice, but many lay people use moxa on this point with instruction from an acupuncturist. Under this supervision, moxa is usually applied to the point for 15 to 20 minutes, two times per day.[7,10] Some women use fingernails, a clothespin, the point of a paperclip, or a rounded stick to press into this point.

hydrotherapy and massage while preserving the wrists and fingers is to use a massage tool (Figure 10.6). Some people like to have rolling pins filled with ice rolled over the buttocks. Cover the skin with a towel first to soften the touch of the rolling pin and be sure to roll only over soft tissue areas and not directly onto bones. Frozen oranges, frozen juice cans, and frozen bags of peas or corn have also been used if no other cold pack is available.

Heat Therapy

Showers can "wash away" the pain, stimulating touch receptors that can override the pain messages. Spray warm water over the back, thighs, and belly. Warm packs can be made by putting damp towels or flax seed bags into a microwave for 1 minute at a time until warm. Apply to the low back as desired. ***

 CAUTION: If you use the microwave method of heating, test your item carefully to avoid starting a fire! Warm for 30 seconds at a time until you determine the appropriate length of time to heat that particular flax pack or towel. Do not apply *hot* packs to the abdomen; use gentle warmth that feels comforting to the touch with the hand or wrist.

Cold Therapy

Cold compresses to the low back and sacral area can offer relief. An alternate way of combining

Sacral Foramen Stimulation

Apply pressure with your palm to the mother's sacral foramen as in Figure 7.4. She can push back into your

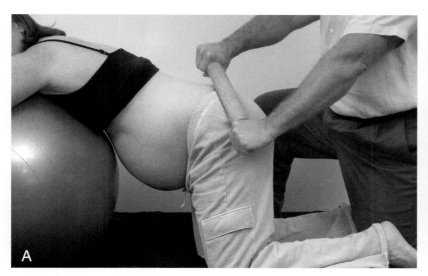
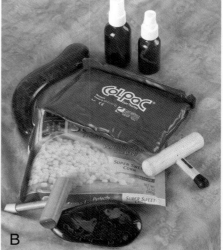

FIGURE 10.6   Massage Tools can be used to save tired hands.
(A) A rolling pin is a great tool to relieve the hands while still helping relieve muscular tension. (B) A variety of tools, such as heat and ice packs, aromatherapy, and deep tissue stones can be used as an alternative to providing touch with tired hands and fingers.

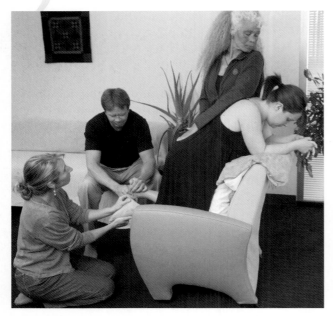

FIGURE 10.7   Ankle squeeze.
*Two people can hold onto either side of the foot directly
posterior to the medial and lateral malleoli while simultaneously
squeezing firmly around the edge of the heel. Encourage the
client to breathe deeply, imagining her breath flowing down the
length of her back and into her feet and relaxing with each
exhalation.*

pressure to help increase it and lessen your own
efforts. Reposition if she experiences sharp pain when
you do this. It should feel relieving, not painful.
Sometimes you may find a "sweet spot," a pressure
point in the sacrum that can totally relieve all the discomfort, without needing full palm pressure.

 CAUTION: Be aware of your own body positioning while giving sacral pressure — if it
helps her, you may find yourself doing it for
hours with every contraction. If you forget to
attend to your own posture, you could end up
with your own low back pain!

Ankle Squeeze

Two of you can work together to hold directly posterior to the mother's medial and lateral malleoli while
simultaneously squeezing firmly around the edge of
the heel (Figure 10.7). Envision grounding while
you encourage the client to breathe deeply, imagining
her breath flowing down the length of her back and
into her feet and relaxing with each exhalation.
Acupressure and reflexology are also helpful for
releasing the whole back and low back pain.

Sacroiliac Relief

1. With the client on hands and knees, stand
   behind her and press into her sacrum with
   both hands or forearms, sliding across the
   buttocks toward the belly using firm pressure, as though you are spreading open the
   sacroiliac joint (Figure 10.8A).
2. Continue sliding all the way around the ilium
   with the hands, pressing in as though closing
   the symphysis pubis, until coming to the center of the belly just above the pubic bone
   (Figure 10.8B).
3. Slide gently back to the starting point and
   begin again.

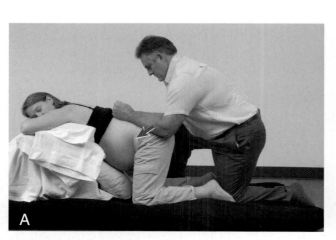
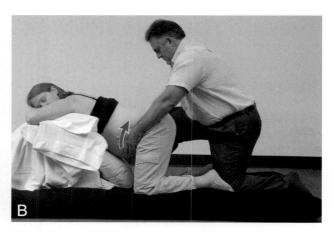

FIGURE 10.8   Sacroiliac relief.
*(A) Press into her sacrum with both hands or forearms, sliding across the buttocks toward the belly using firm pressure, as though you
are spreading open the sacroiliac joint. (B) Continue sliding all the way around the ilium with the hands, pressing in as though closing
the symphysis pubis, until coming to the center of the belly just above the pubic bone.*

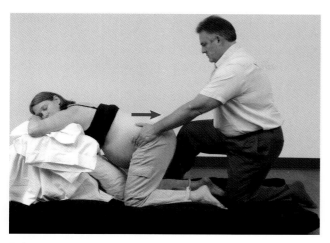

FIGURE 10.9   Hip pull.
Place your palms on the top of her iliac crest, wrapping your fingers around anteriorly. Pull back on her hips. This can help to open the front of the pelvis and relieve some hip and sacral pain.

4. Alternatively, begin at the center of the belly just above the pubic bone, and slide up and around to the sides, squeezing into the buttocks toward the sacrum, as if opening up the symphysis pubis area. This can help open the symphysis pubis joint as well as relieve sacral pain. Depending on the alignment of the pelvis and hips, one direction may feel much better than the other.

If one of these moves is uncomfortable for her, try the opposite one.

 CAUTION: If she has a separation of the symphysis pubis already, the second technique may

Complementary Modalities:
Acupressure on Large Intestine 4

Large Intestine 4 (Figure 4.3) is a point commonly used for labor pain. There are numerous ways to stimulate the point in labor. Commonly, the point is stimulated with finger pressure, but in one study, Large Intestine 4 was massaged with ice for 30 minutes in the beginning of active labor. The results were impressive: 86% of the twenty women studied had a significant decrease in pain intensity. More than half the women continued with the ice massage after the first 30 minutes because it helped so much.[13]

In the active phase of labor, put an ice cube in a bag or wrap in a cloth. Use the ice to massage Large Intestine 4 on one of the client's hands. Use strong pressure during each contraction over a period of at least 20 to 30 minutes. Repeat on the opposite hand.

not be appropriate, as it can pull on the pubic area. Stop either technique if it increases pubic pain.

Hip Pull

If the woman is in the hands and knees position, stand behind her and place your palms on the top of her iliac crest, wrapping your fingers around anteriorly. Pull back on her hips. This can help to open the front of the pelvis and relieve some hip and sacral pain (Figure 10.9).

MASSAGE THERAPIST TIP   Supporting Your Hands During Labor

Hands and fingers can become very tired if they are in service for hours. Remember the following tips to help save your fingers when doing thumb pressure or friction.

- Hold one thumb by wrapping the fingers of the other hand around the thumb to support it. Place one thumb pad on top of the nail of the other thumb to help press. Lean into the thumb with the center of your body, as opposed to pressing solely with the thumbs.

- Instead of using thumbs to work a specific spot, use a knuckle and roll the hand slightly downward to apply pressure into the spot.
- Remember to initiate work from your belly and your whole body rather than from the hands only.
- Shake your hands out between contractions and run cold water over your hands if they are getting sore. Watch the stress flow down the drain.
- Use elbows, forearms, a rolling pin, a tennis ball, or special massage tools as in Figure 10.6 to help soothe the woman in labor.

GENERAL LABOR PAIN

The pain of contractions can occur with or without back pain. It may be felt as intense energy; sharp squeezing; or unrelenting, overall, nonspecific pain. All tools described in Chapters 9 and 10, which relieve tension, free emotions, and offer support, are the techniques of choice. In addition, see "Complementary Modalities: Acupressure on Large Intestine 4."

CHAPTER SUMMARY

Support during labor typically requires that a variety of tools be used in conjunction with nurturing touch. Remember to explore and implement, when appropriate, tools and techniques from other modalities if you are trained in them. Hydrotherapy, acupressure, visualization, emotional processing, position changes, and positive encouragement all offer additional means of helping a woman relax and flow with the birthing energy. Remember that some women will not find any bodywork techniques helpful during labor. Some will choose to be alone and focus in their own way on contractions, while others will prefer to have medically initiated pain relief, such as narcotics or an epidural, instead of, or in addition to, touch. Engage willing birth companions in the process of touching whenever possible and appropriate, giving yourself a break and time for renewal.

CHAPTER REVIEW QUESTIONS

1. Discuss reasons why a woman may develop anxiety during labor and name four tools and techniques for addressing it: Describe two physical-body methods, one energy-body method, and one method of helping a client use her mind to calm anxiety.
2. Describe two ways massage can stimulate energy, and two ways it can be relaxing or sedating. Explain how each can be of benefit to a woman in labor.
3. Consider how long women have been giving birth, and describe how learning about traditional birth practices and the history of touch traditions could possibly help or influence your work with pregnant and laboring women.
4. Describe in what ways massage to the jaw might influence a slow labor.
5. Describe techniques/steps/actions that a laboring mother might take to stimulate contractions.

How could a massage therapist be of assistance with these?
6. In what ways might a woman's partner be especially effective in helping a woman alleviate fear or stimulate labor progress?
7. Explain how changing a mother's position could help a baby to reposition. Should a massage therapist help move a baby with massage?
8. Name four common reasons for back pain during labor. Describe three general bodywork techniques to help decrease back pain that is not due to the baby's position.
9. What types of techniques or movements are inappropriate for a client with a symphysis pubis separation?
10. Describe two hot/cold therapies that may help relieve pain during labor.

REFERENCES

1. Simkin P, Ancheta R. The Labor Progress Handbook. Malden, MA: Blackwell Publishing, 2000:73.
2. Hedstrom LW, Newton N. Touch in labor: a comparison of cultures and eras. Birth 1986;13(3):181–186.
3. Flint M. Lockmi: An Indian midwife. In: Kay MA. Anthropology of Human Birth. Philadelphia: F.A. Davis, 1982:211–219.
4. Drew CG. A child is born. She December 1988.
5. Jordan B. Birth in Four Cultures: A Cross-Cultural Investigation of Childbirth in Yucatan, Holland, Sweden and the United States. Prospect Heights, IL: Waveland Press, 1993:165.
6. Johnson B. We Know How to Do These Things: Birth in a Newar Village. Watertown, MA: Documentary Educational Resources[DVD]. 1997.
7. Deadman P, Al-Khafaji M, Baker K. A manual of acupuncture. Hove, UK. Journal of Chinese Medicine Publications, 2001.
8. Neri A, Kaplan B, Rabinerson D, et al. The management of persistent occiput-posterior position. Clin Exp Obstet Gynecol 1995;22:126–131.
9. Kitzinger S. Rediscovering Birth. New York: Pocket Books, 2000.
10. West Z. Acupuncture in Pregnancy and Childbirth. Oxford: Churchill Livingstone, 2001.
11. Neri I, Airola G, Contu G, et al. Acupuncture plus moxibustion to resolve breech presentation: a randomized controlled study. J Matern Fetal Neonatal Med 2004; 15(4):247–252.
12. Bahasadri S, Ahmadi-Abhari S, Dehghani-Nik M, et al. Subcutaneous sterile water injection for labour pain: a randomised controlled trial. Aust N Z J Obstet Gynaecol 2006;46(2): 102–106.
13. Waters BL, Raisler J. Ice massage for the reduction of labor pain. J Midwifery Womens Health 2003;48(5): 317–321.

PART III

THE POSTPARTUM PERIOD

The most important element of postpartum care is willingness to listen, which includes willingness to go to the mother on her schedule, when she needs you. Attention to physical healing is of course important, but more important in the long-term is that the mother feel well-nurtured and well-taken care of in the vital first days of motherhood.

JENNIFER ROSENBERG, PARENT EDUCATOR AND COFOUNDER OF NINO. IN: MIDWIFERY TODAY E-NEWS. SPRING 2002; ISSUE 61.

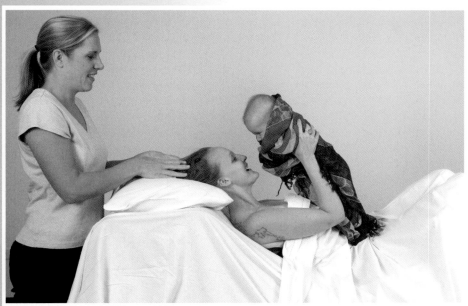

CHAPTER 11

REINCORPORATION: THE POSTPARTUM PERIOD

LEARNING OBJECTIVES

After reading this chapter, you should be able to:

- Describe physiological and structural changes occurring during the postpartum period.

- List and explain the benefits of massage during the postpartum period for both baby and mother.

- Describe the contraindications and precautions relevant to the postpartum client.

- Describe what areas of the body experience strains specifically related to mothering demands and how bodywork can help decrease associated discomfort.

- Explain five ways that a postpartum client's needs and bodywork precautions are unique to the postpartum period.

- Explain what kinds of concerns you'd be listening for during a postpartum health intake.

- Cultivate respect for the physical and emotional challenges of motherhood.

For 9 months your client imagined the day her baby would be in her arms. Now she has birthed the baby and perhaps a part of herself as well; all her attentions are focused on the new member of her family. The invisible mystery that grew inside—the placenta, the extra fluids, and of course, the baby—has entered the world outside the womb, and the mother is now face-to-face with a whole new life of challenges and changes both psychologically and physiologically.

Physiological shifts are dramatic and quick over the next 6 weeks of what western medicine considers as the **postpartum period** or *puerperium*, but subtle transformations continue for the next year or more. Massage for the new mother can help her to acclimate more easily to this new life and its accompanying demands for adaptation. The first half of this chapter describes fundamental concerns of the postpartum period and examines the areas of the body that undergo the most significant changes, while the second half addresses the benefits of massage and contraindications and precautions for bodywork.

PHYSICAL AND EMOTIONAL CHANGES

In the first weeks after birth, the areas of a woman's body that were most stressed during pregnancy and birth need special attention to readjust to the new demands of mothering. The perineal and abdominal muscles have been stretched and strained. Tonifying Kegel exercises, abdominal strengthening, and release of trigger points and fascial distortions will help restore full function of these muscles. The uterine ligaments have stretched to their maximum and now are finding their way back to their pre-pregnant size and job of holding the uterus at an appropriate level in the pelvis. Ligaments throughout the body have been affected by the hormone relaxin will gradually redevelop their stabilizing strength. A woman's core energy is often depleted and needs various forms of nourishment to replenish itself. Bodywork can help facilitate healing and recovery when addressing any of these concerns.

An average time for a woman's body to return to "normal" after birth is 6 to 8 weeks. By then, her postpartum bleeding should have stopped, her milk will have come in fully if she is nursing—or dried up completely if she is not nursing—and the postpartum cramping that helps the uterus **involute**, or shrink back to its nonpregnant size, should have diminished. Stitches from a laceration or episiotomy at delivery are likely healed, and any acute perineal pain gone. However, it may take much longer than 6 weeks to adapt to other changes and feel a complete recovery from pregnancy and birth! Your client will have ongoing fluctuations in her breast tissue if nursing. She may have a misalignment of her hips, a broken tailbone from delivery, or lingering aching in her muscles from a marathon labor. She may still be exhausted if she has not had adequate support or had space and time for rejuvenation. Though she had an immediate loss of weight after the delivery of the baby, placenta, and some of the extra body fluids from pregnancy, she may need 9 months or more to find her pre-pregnant shape, weight, and comfort in her body.

Helping relieve the strains related to labor, nursing, and/or possibly surgery is a massage therapist's first priority when working with a new mother. Attentive massage can address critical areas and help to prevent future complaints. Initially most problems occur in the area of core structural support: the pelvis and pelvic floor, the abdominals, and the low back. The midback and upper back and neck also develop strains as a mother spends time feeding, holding, lifting, and carrying her baby. Your client's vital energy will likely be depleted and need nourishing as well. A full-body relaxation massage will often be a welcome gift during this time to help work out the kinks and strains from labor. Swedish massage, deep tissue massage, neuromuscular therapy, myofascial release, and craniosacral therapy are all helpful during the postpartum period.

Remind your client of simple therapeutic self-care stretches that she can do regularly to help relieve strains and aching muscles, such as shrugging her shoulders, rolling her head and neck in circles in both directions, pelvic tilts, yoga, and walking.

Uterus

Immediately after delivery, the uterus shrinks from a size capable of holding a full-term baby, a placenta, and a quart of amniotic fluid, to the size of a small cantaloupe. Within the next 2 days, it will shrink even more, and after 2 to 3 weeks, it will be nearly back to its pre-pregnant size and will be difficult to palpate through the abdomen. In some cases, after delivery, the uterus may have dropped low down into the pelvic cavity or even prolapsed out of the vagina after delivery.

Bleeding from open vessels at the site of the former placental attachment continues for several weeks, gradually diminishing as the site scars over and is healed.

Many pregnancy hormones stop being produced immediately after the delivery of the placenta. Some postpartum depression can be expected due to this hormonal shift.

Cramping after delivery and during breastfeeding is caused by the uterine effort to constrict these vessels, prevent hemorrhage, and return the uterus to its pre-pregnant size.

Take note of the following regarding this area:

- Kegel exercises to strengthen the pelvic floor and therapeutic strengthening of the transversus abdominus help to minimize or prevent organ prolapse. These exercises can be taught to a client starting on the second postpartum day if she had a normal delivery and is ready to begin.
- Be aware that your newly postpartum client will likely want to wear menstrual pads during massage sessions to prevent leaking of vaginal drainage. She may also have painful, but normal, uterine cramping if she has just nursed the baby.

Perineum

In the first couple of weeks after birth, a woman may feel quite sore in her vagina and perineum. She may have micro-tears, lacerations, or stitches for an incision from an episiotomy. Her perineal muscles have stretched and her pelvic bones separated, and she may be experiencing swelling and stinging sensations when urinating.

Take note of the following regarding this area:

- Use caution with gluteal work and joint mobilizations that may pull on the perineal area and strain stitches.
- Healing of this area may be optimized with self-care hydrotherapy, such as sitz baths, and perineal exercises.

Ligaments, Low Back, and Pelvis

Relaxin continues to be produced for at least 6 to 8 weeks after birth or possibly longer. Relaxin's effect of softening ligaments can continue for months after birth and prolong the process of regaining her pre-pregnancy stability. The woman's pelvis and low back may ache from awkward positions in labor, pelvic expansion at birth, and poor posture throughout pregnancy, as well as from receiving epidural anesthesia, which can be a cause of lingering discomfort at the epidural insertion site.

Take note of the following regarding this area:

- A new mother's joints will still be hyper-mobile (see Chapter 2). Avoid excessive passive stretching.
- Address general areas of discomfort.

Abdomen

Some women will feel a loss of muscle tone and sagging in the abdomen and have concern about visible stretch marks. Stretch marks may stay for a lifetime; there are no cures for stretch marks, despite the marketing of special oils and salves. Any minor diastasis of the rectus abdominus from pregnancy will begin to return to a realigned state in the postpartum period.

Take note of the following regarding this area:

- If your client has more than a 2- or 3-finger-width separation of the recti, encourage her (with her PCP's approval) to explore abdominal exercises that can help correct this separation (see Chapter 3).
- Strengthening the transverse abdominus will improve core stability and tonify the abdomen.

Energy

The new mother has just had an extensive output of energy. During pregnancy, she was feeding an extra person within her body. At birth, she lost cellular fluids and blood and now is having rapid hormonal adjustments, placing her in a vulnerable and depleted state physiologically, though she may feel emotionally energized or euphoric. The baby now requires all her energy and attention, yet she also must cope with new body sensations, having family and friends visiting, and learning how to mother this particular and unique baby. This all may consume what little extra energy she may have.

Take note of the following regarding this area:

- Massage can help in the crucial regeneration of vital energies and a mother's reintegration process.
- Receiving massage can be a time of sanctuary for a new mother, a time for being nurtured and taking a short break from caring for others.

Emotional Changes

No longer the woman she was before birth, a new mother has been transformed through her birthing rite of passage. While often feeling overjoyed and inspired by her encounters with her new baby, a first-time mother is also adapting to her new roles as mother to this child, mother within the context of her society, mother within a significant relationship, and mother in relation to her own parents. It took 9 months for the woman to create and nurture the baby; it may well take another 9 months for the transformation and birth of her mother-identity to complete itself. Be aware that when your client comes for a massage, she may bring with her overwhelming feelings related to these adaptations, as well as from getting too little sleep and having constant anticipation about the needs of the baby. In addition, any of the following dynamics may be plaguing her in the midst of her birth euphoria: her relationship is likely shifting with her partner; older siblings may be resenting the loss of attention and begin acting out; she may be processing disappointment in her birth experience; or she may be falling into an overwhelming love and growing attachment for this new little life, leaving little room for any others in her life, including herself. She may have problems with lactation and feel frustrated, sore, or despairing about her difficulties in nourishing her baby. She may be missing the comfort and anticipation of the child growing inside her belly and feeling an inner emptiness. She may feel suffocated or trapped being at home alone and caring constantly for a demanding and helpless baby. She may be processing unresolved issues and unanswered questions about the birth. While the overriding feeling many women have is one of excitement and love, any of these factors mentioned above can contribute to her psychological-emotional status as her pregnancy hormones diminish.

Take note of the following regarding this area:

- Create nurturing space for your client and for whatever emotional state she is in; create a place where she can receive nurturing and ease herself through the adjustments to her new world.

BENEFITS OF AND PRECAUTIONS FOR POSTPARTUM MASSAGE

Below are discussed some of the benefits of postpartum massage for both mothers and babies. Also discussed are special considerations, preparation, and precautions for postpartum massage.

Traditional Birth Practices:
Postpartum Care

"Ilocanos mothers in the Philippines are given a ritual bath . . . and regular abdominal massages. Moroccan mothers are massaged with henna, walnut bar and kohl; traditional Hawaiian midwives give a vigorous circular lomi-lomi massage with their fingers, elbows and thumbs. . . . " [1]

Many traditional communities around the world have time and space built into their lives for women to care for one another. A new mother and baby are coddled and cared for, often isolated from the world at large for weeks or sometimes months after delivery. The postpartum period is considered a critical time of recovery and bonding. The mother must get to know the baby. She must allow the psychic and physical energy gates that opened during labor to close once again before she re-enters the demands or activities of the world or her community. Special nurturing foods and daily massage are given to the mother; if she is a first-time mother, she is taught how to care for her baby.

In Tibet, a new mother rests and recovers while she and the baby are cared for by her family. No visitors are allowed for days.[2] Acknowledging that the mother is newly born as well, the Mexican Maya wrap up the baby and mother and care for both for weeks with an attention and nurturing that we often devote only to newborns.[3]

In Sweden, for up to 8 years after the birth of her child, a woman has the option of taking as much as 21 weeks of paid leave during pregnancy and postpartum. This is followed by 18 months of parental leave during which fathers must also take at least 2 months off from work. In Norway, this leave lasts for 52 weeks. In Italy, new mothers who work full time in their first year postpartum are given a rest period at work of 2 hours per day.[4]

Benefits for the Mother

Postpartum bodywork is focused on helping a client regenerate, renew, and release. Whether or not she feels a need for special care, her body is still making numerous and rapid changes and she is still quite vulnerable to external influences. Most of those who will use this book do not live in a traditional culture, which may offer a new mother intensive caregiving (see "Traditional Birth Practices," above), but massage can at least address some of the client's needs during her recovery time.

One primary concern of a new mother is that she has opened and been exposed both psychically and physically to bring forth new life. Now, she needs support to gently close this expansion from birth. Physically, her ligaments must tighten, her pelvic bones close and realign, and her core support structure—the spine and supporting muscles, the pelvic floor, and the abdomen—must be strengthened. She must tend to her postural alignment as she adjusts to a nonpregnant shape and weight. Her internal organs—bladder and womb—need support through muscular toning of the perineals and abdominals, as well as uterine massage. (See Appendix B, "Mayan Abdominal Massage.") New discomforts related to mothering are developing and can be mediated with massage. With all these changes occurring musculoskeletally, hormonally, emotionally, and psychically during the postpartum period, bodywork is vital to assisting a woman's return to equilibrium by increasing the release of endorphins; rebalancing hormones; increasing blood flow; and reducing stress, anxiety, and depression. Massage can be a reminder to a woman that *she* needs nurturing as much as her baby does. Meaningful touch will help her to transfer that touch to her own child.

Benefits for the Baby

Postpartum massage benefits not only a mother, but her baby as well. Women who are massaged during pregnancy or the postpartum period touch their babies more often. Babies respond to this touch overall with faster development, greater social skills, stronger immune systems, and increased weight gain. One study asked new mothers during the first day after birth to touch their babies with skin-to-skin contact for 1 hour longer than they would have normally and to add an extra 5 hours of touching over the next 3 days. When these mothers were observed 1 month later, they were found to make much more frequent nurturing contact with their infants than mothers who only gave the routine contact. The researchers returned 5 years later to test the children; those who had received the extra touch were uniformly found to have higher IQ and language test scores than the children who did not have the extra touch.[6]

See Table 11.1 for a list of benefits of bodywork during the postpartum period.

Special Considerations

A client who has given birth within the past 6 to 12 weeks will need the therapist to do a thorough health

BOX 11.1 | Attending to the Postpartum Client

When seeing postpartum clients, the massage therapist might:

- Review pregnancy and birth health history
- Assess posture and hip alignment
- Assess abdominal muscles for diastasis recti and need for abdominal strengthening
- Offer tonifying and renewing bodywork appropriate for the postpartum period

- Assess need for psoas strengthening or strengthening
- Create a safe space where the client may find relief from daily stresses
- Encourage the use of well-fitting, supportive nursing bras to help relieve and prevent upper back strain

intake and to observe special needs and issues relevant to the postpartum period. Review the following considerations before beginning work and see Table 11.2 for a list of five basic postpartum concerns for bodyworkers.

Positioning

A general full-body massage can be appropriate for the healthy postpartum woman, but she may need to use the sidelying position if her breasts are large, sore, or leaking or if she wants to hold or nurse the baby during the session. If she prefers to be prone, try a pillow under the ribs and abdomen to help take pressure off her breasts or use special foam cushions with cutouts for the breasts.

Baby and Mother

Women in the early postpartum period may want to or may only be able to receive a massage by bringing the baby with them or by receiving house calls. Be aware of a new mother's concerns and challenges in making time for her personal nutruting and realize that it is not unusual for a mother to be late for a session due to last minute nursing, diapering, emotional nurturing, etc. Just as it is recommended to allow extra time for your pregnant clients, you may want to do the same with your postpartum clients as well.

Be prepared to work with your client in adapted modes so that the baby can accompany her. You will need to allow extra time for positioning and your

Table 11.1	Benefits of Postpartum Bodywork
Reduces Aching Muscles	• Reduction of aches and stress accumulated during pregnancy and labor, including headaches, backaches, sore muscles, neck and shoulder discomforts, and abdominal discomforts
	• Decrease of muscle tension associated with nursing and other mothering activities
Improves Posture	• Assists return to pre-pregnant physiology and posture, including realignment of the pelvis
Provides Emotional Support	• Can be a source of emotional and physical support during a possibly stressful time
	• Possible decrease in risk of postpartum depression[9,10]
	• Can be an encouragement and reminder for a mother about self-care and self-honoring, in a time when most attention is being focused on the baby
Hastens Recovery	• Offers nurturing while in recovery from cesarean section
	• Decreases formation of adhesions [11]
	• Uterine massage helps decrease risk of excessive postpartum uterine bleeding[8] and uterine or bladder prolapse
	• Exercises taught by massage therapists help mothers tone and strengthen their abdominals, perineals, and psoas
• Benefits Breastfeeding	• May increase lipids, solids, and casein in breast milk[12,13]
	• Decreases risk of clogged ducts and mastitis[14-16]
• Benefits Intestines	• Can encourage bowel evacuation, decreasing constipation[17,18]
• Benefits Baby	• Nurturing touch to the mother leads her to touch her infant with more awareness and confidence
	• The mother and family can be taught infant massage skills, to enhance, promote, and increase meaningful contact between the infant and family [9]

Table 11.2	Five Postpartum "Bs" for the Bodyworker to Consider: Baby, Belly, Blood, Bottom, and Breasts
Baby	• The new postpartum mother may need to bring her baby with her to receive bodywork, or she may need house calls if she cannot get away.
	• Lifting, nursing, and carrying the baby are activities that will impact and strain her musculoskeletal system, so teach posture correction and proper body mechanics, and address muscular tension with bodywork.
Belly	• A woman's belly was stressed and stretched in pregnancy and birth: check for diastasis recti, encourage abdominal toning, and address scarring if she had a cesarean section or tubal ligation postdelivery.
Blood	• Vaginal bleeding may continue for several weeks after birth. Be aware that newly postpartum clients will likely want to keep their underwear on during massage sessions and will be wearing a menstrual pad.
	• Use universal precautions (gloves) when handling linens that have become soiled with milk or leaking blood if her absorbent pads were inadequate.
	• Maintain blood clot precautions for at least 6 weeks postpartum when working on the legs.
Bottom	• Your client may have stitches in the perineal area from lacerations or episiotomy. Avoid moving gluteal muscles and hip adductors in such a way that might pull on perineal stitches or lacerations.
	• Encourage toning exercises for the pelvic floor to promote healing and prevent organ prolapse.
Breasts	• Sore and leaking breasts may affect positioning during massage.
	• Have towels available to help absorb leaking breast milk.

client's attendance to the baby's needs. If necessary, your client can lie on the table in the sidelying position and hold or nurse the baby there (Figure 11.1A). This may be the best option for a woman to receive a massage if the baby will not rest quietly without being held close or nursed. While having the baby present at a massage can be fun, it may not be the most relaxing experience for the mother, especially if the child does not sleep through the session. A good option is to have a helper along to care for the baby in the waiting room while mother receives her massage.

Other options include having the client in the semi-reclining position, with the newborn on her knees and lap. (Make sure her knees are spread slightly and supported on a bolster to make a space for the baby to rest as in Figure 11.1B.) Or, a mother may choose to have the baby napping near the massage table.

House calls are particularly welcome during this period, when it may be difficult for a mother to get away.

When the baby comes with your client to a session, use the opportunity, if appropriate, to share with your client ways of offering nurturing touch to her infant. Whether or not you have studied infant massage, general effleurage is normally beneficial, and simple strokes along the extremities, back, and abdomen can be demonstrated if the baby is in a relaxed, alert state. More advanced infant massage is currently offered in a variety of certification programs.

Preparation

After a client has given birth, ascertain the client's birth history and appropriateness of bodywork by conducting a thorough health intake before commencing work with her.

How Soon to Begin Massage

Gentle massage can be initiated 24 hours after delivery, assuming that there have been no complications during delivery or afterward. Adhere to all precautions, especially using clot precautions for at least 6 weeks after delivery (see "Embolism" below).

Know the Birth History

Be aware of any complication that may have occurred in pregnancy or labor and the consequent physical and emotional problems that may still be lingering because of it. This could include conditions such as preeclampsia, emergency surgery, infection, retained placenta, deep laceration or episiotomy, or prolonged bed rest before labor.

 CAUTION: Get a doctor or midwife release before beginning postpartum massage if the client is still in the hospital for observation or if she had complications during pregnancy or birth.

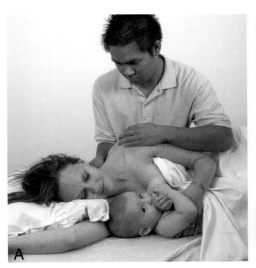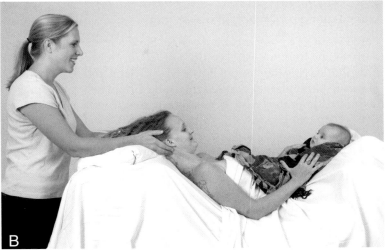

FIGURE 11.1   Positioning for a mother holding her infant during massage.

Be prepared to work with your client in adapted modes, so that the baby can accompany her if necessary. (A) Sidelying position. If the baby is fussy when not held, the mother can hold or nurse the baby in the sidelying position. (B) Semi-reclining position. If the sidelying position is not comfortable, the client can try the semi-reclining position, with the baby resting on her bolstered knees.

Health Intake

The following health intake questions can help assess risk factors in the postpartum period that might require precautions or medical release for bodywork. Following each is the associated concern or action that the therapist should have or take.

- *Did she have any problems or high-risk conditions during pregnancy, labor, or birth (preeclampsia, high blood pressure, postpartum hemorrhage, etc.)?* If so, obtain a release from the primary care physician if she is less than 3 weeks postpartum or is still being observed by her health care team.
- *Did she have a postpartum surgery: tubal ligation, cesarean section, or perineal lacerations or episiotomy?* Be aware of scarring, stitches, or other postsurgical concerns.
- *Is she currently breastfeeding? Is she having any related problems?* She may be leaking milk, wanting breast massage, or having emotional tension or anxiety related to nursing difficulties or waiting for her milk to dry up.
- *What are her current complaints?* Current muscular strains and tension may indicate the need for instruction in proper body mechanics and postural correction for standing, sitting, and nursing.
- *Does she have a diastasis of the recti muscles or of the pubic symphysis?* Encourage abdominal

strengthening. Specific corrective exercises can be taught by a qualified physical therapist. Your client can be referred to a chiropractor for a pubic symphysis separation.
- *Does she have varicose veins, phlebitis, or known deep vein thrombosis (DVT)?* Caution must be maintained with regard to blood clots and varicosities.
- *What is the baby's current condition?* If the baby was born premature or has other problems, your client will generally have more emotional stress as well as muscular tension.

Precautions

Know the contraindications and warning signs listed below that might indicate alterations in your work with postpartum women. *Note:* All standard massage precautions and contraindications are applicable in the postpartum period.

Essential and Scented Oils

Essential oils and scents used topically in massage oils, creams, or soaks and compresses are absorbed through the skin and could be absorbed by a nursing baby from a mother's skin or theoretically from her breast milk.

Case Study 11.1:
MASSAGE FOR THE MOTHER AND BABY

Paula wanted a postpartum massage. However, as a first-time mother, she could not comfortably imagine leaving her infant for 2 hours. Sara, the massage therapist, suggested that she bring her newborn daughter with her. Paula arrived with Zoe asleep in a car seat.

Sara positioned Paula on the massage table in the sidelying position, as Paula did not want to be prone on her breasts, which were sore and full with milk, and she wanted to be able to see Zoe easily if she stirred. Within moments after Paula lay down on the table, Zoe awoke and began to fuss, and Paula got up to make her comfortable. Moments after Paula got on the table again, Zoe began to cry. Paula brought Zoe onto the massage table with her and held and nursed her in the side-lying position, while Sara massaged Paula's feet and legs. Zoe soon fell asleep again, but Paula did not want to move her back to the car seat, fearful that she would awake. She also felt nervous holding her while in the sidelying position, worried that if she relaxed too much, she might let the baby fall off the side of the table.

Sara suggested they change position to the semi-reclining. In this position, Paula was able to let Zoe sleep on and between her thighs, without feeling that she had to hold onto her so tightly. Sara was able finish the session for Paula by working on her head, neck, shoulders, and arms. By then, Paula was relaxed enough to allow Sara to

move Zoe, now sound asleep, to a blanket on the floor. Zoe slept for the next 30 minutes while Sara finished massaging Paula in the semi-reclining position, working on her legs and abdomen and reaching around her belly and her sides to work on her low back. Toward the end of the session, when Zoe awoke again, Sara took the opportunity to demonstrate to Paula a few infant massage techniques with Zoe.

Sara had worked with many postpartum women, some of whom chose to bring their babies with them to the massage. Each situation was unique in how to manage the needs of the child and mother, as well as those of the massage therapist. Sara always suggested that the mother bring someone to take care of the infant while she received a massage, so that the client could have the optimal relaxing experience. When this was not possible, she would encourage the mother to bring her child into the massage office and adapt her positioning so the client could hold the baby during the massage, or have him or her close by. Sara was interested in providing massage for the new mother in whatever way would most optimally suit her and her new baby, knowing that any nurturing touch would be beneficial for both mother and infant. The sessions were not always as relaxing as a massage would have been without the infant present, but clients appreciated Sara's flexibility.

 BODYWORK PRECAUTIONS:

- Avoid the use of any scented oils or lotions on breastfeeding mothers unless you have been educated as to which essential oils are appropriate or beneficial during the postpartum period.
- Instruct your client to wash her breasts prior to nursing to remove all oils, lotions, and scents used for massage and prevent the baby from ingesting the oil directly from her skin.
- More detail of the use of aromatherapy and appropriate oils during the postpartum period is beyond the scope of this book. For resources, see Appendix B.

Embolism and Varicose Veins

Embolism, or the blockage of a blood vessel by a migrating blood clot or other foreign material (such as an air bubble or amniotic fluid), is the leading pregnancy-related cause of maternal death in the United States. The majority of these deaths occur during the *postpartum period*. While the occurrence of DVT is still rare, the postpartum period, as compared to pregnancy, has a 5 times greater risk for the development of DVT and a 15 times greater risk for the occurrence of a pulmonary embolism.[5,6]

Blood clots continue to be a concern for at least 6 weeks after delivery while the fibrinogen and blood clotting factors are readjusting. Risks are especially increased for women who have undergone cesarean or other surgery during, or immediately after, birth.[7] Women who have had a previous blood clot are at a higher risk for developing another clot during pregnancy or in the postpartum period.

 BODYWORK PRECAUTIONS:

- Continue all the contraindications related to varicose veins and DVT, including medial leg massage contraindications, for at least 6 weeks after delivery. This may be longer if she has pregnancy-related medical issues and is still being watched by her PCP for more than 6 weeks postpartum. (See Chapter 4, Precautions and Contraindications for Bodywork During Pregnancy).

Postpartum Hemorrhage

A postpartum woman is at risk for hemorrhage up to 1 to 3 days after delivery. Hemorrhage most commonly occurs due to uterine atony, or the inability of the uterus to contract effectively. Those at highest risk for atony include those with multiple gestation, those who have had more than five children, or had a very long labor or a very large baby. Uterine massage is one of the first actions used for preventing or stopping excessive bleeding.[8] A mother usually is taught how to massage the top of her uterus, or fundus, by her midwife or doctor.

 BODYWORK PRECAUTIONS:

- If a woman did have a hemorrhage, or is at risk for one, avoid deep, circulatory-stimulating full-body massage in the first 3 to 4 days postpartum, utilizing instead gentle Type II work and focused techniques addressing specific areas of tension.
- A woman who bled significantly at or after birth may be anemic and experiencing fatigue or dizziness. Be aware of the possibility of dizziness from postural hypotension when having this client stand after a massage. Have her sit for a moment before standing.
- Keep passive stretches and self-care exercises simple and slow until the client recovers her strength and blood!

Surgical Incision

A woman may have incisions from a cesarean section, postpartum tubal ligation, or episiotomy.

 BODYWORK PRECAUTIONS: See Chapter 13 for details about care after surgery.

Gestational Hypertension/Preeclampsia

If the mother had special attention during labor because of preeclampsia or very high blood pressure, she may need to be monitored for up to 3 weeks after birth as preeclamptic conditions can still progress to eclamptic seizures during the postpartum period (see Chapter 4).

 BODYWORK PRECAUTIONS:

- A client may remain on bed rest after delivery if her blood pressure and laboratory test results indicate she is still at risk. Bodywork in this situation requires a medical release and should be gentle and cautious: breathing and visualizations, reflexology, gentle acupressure, and Type II bodywork are all helpful during this time.
- Simple stress-relieving activities, such as foot rolls and shoulder shrugs, are useful to help relieve some body aches, but more strenuous activity should be avoided until the client's blood pressure has returned to normal and she has been cleared from danger by her health provider.

Separated Symphysis Pubis and Unstable Joints

The effects of the ligament-relaxing hormone, relaxin—such as sacroiliac joint hypermobility—are present for months after delivery. Due to relaxin's effects on ligamentous structures, some women can experience a separation of the pubic bone during pregnancy or the postpartum period.

 BODYWORK PRECAUTIONS:

- Be aware of current symphysis pubis separation before beginning stretches or bodywork that involve abduction of the legs or hips or that may stretch the pelvic area.
- Avoid excessive stretching of the joints.
- A separation may realign itself weeks or months after delivery or may need referral for chiropractic or osteopathic attention.

Body Fluids

A new mother may be leaking breast milk and still bleeding from her uterus for several weeks after delivery.

 BODYWORK PRECAUTIONS:

- Your client will likely keep on her underwear and wear a menstrual pad to avoid leaking during a session. Use universal precautions

(wear gloves) when handling linens that have soaked up body fluids, particularly bloody discharges.
- Have towels available to put between the breasts and sheets to absorb leaking milk.

Uterine Infection

If the client had a retained placenta, cesarean section, or other condition, she could develop an infection after delivery, resulting in fever and abdominal pain.

 BODYWORK PRECAUTIONS:

- Type I bodywork is contraindicated with any infection and fever.
- Type II gentle energy work may be nourishing and healing.

Mastitis

During the postpartum period, it is not unusual for some mothers to develop a breast infection called mastitis.

 BODYWORK PRECAUTIONS:

- Breast massage and Type I bodywork is contraindicated during inflammation and infection of the breast.
- Type II gentle energy work may be nourishing and healing.

CHAPTER SUMMARY

Perhaps now during the postpartum period, more than ever, women need to be nurtured with healing touch as they face the joys and stresses of mothering. For many women, finding the time for relaxing and focusing on their own recovery from pregnancy and birth may be quite difficult in the midst of baby care. With respect for the challenges of the new mother, consider making special provisions for her care, such as: allowing more time for a standard session; making it possible for her to have her baby with her during massage; offering house calls; being aware of breastfeeding considerations such as the likelihood of leaking milk or possible breast discomfort in the prone position; being prepared to stop in the middle of a session to reposition your client so she can nurse her baby. Both baby and mother will benefit from the relaxation, support and nurturing care that you can offer at this time.

CHAPTER REVIEW QUESTIONS

1. List five benefits of postpartum bodywork for the mother, and two for the baby.
2. Describe how you might ask about a client's birth story and assess the appropriateness of massage at this time. What particular concerns might you have with a client who is 48 hours postpartum, had a long labor, pushed for 4 hours, and had a large perineal laceration?
3. Describe what kind of positioning considerations might be necessary with a client who has brought her baby to a session along with a caregiver.
4. Name common areas of muscular strain that can cause discomfort in the postpartum period and that can be addressed with bodywork.
5. Describe the postpartum client's needs and bodywork precautions that are different than those for other clients.
6. Discuss the ways other cultures care for and honor a new mother. How have you seen, or not seen this manifest in your culture or community? In what ways could a massage therapist perhaps support a special honoring of the mother?
7. In what ways can nurturing touch to a postpartum client also impact her baby positively?
8. Explain what kinds of concerns you would watch for when doing a postpartum health intake.
9. Explain what concerns you would have for a postpartum client who, 10 days ago, had labor induced due to preeclampsia.
10. Name two conditions that most postpartum women have at least a little risk for in the first 2 days after birth. For what reason should a massage therapist be aware of this?

REFERENCES

1. Jackson D. With Child: Wisdom and Traditions for Pregnancy, Birth and Motherhood. London: Duncan Baird Publishers, 1999:72.
2. Farwell E, Maiden, AH. The wisdom of Tibetan childbirth. In Context: A Quarterly of Humane Sustainable Culture Spring 1992;(31):26–31.
3. Jordan B. Birth in Four Cultures: A Cross-Cultural Investigation of Childbirth in Yucatan, Holland, Sweden, and the United States. Prospect Heights, IL: Waveland Press, 1993.
4. Lund K. International Best Practices for Maternity and Parental Benefits. An Atlantic Canada Project. Funded By: Status Of Women Canada. Sponsored By: Women's Network Pei. Dec 2004.
5. Anderson S. Blood clot problems in pregnancy and soon thereafter are infrequent but can be life-threatening. Medical News Today, online at

http://www.medicalnewstoday.com/medicalnews
.php?newsid = 33624. [Main Category: Pregnancy
News. Article Date: 17 Nov 2005.]

6. Pabinger I, Grafenhofer H. Thrombosis during pregnancy: risk factors, diagnosis and treatment. Pathophysiol Haemost Thromb. 2002;32(5-6):322.

7. Gherman RB, Goodwin TM, Leung B, et al. Incidence, clinical characteristics, and timing of objectively diagnosed venous thrombo-embolism during pregnancy. Obstet Gynecol 1999;94:730–734.

8. Anderson JM, Etches D. Prevention and management of postpartum hemorrhage. Am Fam Physician 2007;75(6):875–882.

9. Field T, Hernandez-Reif M, Diego M, et al. Cortisol decreases and serotonin and dopamine increase following massage therapy. Int J Neurosci 2005;115(10): 1397–1413.

10. Field T, Grizzle N, Scafidi F, et al. Massage and relaxation therapies' effects on depressed adolescent mothers. Adolescence 1996;31(124):903–911.

11. Lowe W. Orthopedic Massage: Theory and Technique. New York: Mosby, 2003.

12. Foda MI, Kawashima T, Nakamura S, et al. Composition of milk obtained from unmassaged versus massaged breasts of lactating mothers. J Pediatr Gastroenterol Nutr 2004;38(5):477–478.

13. Hongo H. The issue of breast massage and milk quality in japan: when cultural perspectives differ. Leaven 2007;43(1):10–12.

14. Wilson-Clay B, Hoover K. The Breastfeeding Atlas. Austin, TX: LactNews Press, 1999.

15. Smith MK. New perspectives on engorgement. Leaven Dec1999-Jan 2000;35(6):134–136.

16. La Leche League. Online at http://www.llli.org/.

17. Ernst E. Abdominal massage therapy for chronic constipation: a systematic review of controlled clinical trials. Forsch Komplementarmed 1999;6:149–151.

18. Ayas S, Leblebici B, Sozay S, et al. The effect of abdominal massage on bowel function in patients with spinal cord injury. Am J Phys Med Rehabil 2006; 85(12):951–955.

CHAPTER 12

BODYWORK FOR THE POSTPARTUM CLIENT

LEARNING OBJECTIVES

After reading this chapter, you should be able to:

- Describe techniques for assessing the spine, posture, abdominals, and psoas during the postpartum period.

- Explain reasons for 10 common complaints of postpartum and describe bodywork techniques for each.

- Describe specific bodywork techniques for addressing the postpartum abdomen.

- Describe the etiology of and treatment for certain musculoskeletal conditions that frequently develop during the postpartum period.

- Describe breathing techniques that can be used to help support a woman experiencing postpartum depression.

- Explain postpartum breast massage techniques and precautions.

*T*his chapter begins with a few techniques to address a mother's condition in the first hours after birth. This is followed by assessments of the spine, abdominals, and psoas which have all been compromised during pregnancy. The majority of the chapter is focused on common complaints during the postpartum period and methods of addressing these complaints with a wholistic bodywork approach.

BODYWORK FOR THE IMMEDIATE POSTPARTUM PERIOD

The baby is born and the room is filled with excitement, relief, and exhaustion. Sooner or later, the mother is going to need to get up and walk around. If appropriate, before she does get up, take a few moments to help her attune to her body and breath, to the joints and bones that may be stiff or misaligned, and to the muscles that may have been strained. The following practices can help alleviate accumulated stress from labor and realign the hips, pelvis, and spine.

Low Back Release

Benefits: This technique may relieve some backache due to sacral misalignment from pushing during birth.

Technique: The client is supine on a firm surface with legs straight and with no pillow or just a small pillow under her head.

1. Gently flex one knee at a time up to her chest.
2. Have the client push against your pressure as she attempts to extend her leg with 1/4 of her effort.
3. Lower the leg slowly again to an extended position. Do not have her assist you—do it for

her—as a passive flexion will enable more adjustments to occur naturally in the low back and pelvis.

4. Repeat on the opposite leg.

Sacroiliac and Pelvic Rebalancing

Benefits: Relieves misalignments of the hips and pelvis, which may have occurred during birth.

Technique: See Chapter 6.

ASSESSMENTS

After doing an initial health intake with your new postpartum client to determine her pregnancy and birth history, assess for potential dysfunctions and stresses by examining her spinal, pelvic, and abdominal support. This can provide useful information as you determine your treatment plan or focus for your bodywork.

Spinal Assessment

Benefits: To locate areas of stress in the spine.

Technique: Have the client sit in a chair, with her back straight, feet flat on the floor, and thighs horizontal to the floor. This can be assessed at any time during the postpartum period.

1. Stand behind the client. Observe her spine as she sits, and take note of any raised areas on either side of the spine, often indicating a vertebral subluxation that might return to its aligned state after massage and the release of myofascial restrictions in the area.

2. Ask her to inhale, and on her exhale, have her slowly roll forward, one vertebrae at a time, from the top of the spine to the bottom, first letting the head fall forward, then the shoulders, then the mid back, etc., until she is resting over her knees as far as she is able, with arms relaxed down at her side.

3. On her next exhale, ask her to unfurl her spine from the waist back up the spine, with the head being the last to uncurl. Gently touch each vertebra as she rolls up, helping her feel which vertebrae are moving. Notice as she rolls (and have her notice also) where the spine catches and moves as a segment rather than as individual vertebrae. Ask her to inform you at any point that she notices a restriction in or tension with in her movement. Address these areas later with massage.

Diastasis Recti Assessment

Benefits: Assessment of a rectus separation will help determine one possible correctable cause of low back pain and will initiate the process of teaching your client strengthening exercises.

Technique: Review assessment of diastasis recti in Chapter 3.

Postpartum is an important time for correcting separations of the abdominal muscles which may have occurred during pregnancy. A mild diastasis recti will begin to naturally correct itself in the weeks postpartum, but if your client has a gap greater than 3 finger-widths, exercises to correct the gap should be started as soon as the client is ready to focus, in days or at least within a couple weeks after birth. If you have been trained in appropriate abdominal strengthening and toning exercises, such as sit-backs or curl ups, with a focus on postpartum clients, you may teach these exercises to your client. If not, refer your client to a local physical therapist or trained Pilates instructor.

Psoas Assessment

Benefits: A tight or weak psoas can cause low back, sacral, and pelvic discomfort. This can be assessed 4 to 6 weeks after a normal vaginal birth. Until then, the postpartum body is still adjusting to changes in weight distribution and mothering demands. Psoas assessment is discussed in Chapter 6 and determines the tightness and balance of the iliopsoas and the need for therapeutic stretching. If the psoas is weak, the abdominals are most likely weak, which is typical after pregnancy. Many abdominal strengthening exercises prescribed by a physical therapist will strengthen the psoas as well.

Position: The client is supine with one knee flexed. The other leg is extended with the lower leg hanging off the table end.

Technique: See Chapter 6 ("Assisted Psoas Stretch") for instruction on assessment and treatment. *Note:* In the process of psoas assessment, you might find any of the following conditions:

- If the hamstrings of the extended leg do not lay flat on the table, the psoas of that side is tight and may need to be stretched (Figure 12.1). If one or both sides are tight, do the Assisted Psoas Stretch described in Chapter 6.
- If the hamstrings lay flat on the table but the lower leg extends when hung off the table, the quadriceps may be tight and could be stretched. Stretch, if indicated, with the client

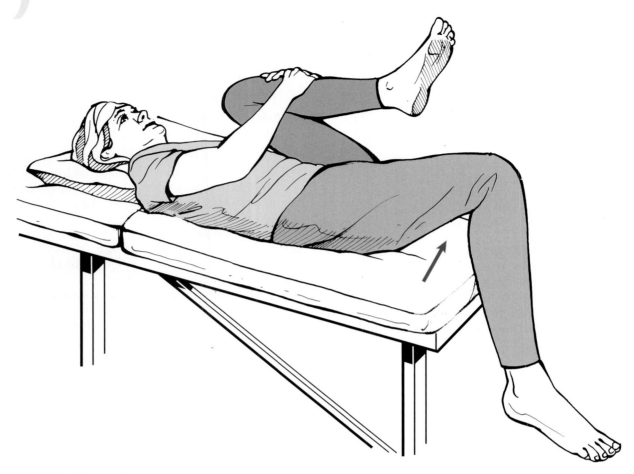

FIGURE 12.1   Psoas assessment.
A tight psoas prevents the thigh of the extended leg from resting on the table.

in a prone position. Flex her knee and push her foot toward her buttocks. Hold in a stretched position and instruct her to extend her knee against your pressure with 1/4 of her effort for 7 seconds. After she relaxes her effort, flex her knee further and repeat.

- If the hamstrings lay flat on the table, and the leg and foot stretch easily off the table toward the floor, the psoas does not need stretching, but may require strengthening. If she has little strength to flex her hip, her psoas is likely weak. To assess with less stress, have her move back up on the table and keep her leg extended on the table, rather than dangling off the end. Place your hand on the knee of her extended leg and instruct her to press her knee up against your hand pressure, keeping her back flat on the table. As she slowly raises her extended leg about 8 inches off the table, determine the level of difficulty and weakness. Compare each side.

COMMON COMPLAINTS

By the third postpartum day a woman's most immediate needs are often resolved. At this time, massage can begin to address other common complaints and concerns that are residual from pregnancy and birth or that develop from postpartum activities such as nursing, lifting, and carrying the baby.

Pelvic Misalignment and Sacrolliac Pain

The pelvis can become poorly aligned at any time during pregnancy. Now, in the postpartum period, it is important to ensure that good alignment is cultivated as the ligaments begin to tighten again and the hypermobility of the joints slowly decreases. Many women experience low backache or sharp pains in the sacroiliac area when the pelvic and sacral joints are misaligned.

General Treatment

Below are some suggestions for general treatment of pelvic misalignment and sacral-iliac pain:

- To help stabilize the pelvis, encourage strengthening exercises, particularly of the back, psoas, and abdominals. Use compression, friction, and cross-fiber friction techniques for the sacrum and sacroiliac joint area.
- Work with postural education and teach proper body mechanics to prevent aggravation of her condition.
- She may find a sacroiliac joint support brace to be helpful.

Specific Techniques

In addition to the general treatments listed above, a number of specific techniques may be used to address this condition. These are presented below.

Abdominal/Perineal Connection
Benefits: An attunement to the area of her body that was just recently very active and which will soon need tonifying for recovery.

Technique: The client is supine.

1. Ask your client to breathe slowly into her belly.

2. On an exhalation ask her to contract her perineal muscles, as in a Kegel exercise. Simultaneously, she should contract her abdominals, flattening or pulling them in toward her spine.
3. As she inhales again, ask her to release and relax her abdominals, psoas, and perineum, letting the belly expand up and out with her breath. Repeat 2 to 3 times.

On her next inhalation, ask her to breathe into her belly and allow it to soften completely, giving thanks for all that her body has accomplished through birth.

Sacroiliac and Pelvic Rebalancing
Benefits: Relieves misalignments of the hips and pelvis.

Technique: See Chapter 6.

Sacral Push
Benefits: Flattens and helps realign the sacrum and relieves low back pain and sciatica.

Position: The client is supine with her knees bent. Stand at her feet.

Technique:
1. As the client exhales, press slowly into her knees through her femur toward her sacrum to flatten her back (Figure 12.2).

Self Care Tips FOR MOTHERS:
Re-Stabilizing After Birth

It may be advisable for a new mother to perform the simplest of exercises to help rebalance, strengthen, and stabilize the joints, abdominals, and psoas. One such exercise of leg sliding is described below. This can be initiated in the immediate postpartum period if desired.

Benefits: Initiates rebalancing of the abdominals and psoas and brings the client's attention to her posture and body sensations; strengthens the transverse abdominals and stabilizes the psoas.

Position: The client is supine on a firm surface with her knees bent and feet together and flat on the floor.

Technique:
1. As the mother exhales, instruct her to flatten her abdominal muscles and low back, contract her per-

ineal muscles and slowly let the legs slide out toward a straight position.
2. Instruct her to stop as soon as the low back begins to arch.
3. Have her pull the legs back to the point right before the arching of the back began, and then have her hold, breathing in and out slowly for 2 to 3 breaths, maintaining a flattened low back.
4. On her inhale, have her bring her knees back up to original position.
5. Repeat 2 to 5 times.
6. If she is unable to feel the arching of her back, she may be more successful with your help. Place your hand lightly under her low back and one on her belly, and ask her to press her back down against your lower hand. Feeling your hand will help her to sense the flatness of her back.

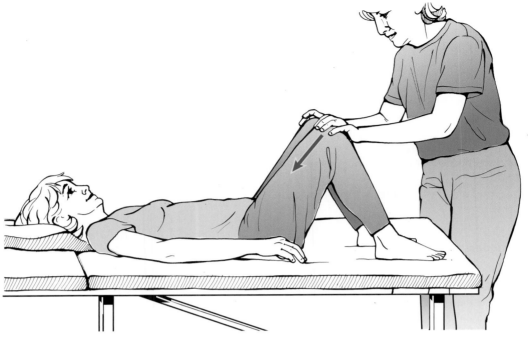

FIGURE 12.2   Sacral push.
Press slowly into the client's knees as she exhales, directing pressure through her femur toward the sacrum to flatten her back and sacrum.

2. Hold there as long as it is comfortable for her.
3. Slowly release and repeat.

Supine Pelvic Unwinding

Benefits: Releases sacral tension, torqued sacrum or pelvis, low back pain, and QL tension; lengthens the low back and releases the anterior tilt of the pelvis; unwinds the spine, decreasing low back discomfort.

Technique: The client is supine.

Note: This requires at least 5 to 10 minutes of holding under the woman's sacrum in a position that some practitioners may find awkward or straining. Relax your hand and arm while you work.

1. Ask your client to lift her hips up slightly to allow you to slip your hand under her sacrum, palm facing up, with your other hand resting gently on her lower abdomen over the sacral hand (Figure 12.3).
2. Hook your fingers on top of her sacrum or in the lumbar region, and begin a sacral traction, pulling caudally. There is very little movement from your hand, but as you attune to the subtle energetics of the sacrum it will begin to unwind and release; your hand may move slightly downward as the sacrum and spine extend. This is subtle but very effective work.
3. This can be done with less strain, but with a different depth of effectiveness, with the

client in the sidelying position. Apply traction and pressure onto the sacrum in this position. (See "Pelvic Compression and Unwinding" in Chapter 5.)

Edema

Edema that was present during pregnancy, especially associated with gestational hypertension, can continue for days after delivery until the body has regained its equilibrium. (See "Edema" in Chapter 6.)

Uterine and Abdominal Concerns

During pregnancy, the abdomen is maximally stretched. In the postpartum period, the abdominal fascia will begin readjusting itself to support a non-pregnant belly. Abdominal massage can help prevent restriction and distortion of the fascia as it reorients. By one week after delivery, focused superficial abdominal work can be implemented.

General Treatment

Below are some suggestions for general awareness or treatment of the uterus and abdomen after birth:

- Before doing abdominal work, review "Honoring" in Chapter 5.
- General abdominal work can help a woman connect with her belly that may seem new

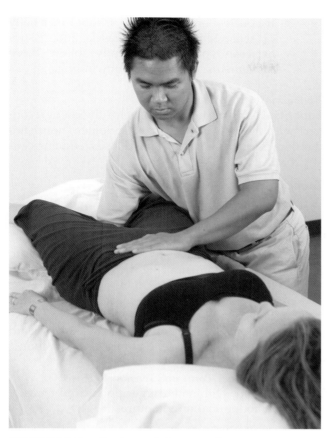

FIGURE 12.3   Supine pelvic unwinding.
One palm is under the client's sacrum and the other hand rests gently on her lower abdomen over the sacral hand. Hook your fingers at the top of her sacrum and traction caudally. There is very little movement from your hand, but slowly the sacrum will begin to unwind and release.

Case Study 12.1
MASSAGE FOR EDEMA

During a hot summer in the third trimester of pregnancy, Rose began to develop an uncomfortable level of edema in her legs and hands. During the first day in the hospital after the birth of her baby, she had a visit from a massage therapist, who noted that the edema was still present in Rose's lower legs. The massage therapist had Rose lie supine and placed her legs on pillows. She wrapped her lower legs in moist, cool cloths, and while Rose relaxed, the therapist massaged her neck and shoulders. After 5 minutes, the therapist went back to the legs, removed the cloth on one leg, and began to perform light lymphatic drainage stroking. She began on the proximal end of the edema at the mid-calf area and stroked toward the torso. Using just her fingertips with featherlight touch, she stroked hand-over-hand around each leg, gradually working her way down to the feet. Between the light strokes, she occasionally did a gentle C-clamp stroke up the leg with her hand. She worked on each leg for 10 to 15 minutes. When she was done, there was a visible reduction in the depth of the swelling on both legs. Rose used the bathroom soon after the massage. Her urine was being measured and so she knew she had voided 1200 cc of urine. This was a surprisingly large amount, indicating that her body was releasing the excess fluids that had accumulated during pregnancy, including those extracellular fluids that were causing edema in her legs.

and unfamiliar with stretch marks or sagging skin.

- After warming the tissue and cultivating trust with your client, begin work on the attachments of the rectus abdominus at the ribs and on the pubic symphysis. Use friction, cross-fiber friction, and direct pressure to help release trigger points that may have developed during the pregnancy. (See "Specific Bodywork Techniques for Groin Pain" in Chapter 6 for instruction.)
- Address the rectus and transversus abdominal muscles with myofascial release and the release of trigger points, which may be found along the lateral edges of the rectus, as well as at their attachments on the ribs and pubic bone.

Specific Techniques

Several specific techniques may be used to support and nourish the uterus and abdomen. These are presented below.

Energizing the Abdomen
Benefits: Sends healing energy to the uterus and abdomen. Helps a mother connect with her belly and inner-self or release abdominal tension and emotions related to pregnancy, birth, and motherhood.

Technique: The client is supine or sidelying. Stand or sit at her side.

1. Keeping one hand on the belly just below the navel, slide your other hand underneath the client's lumbar spine and waist so that her belly rests between your two hands.

Traditional Birth Practices:

Soothing the Womb

Massage of the uterus is the most common postpartum massage practice found around the world. Uterine massage is typically used immediately following the expulsion of the placenta. This massage causes the uterus to contract, releasing any developing blood clots collecting at the opening of the cervix, and ensuring no placental fragments remain. Worldwide, uterine massage practices include using a hand, a knee, or someone's oiled head to press and rub into the mother's belly to help push out blood and clots.[1]

In Thailand, a midwife gives daily uterine and abdominal massage to the postpartum woman for up to 1 week after birth to help reposition the uterus correctly in the pelvis or "restore the belly" and assist with uterine involution and "sooth(ing) the womb."[1]

This type of uterine massage is also practiced daily in Malaysia, Tahiti, Java, the Philippines, and India for up to 1 month after delivery, along with full-body massage, to help a woman's recovery from birth.[1,2]

Postpartum Mayan women also may receive up to 3 weeks of uterine massage during midwife visits. The new mother will likely wear a rebozo, or long shawl wrapped around her belly and hips, to help hold the uterus in place.[1-3]

Traditional postpartum practices of the Hawaiians, Haitians, Japanese, and Mayans include binding the belly with cloth or leaves to help support the uterus until bleeding decreases and stops.[2-6] Many women wear abdominal binders, not only to prevent postpartum hemorrhaging, keep the uterus supported, and help regain a pre-pregnant shape, but also as a layer of energetic protection and to help "close the bones"—bringing the hips together and aligning the pelvis.

Only in birth does the cervix open so completely, the pelvis and perineum open to release the baby, and the mind, psyche, and spirit open so wide to new possibilities of creativity. Many cultures take measures to help the mother "close" again, energetically and physically, before her re-entry into the world at large.

All mothers can support and protect their abdomen and uterus by wrapping a long sash or elastic abdominal binder tightly around the hips and belly.

2. Visualize, and help her envision too, energy spreading like warm morning sunlight from your hands, through her belly, softening, healing, and clearing unresolved feelings, resistance, or pain.

3. If you feel energy moving through her belly or sense shifting of the fascia and tissues between your hands, gently follow those movements, encouraging unwinding.

Abdominal Effleurage Warm-Up
Benefits: Helps the belly relax; helps the client reconnect with her new nonpregnant abdomen; nourishes the skin; improves intestinal peristalsis, reducing constipation.

Technique: The client is supine. Stand at her side.

1. Using the soft palms of the hands, stroke the abdomen in a clockwise circular direction with slow, firm strokes.
2. Begin at the navel and spiral out to the width of the abdomen, using the flat palms of your hands or fingertips.
3. Rake hand-over-hand, reaching over to her far side and stroking toward her navel.
4. Scoop up from the pubic and groin area toward the navel, hand-over-hand for several minutes.

Abdominal Trigger Point and Tension Release
Benefits: Helps eliminate trigger points and areas of tension in abdominal musculature.

Technique: The client is supine and her knees supported on a bolster. Stand at her side.

1. Beginning at the client's solar plexus area with the fingertips of one hand, gently making small circles, pressing through the fascia and fat to the muscles.
2. Move slowly around the belly, in a clockwise direction, making the small circles and working more deeply into areas where the muscles are especially tense. If there is an area that feels particularly sore to her, focus there with gentle touch, holding and breathing, encouraging the tissues to relax.
3. You may feel or even see a strong blood pulse in parts of the abdomen. Often this is an area where there is more intensive muscular or emotional holding with restrictions of blood flow. Avoid pushing deeply or suddenly into these areas, but do address the musculature around the pulsing.
4. Emotions are bound into contracted musculature, in adhesions, and in trigger points; work sensitively and with a listening heart and mind to emotions that may emerge.

Skin Rolling / Fascial Lift
Benefits: Helps break up and loosen distorted and restricted fascia on the abdomen; creates space in

areas of congestion. This technique is especially useful after surgery, but is not to be done after a cesarean section before the scar is well-approximated and the internal sutures absorbed—at least 4 to 6 weeks.

Technique: The client is supine with knees on a bolster. *Note:* This is done *without* oil to ensure a better grip of the skin.

1. Pick up a fold of the abdominal skin between the fingers and thumb.
2. Walk the fingers along the belly while holding and rolling the skin away by pushing and stretching with the thumbs as the fingers walk (Figure 12.4A).
3. Do this across the whole belly, working from the navel in outward rays, moving vertically and horizontally across the abdomen.
4. Take hold of as much low abdominal skin and subcutaneous fat that you can grasp with your palms and fingers.
5. Lift up, as though lifting the belly skin away from the abdominal contents (Figure 12.4B).
6. Hold. The client should not feel pinched; instead, she should feel as though space was being created in her abdomen.

Abdominal Myofascial Release

Benefits: Releases abdominal restrictions.

Technique: The client is supine. Stand at the client's side.

1. Place the flat palm of your hand that is closest to the client's head on her belly with your palm resting on her anterior superior iliac spine (ASIS) of the opposite side from which you are standing.
2. Place your other hand on the closer side of the client's upper belly, just below her ribs.
3. Hold for a moment, as the client relaxes. Breathe together to increase relaxation.
4. Allow your hands to slowly sink into her abdominal fascia.
5. Apply traction to stretch the fascia, holding for several moments until the tissues begin to release and unwind (Figure 12.5).
6. Repeat on the other side.

Womb Massage

Benefits: Encourages uterine ligaments to hold the uterus in place; helps a low-lying uterus move back into appropriate positioning within the abdomen; relieves low pelvic pressure or aching. This technique is beneficial anytime *after* heavy bleeding has stopped.

Note: Many women have felt their uterus in the first 1 to 3 weeks postpartum, when it can still be located

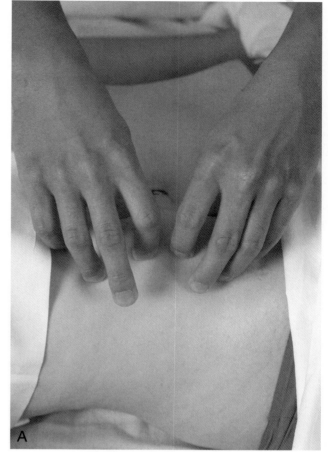

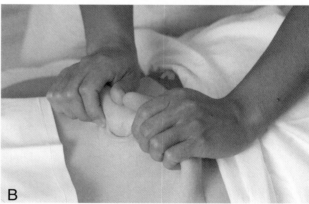

FIGURE 12.4   Skin rolling/fascial lift.
(A) Pick up a fold of the abdominal skin. Walk the fingers along the belly, rolling the skin by pushing and stretching with the thumbs as the fingers walk. *(B)* Lift up the abdominal skin and fascia away from the abdominal contents.

easily above the pubic bone. Carefully pushing into the low abdomen with soft fingertips against the uterus and rubbing in a circular motion can stimulate it to contract. This will decrease bleeding and help it return to a smaller, nonpregnant size.

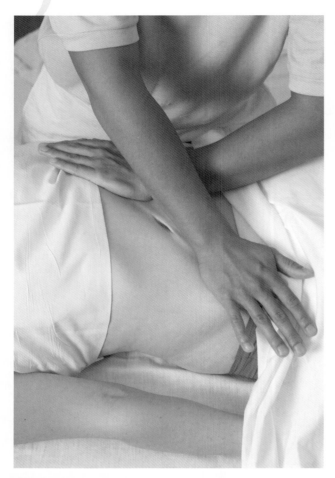

FIGURE 12.5   Abdominal myofascial release.
As the client relaxes her abdominals with an exhalation, allow your hands to sink into the fascia. Apply traction holding for several moments until the tissues begin to release and unwind.

![!] **CAUTION:** Do not do womb massage during uterine or other infections, fever, or heavy bleeding. Avoid womb massage on women who have an intrauterine device in place. Avoid pushing the uterus down toward the perineum. Instead, use any of the following techniques to help the uterus move upward in the abdomen, rather than down.

Technique: The client is supine, with knees bent and feet flat on the floor. Stand at her side, facing her feet.

1. Place your fingertips on top of the client's pubic bone, or ask her to locate her pubic bone for you.
2. Push your fingers into her abdomen just above the superior edge of her pubic bone firmly enough to go deep but remaining comfortable for her.

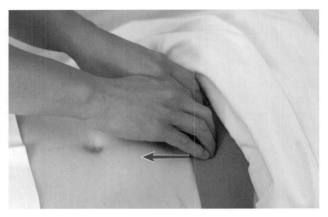

FIGURE 12.6   Womb Massage.
Using fingers like a hoe in the earth, sink carefully down into the abdomen just superior to the pubic bone and then stroke up toward the navel on the midline as well as from the sides. Envision lifting and supporting the uterus as you work.

3. Have the client exhale as you push in, allowing the belly to relax more easily. You may feel a lump there—it is likely the uterus.
4. Palpate with your fingers around the uterus to find the sides and top edge. Then, from the pubic bone, make strokes up toward the navel from just superior to the pubic bone as well as from the lateral edges of the uterine area. Always move up toward the midline, envisioning lifting and supporting the uterus as you work (Figure 12.6).
5. Move slowly and with honor. The client can also do this herself. Either way should be relaxing.

Uterine Cramping Relief The uterus must continue contracting after delivery to help constrict open blood vessels left after placental detachment and to help the uterus return to its nonpregnant size. Without these contractions, the mother would hemorrhage from the placental site. Despite their beneficial effects, the contractions can at times be quite painful. This may be especially true for those with previous births, as the uterus must work harder to contract a uterus that has been stretched previous to this time.

Benefits: Massage can help to relieve some of the cramping, at least temporarily. If cramping is occurring during a massage session, try the following techniques.

Technique: The client is supine.

1. Perform energizing the abdomen, as described earlier in this chapter.

Complementary Modalities:
Hydrotherapy for Postpartum Renewal

A perineal and womb steam, similar to those described in Traditional Birth Practices later in this chapter, can be done using common items from your home.

Benefits: Softens and regenerates the tissues that have been injured and stressed in birth, helping to support and nourish the womb and cleanse the remaining residues from pregnancy and birth.

Technique: Steep several handfuls of fresh herbs or 1 cup of dried herbs of calendula, plantain, yarrow, motherwort, or rosemary in 2 quarts of boiled water. Alternatively, use 6 to 10 drops of any of the following essential oils: sandalwood, vetiver, cypress, geranium, or rosemary. The herbed water is placed in a bucket, commode, or bedpan with cushioned edges so the mother can sit comfortably over it. If that is not possible, a pot of boiling water can be placed under a chair that has slats or reeds that will allow the steam to come through. The mother then sits for 10 to 20 minutes above the steam, naked from the waist down with towels wrapped around her waist and legs to keep the steam directed toward her perineum and vagina. Only one steam is typically done during the postpartum period, but it can be used at other times of a woman's life, between menses.

 CAUTION: Steaming should not be done if a woman is seriously depleted of energy or blood, has an infection or fever, or has other high-risk conditions after birth, as excessive heat may exacerbate these conditions.

2. Place a warm compress on her abdomen.
3. Perform supine pelvic unwinding, as described earlier in this chapter.
4. Make repetitive, long, slow, firm strokes from her abdomen down the medial and lateral sides of her legs to her feet, imagining pulling the cramps out of the womb and into the earth through the feet.
5. Massage the ankles and soles of the feet. Press and hold your thumbs in the center of the sole of her foot, while also pressing your fingers on the dorsal side of the foot between the great toe and the next toe. Imagine opening a door in the feet to allow the cramps to flow out and healing energy to flow in to the womb.

Nursing Neck

A common complaint in the postpartum period is upper back, shoulder, and neck tension, sometimes called "nursing neck." This is often caused by a mother sitting with one arm contracted, holding the baby to her breast while tilting her head down and slightly to the side as she stares into the eyes of her new love. It does not take long for this posture to cause tension in her neck. Neck tension reduces blood circulation to the brain and can cause fatigue, shoulder pain, and headaches. If a woman pays attention to how she holds her neck for extended periods of time, she can adjust her posture when nursing, so as to support her arms and back. The massage therapist may encourage postural awareness in addition to offering massage for relief of tension.

General Treatment

As a massage therapist, you may hear of your client's discomforts or you may have the opportunity to observe her as she nurses her baby. Some women may not have tried the following type of supportive posture while nursing, and may find it relieves their complaints.

While sitting, her feet may need to be raised on a stool so the knees are at least at a 90-degree angle from her hips. Both the mother's arm and baby should be on a pillow, with another pillow behind the mother's low back for lumbar support. Once a mother is situated, she can observe herself regularly to avoid hunching over her baby or developing a crook in her neck from constantly watching the baby with her head turned to the side. She should change nursing sides regularly and practice relaxed breathing to avoid static muscle tension. Below are some other suggestions for general treatment of nursing neck:

- Self-care exercises can be taught, including shoulder shrugging, and stretches for the pectoralis and subscapularis (see Chapter 6).
- General petrissage to the neck and shoulders, along with deep tissue sculpting, muscle stretch and resistance, and myofascial release to the levator scapula, sternocleidomastoid, trapezius, pectoralis, and scalenes is appropriate.

Specific Techniques

In addition to the general treatments listed above, a number of specific techniques may be used to address this condition. These are presented below.

Neck Release
Benefit: Releases the neck and shoulders.

Technique: The client is supine on a massage table. Sit in a chair at her head.

1. Slide your hands under her back and press in to the intercostal space with your fingertips between the medial edge of her scapula and the thoracic vertebrae around the level of T-3 or T-4 (Figure 12.7A).
2. Hold until you feel a pulsing or release of energy.
3. Slide your hands out and press down caudally into the tops of the shoulders. Hold until you feel a pulsing or release of energy (Figure 12.7B).
4. Slide halfway up the neck, and press in carefully into the lateral edges of the erector spinae bundle and hold (Figure 12.7C).
5. Slide up to just under the occiput and press on either side of the spine in the hollow between the sternocleidomastoid and

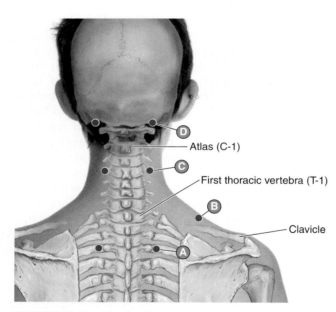

FIGURE 12.7   Neck release.

*Location of areas to press into for neck release. (**A**) Press in to the intercostal space with your fingertips between the medial edge of her scapula and the thoracic vertebrae around the level of T-3 or T-4. (**B**) Press down into the tops of the shoulders. (**C**) Halfway up the neck, press in carefully to the lateral edges of the erector spinae bundle and hold. (**D**) Press in the hollow on either side of the spine under the occiput between the sternocleidomastoid and trapezius origins. (From Clay JH, Pounds DM, Basic Clinical Massage Therapy. 2nd Ed. Philadelphia: Lippincott Williams & Wilkins, 2008.)*

Labels in figure: Atlas (C-1); First thoracic vertebra (T-1); Clavicle

trapezius origins, 3 to 4 fingerwidths lateral to spine (Figure 12.7D).
6. Work all the muscle attachments along the bottom of the occiput, from the spine to the mastoid process.
7. Hold the occiput in the palms of your hands and gently traction the neck.
8. Hold the traction while bringing her head up and chin toward her chest to lengthen the posterior neck.
9. Ask the client to let you know when she feels a full stretch. Ask her to push back with her head with just the lightest pressure against your hands as she exhales. (Remind her to stop if she experiences any discomfort at all.)
10. Stretch further if it is comfortable for her.
11. Relax her head and rock her head side to side with your fingers.

Shoulder Pressure Resistance
Benefits: Helps muscles to lengthen and relax.

Technique: This can be done with the client sitting, supine, or sidelying with work to one side at a time.

1. Place your palms on top of the woman's shoulders and push down gently.
2. On her exhalation have her shrug her shoulders up against your pressure with 1/4 of her effort and hold for 6 to 10 seconds.
3. Ask her to relax and then shrug again, but this time, as you offer resistance, allow her shoulders to come up to her ears.
4. As she holds her shoulders up, place your hand onto the outside of her upper arms and hold and resist as she begins to pull her shoulders back down to a relaxed position again.
5. Once back to neutral, ask the client to relax fully.
6. Press your thumbs into a tight area on the top of the shoulder mid-way between the acromion process and the base of the neck.
7. On an exhalation, have the client push her shoulders up against your thumbs; hold 6 to 10 seconds and then relax.
8. Repeat steps 1 through 7 one or two more times.

Neck Traction
Benefits: Manual traction can help unwind and relieve compression of the vertebrae and muscles.

Technique: The client is supine; her legs may be under a pillow. Sit in a chair at her head.

1. Make a sling from a small towel or thin scarf. Wrap this under the woman's head and hair

behind her neck, with the ends coming up on either side of her head by her ears. Be sure her ears are not folded.

2. When you are certain the towel is secure and will not slip off her head, apply a slight traction to her spine, staying aligned with the length of her spine.
3. Hold the traction for up to 1 minute. Slowly release.

Arm Mobilizations
Benefits: Helps release the upper back and neck.

Technique: See Chapter 6.

Upper Back Pain

There are many causes of postpartum upper back pain, including increased breast size and weight with lactation, improperly fitting nursing bras, poor posture during nursing, and improper lifting and carrying of the baby. Internally rotated shoulders, which develop from these conditions, strain the upper back musculature.

General Treatment

For best overall treatment, a new mother must stretch the muscle agonists and strengthen the antagonists of the involved muscles. Below are some suggestions for general treatment of upper back pain:

- The medially rotating pectoralis major and subscapularis muscles most likely need to be stretched.
- The rhomboids and medial trapezius muscle can be strengthened to counter the anterior pulling muscles.
- Also see "Back Pain: Mid and Upper" in Chapter 6.

Specific Techniques

In addition to the general treatments listed above, a number of specific techniques may be used to address this condition. These are presented below.

Pectoralis Stretch
Benefits: Relieves some discomfort associated with medial shoulder rotation.

Technique: See "Pectoralis Stretch and Resistance" in Chapter 6.

Subscapularis Massage   The subscapularis medially rotates the shoulders. It is located on the anterior surface of the scapula and so is difficult to access. As with the psoas, subscapularis work is not especially

"relaxing" to receive—the therapist must reach up into the armpit to access the lateral edge of the muscle. Use caution and good communication with your client as you massage this muscle, to ensure client comfort.

Benefits: Relieves upper and mid back pain caused by slumping and internally rotating shoulders.

Technique: The client is supine. Stand at her right side to work on her right subscapularis.

1. Abduct your client's right arm slightly, holding under her elbow with your left hand.
2. With your right hand fingers, push up into her armpit posteriorly and medially until you can feel the anterior lateral edge of her scapula (Figure 12.8A).
3. With your left hand, bring her right arm over her chest to create more space for your right hand under the scapula.
4. Feel along that edge for trigger points, holding and pressing or pulling slightly laterally, scooping on the muscle, until the trigger points release. To increase access to the subscapularis, rest the client's arm across her chest and slide your hand under her right scapula on her back. Hook your fingers onto the medial edge of her scapula and pull out laterally on the scapula (Figure 12.8B).

 CAUTION: Avoid pressing straight up into the armpit, which can compress nerves.

Subscapularis Stretch
Benefits: Relieves upper and mid back pain caused by slumping and internally rotating shoulders.

Technique: See Chapter 6 and Figure 6.9.

Low and Mid Back Pain

Back pain is a common complaint in the postpartum time for several reasons: a new mother's body is readjusting and finding its stability again after 9 months of pregnancy, often with strained or improper posture. The birth process itself may have caused misalignment of the pelvic girdle, especially if she labored in unsupported positions. Lifting, carrying, twisting, flexing, and reaching for heavy children and putting babies and children in and out of car seats adds to a woman's complaints of pain.

General Treatment

Strengthening the abdominals, particularly the transverse abdominus, practicing proper body

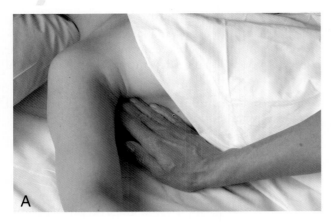
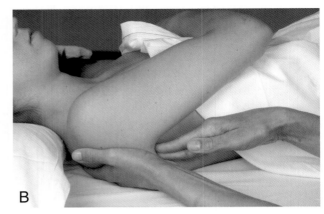
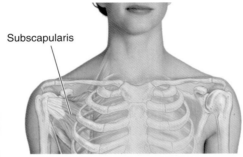

Subscapularis

FIGURE 12.8   Subscapularis massage.
Abduct the client's arm slightly out to the side. **(A)** *Push your fingers up into the back of her armpit and posteriorly toward the table until you can feel the edge of her scapula, between her ribs and scapula.* **(B)** *Bring her arm over her chest if necessary to increase access and pull her scapula laterally while continuing to press up into subscapularis area.* **(C)** *Subscapularis. (From Clay JH, Pounds DM, Basic Clinical Massage Therapy. 2nd Ed. Philadelphia: Lippincott Williams & Wilkins, 2008.)*

mechanics, and reducing stress will help relieve low back pain in the postpartum period. Below are some suggestions for general treatment of low and mid back pain:

- See "Back Pain: Low" in Chapter 6 for more details on bodywork techniques—all are applicable in the postpartum period.
- Address the abdominals, pelvic floor, multifidus, QL, and psoas with your bodywork.
- Assess for diastasis recti and recommend the practice of corrective exercises.
- Help her pursue abdominal strengthening exercises as well as the psoas stretch and assisted psoas stretch described in Chapter 6.

Specific Techniques

In addition to the general treatments listed above, a number of specific techniques may be used to address this condition. These are presented below.

Psoas Release   The psoas worked hard for 9 months to support the anteriorly rotating pelvis as it carried the extra weight of pregnancy. Stretching and strengthening of the psoas can be practiced throughout pregnancy and continued in the postpartum period.

Benefits: Gentle bodywork to the psoas can be started 6 weeks after a normal pregnancy and vaginal delivery to help eliminate trigger points, assist in its stretching, and help alleviate back pain.

 CAUTION: Concern for clots is increased during the first 6 weeks postpartum, until blood volume and clotting factors return to normal. Psoas work should not be done until at least 6 weeks postpartum; however, gentle work can be done on the iliacus just inside the ilium, avoiding deep compression in the abdomen near the aorta and major blood vessels, as well as close to the femoral triangle. The psoas work described below may be started 6 weeks after a normal pregnancy and birth, if it is comfortable for the client.

Follow these guidelines when beginning psoas massage:

- The psoas can be very tender; be sure to communicate with your client throughout your work, explaining clearly what you are about to do before and while doing it.
- Always work very slowly when working on the abdomen, encouraging your client to relax and letting her know through your sensitive and slow touch that she can trust you enough to let down the natural guarding of the abdominal musculature. Never press deeply into the abdomen without working together with your client to ensure her trust and ability to relax with your pressure.
- If you are uncertain about the location of the psoas, learn from another practitioner's demonstration of the work, to ensure proper technique and avoid possible risk of client injury.

Technique: The client is supine with knees bent, a hip-width apart with feet flat on the table. If necessary for her comfort, she can let her knees fall together in a relaxed, supported position. Keeping the knees bent relaxes the abdomen and psoas and allows easier access into the abdominal area. For some it may be easier to work on the side opposite your intended focus. This description starts with the massage therapist on the client's right side.

1. Use soft fingertips to gradually compress through the abdomen lateral to the rectus abdominus and just medial to the right anterior iliac spine onto the psoas. Carefully sink into the abdomen along the iliacus toward the anterior musculature of the back (Figure 12.9).
2. Ask her to pull that knee up slightly until you feel a movement or bulge of the psoas under your fingers, indicating correct position.
3. Have her relax that leg again.
4. Knowing you are on the psoas, compress gently and hold, allowing the muscle to relax under your touch. When it does, slide your hands slowly down 1 inch and repeat.
5. Holding pressure on a tight area of the psoas with your left hand, place your right hand on her right knee. Ask the client to bend her knee up further with a very slight effort. Give her knee a little resistance with your hand and

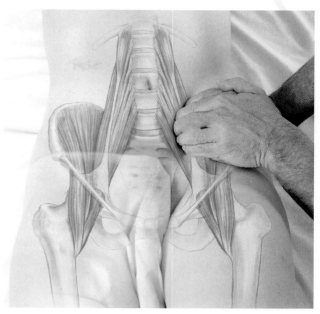

FIGURE 12.9   Psoas release.

Use soft fingertips to gradually compress through the abdomen (the medial side of the ASIS onto the psoas. Compress gently and hold, allowing the muscle to relax under your touch. When it does, slide your hands slowly down an inch and repeat. (From Clay JH, Pounds DM, Basic Clinical Massage Therapy. 2nd Ed. Philadelphia: Lippincott Williams & Wilkins, 2008.)

keep holding pressure on the psoas while it contracts. (Lighten up or release the pressure if your client complains of significant pain or discomfort.) This technique should not be more than slightly uncomfortable for the client, provided you encourage her to relax using focused breathing and provided you work very slowly, encouraging feedback regarding pressure and her sensations.

6. Instruct her to relax the knee, and then slowly slide your palpating fingertips to a new area of the psoas, and repeat. Do not release pressure fully to move to new areas. It is better to maintain the pressure, now that your client's muscles have relaxed enough to let you in the abdomen, and slide along the psoas as you move. Ensure that compression into the abdomen occurs as she is exhaling. Always do slow, gentle touch and effleurage on the abdomen prior to pressing in deeply, so that she can develop trust with your touch and sensitivity. Instruct her to contract her perineal muscles in conjunction with your work, which can help relax the psoas.

Quadratus Lumborum Work
Benefits: Relieves low backache.

Technique: See Chapter 6.

Quadriceps Work
Benefits: Due to chronic anterior pelvic rotation during pregnancy, the hamstrings become stressed, tight and lengthened and the quadriceps becomes tight and shortened. Releasing the quadriceps may help the pelvis recover optimum positioning in the postpartum period. Sometimes the hamstrings need to be released as well.

Technique: The client is first supine, then prone. Stand close to her knee, facing her head.

1. First warm the quadriceps with effleurage and petrissage.
2. Starting just inferior to the inguinal area, compress onto the rectus femoris with flat knuckles, forearm or the palmar surface of your hand, and slide slowly toward the patella decompressing and opening the hip joint.
3. Compress into the tendon, just superior to the patella, and slide slowly up the vastus lateralus. Avoid deep pressure on the vastus medialis except near the patella, until 4 to 6 weeks postpartum when the risk of blood clots is resolved.
4. Press carefully onto the tendon at the superior attachment of the rectus femoris near the anterior inferior iliac spine, searching for tenderness or tightness that can be reduced with gentle compression.
5. Feel the tendon of the quadriceps just superior to the patella. Apply cross-fiber friction to the patellar tendon until you feel a softening.

Lateral Hip Rotator Anchor and Stretch
Benefits: Chronically poor posture during pregnancy usually involves tightening of the lateral hip rotator muscles, potentially causing sciaticlike pain, strain on the sacroiliac joint, and referred pain to the low back. Releasing the hip rotators helps relieve low back pain and assists the pelvis to recover to optimum positioning in the postpartum period.

Technique: The client is prone. Stand at her side.

Note: Before beginning deeper work, warm the gluteals with effleurage, petrissage, and myofascial stretching, stripping, and compression.

1. With one hand, compress against the medial edge of the greater trochanter in the area of the piriformis attachment.
2. With the fist or palm of the other hand, compress and slide from the trochanter toward the sacrum along the belly of the piriformis.
3. Return to step 1. Flex the client's knee and hold her leg just proximal to the ankle. Maintaining compression on the attachment at the trochanter, pull the lower leg laterally, to medially rotate the hip and stretch the piriformis (Figure 12.10).
4. Hold this stretch while compressing for 8 seconds. Release.

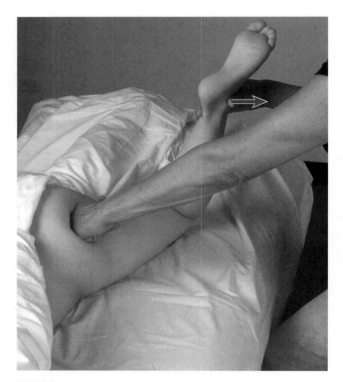

FIGURE 12.10   Lateral hip rotator anchor and stretch.
Flex the client's knee and hold her leg just proximal to the ankle. Maintaining compression on the tendonous attachment of the piriformis at the trochanter with flat knuckles, fist, or palm, pull her lower leg laterally, to medially rotate the hip and stretch the piriformis.

5. Rotate the lower leg in a circle until her hip is again medially rotated and repeat steps 3 and 4.
6. Return the lower leg to a neutral position. Compress gently with your fingertips or fist into the belly of the piriformis.
7. Pull the client's lower leg laterally again to medially rotate the leg and stretch the piriformis.
8. Hold here and ask your client to resist for 7 seconds during her exhalation with 1/4 of her effort against your holding, attempting to bring her lower leg back to neutral.
9. Relax. Increase the medial rotation and repeat step 8.

Pelvic Alignment Rock

Benefits: If there is an excessive anterior pelvic tilt, or if one ilium is rotated causing sacroiliac discomfort, this technique can help align it into proper supportive position.

Technique: The client is prone.

1. Assess balance of the ilium: There are a variety of ways to assess ilium rotation. If one ilium is rotated anteriorly (which you may find more commonly than posterior rotation), stand at the client's side opposite the rotated hip. Have her lie prone and place your thumbs or fingers on both posterior superior iliac spines, assessing if they are level, or if one is higher or lower than the other, likely indicating that one ilium is rotated anteriorly or posteriorly. Have her lie supine, and measure levelness of the ASIS. Next place your two index fingers parallel with and on the superior edge of the pubic bones, to determine if one side is higher or lower than the other.
2. Reach across your client to that hip and slide your hand around and under the ASIS. Place your proximal hand at your client's posterior lower ribs.
3. Pull on the ASIS while simultaneously holding or pushing on the lower ribs and waist area (Figure 12.11). Move up the ribs, pushing or holding them against the table and releasing as you pull and rock the ASIS away from the table.
4. Establish a comfortable rocking motion, pulling and releasing with these holds, rocking the client's hip posteriorly.
5. Continue for 30 seconds to 1 minute.
6. If neither ilium is rotated and both sides are equal, treat both sides as described above. If one side is rotated, first treat the anterior rotated side as above. Treat the opposite side

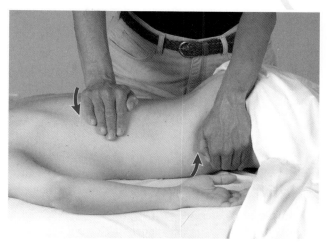

FIGURE 12.11   Pelvic alignment rock.
Reach across the client and hold with your distal hand on her ASIS. Place your proximal hand on the client's lower posterior ribs. Pull on her ASIS while simultaneously pushing on her lower ribs and waist area. Establish a comfortable rocking motion, pulling and releasing with these holds, rocking the client's hip posteriorly.

with the opposite treatment. In other words, push on the gluteal area, while pulling on the lower ribcage. Hold for 30 seconds to 1 minute or again establish a rocking action.

Fatigue

The new mother has been through an enormous life transition and now, after delivery, she may be drained and getting little sleep. Fatigue is common and often continuous for months (or years!) after birth. A woman may also be slightly anemic if she had a large blood loss after delivery, causing a deeper level of fatigue.

General Treatment

Below are some suggestions for general treatment of fatigue:

- Exercise will improve a woman's overall well-being, reduce fatigue, and increase energy.
- Rest is just as important as exercise and is often the most important advice. When the baby naps, so should the mother, to ensure she gets that vital renewing relaxation each day.
- If the woman is breastfeeding, she should drink enough water to keep her thirst quenched, to replenish fluids used for creating breast milk, to prevent dehydration, and to

Self Care Tips FOR MOTHERS:

Therapeutic Strengthening Exercises

*N*ew mothers can be taught certain therapeutic strengthening exercises to reinforce the work you are doing for the psoas and low back.

Supine Bicycle Riding

Benefits: Strengthens the psoas and transverse abdominus.

Technique: The client is supine with her knees bent to her belly and her low back flattened on the floor by contracting the abdominals down toward the anterior spine. The back must remain flattened during exercise.

1. Have your client slowly extend each leg, singly, as though pushing down on the pedal of bicycle, keeping the leg parallel to the floor and about 4 to 6 inches above it.
2. Bringing that knee back to the belly, the other leg extends. The low back should constantly stay flat on the floor, so she should only extend her legs to a height where she can maintain the flattened back.

Transverse Abdominus Strengthening

Benefits: Strengthens the transverse abdominus—a primary support of the abdomen and pelvis—and helping decrease low back pain.

Technique: The client is on her hands and knees or standing erect. Keeping her spine straight, she exhales and pulls her navel toward her spine, without moving the spine while exhaling. (This is different from the "cow and cat" yoga pose, in which the back arches and sags; here the spine stays flat.) While contracting the transversus abdominus, the client can also contract her pelvic floor. Hold for 10 seconds or until needing to inhale. Relax and repeat 5 to 20 times.

---

nourish her general energy. Offer her water after every session.

- A stimulating massage with brisk strokes, tapotement, and deep tissue work increases blood and energy flow. A relaxing massage with long, slow strokes, slow shaking of the extremities, and releasing stuck energy with palming, holding, and breathing can help a woman get a more nourishing rest. Offer full-body massage with an intent of stimulating or relaxing energy.
- Hands and feet massage can be refreshing, renewing, healing, and nourishing. Hand and foot reflexology specifically can help stimulate and reharmonize, especially with focus on the breasts, lymphatics, low back, pelvis, uterus, and neck and shoulders.

Specific Techniques

In addition to the general treatments listed above, a number of specific techniques may be used to address this condition. These are presented below.

"Closing the Bones"
Benefits: Helps close the physical expansions and psychic openings from birth and increase internal energy regeneration.

Technique: The client is supine on a sheet laid out horizontally under her.

1. Pull up on the edges of the cloth, starting at the client's head.
2. Bring the ends of the sheet around her forehead, crossing it over itself, and pulling to tighten so there is a firm pressure around her head (Figure 12.12A).
3. Squeeze gently, imagining compressing any openings. Be sure her ears are not bent forward. Hold for 30 seconds.
4. Move the cloth or pick up the edges of the sheet further down to her shoulders, then to the abdomen, hips, low back area, legs, and feet (Figure 12.12B).
5. Repeat the treatment, starting again at the client's head and moving down her body.
6. If there are 2 to 4 people available, you may be able to wrap all of her body at once.
7. Alternatively, without a cloth, press hands on either side of the mother's hips, pushing inward firmly and imagining the pelvis "closing."

Cradle Rock
Benefits: Relaxes and rocks the mother, bundling the mother as she bundles her baby.

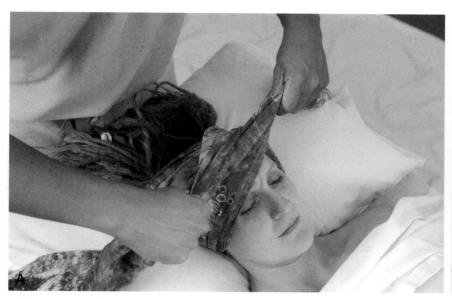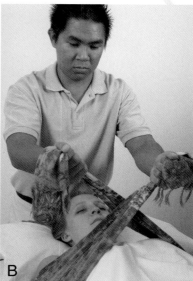

FIGURE 12.12   Closing the bones.
(A) Tighten the ends of the sheet around her head to give a firm pressure. (B) Gradually squeeze all the way down her body.

Technique: The client is supine on a sheet. Have a helper available. Stand at the client's sides, each of you holding onto one side of the sheet.

Note: If you are alone and it is appropriate to do so, stand over the client, holding the edges of the sheet on either side of her hips.

1. Ask the client to breathe into her abdomen, relaxing her entire body with one big exhalation.
2. Lift up on the sheet so it is tight against the mother's body. Roll her back and forth gently on the sheet.
3. Adjust your hold to move your pressure up the client's body, repeating the gentle rocking (Figure 12.13).

Postpartum Blues

Recovery from pregnancy and birth is a physiological process, but it is also a spiritual, psychological, and emotional one. The experience of **postpartum "blues"** is not unusual, and is most likely due to the sudden shift in hormonal production immediately after delivery. Symptoms of the blues include fatigue, irritability, and frequent, sometimes incessant, crying. Transculturally, rates for the blues are estimated to range from 40% to 85%[8-12] of postpartum women typically begin in the first days after birth, lasting for up to 2 weeks. Fewer women (10% to 20%) experience a more involved, but nonpsychotic depression which

may develop within the first month after birth.[12,13] This can be caused by chemical imbalances, as well as social isolation and confusion about identity and new roles as a mother.

Touch may have a positive effect on the frequency and level of postpartum depression. One study done at the Touch Research Institute looked at teenage mothers who received massage in the postpartum period. They were found to have lower urinary cortisol levels (stress hormones) and higher serotonin levels (which relate to stress and relaxation) than those who received other relaxation therapy. The young women described feeling a decrease in anxiety and depression after massage.[14] Women who are massaged have brainwave changes that can be identified on electroencephalograms, and which represent an improvement of postpartum depression.[15] Studies also indicate that an increase in postpartum and prenatal support reduces the risk of postpartum depression.[16,17] The massage therapist can play a role in postpartum support by offering caring touch.

General Treatment

Below are some suggestions for general treatment of postpartum depression:

- Full-body relaxation massage helps women integrate mind and body and stimulates release of serotonin, oxytocin, and dopamine.[20,21]

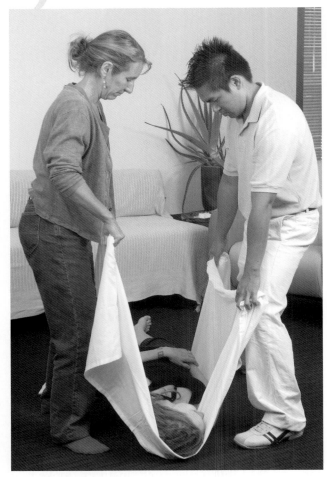

FIGURE 12.13   Cradle rock.

Lift up on either side of the sheet so it is tight next to the mother's body and roll her back and forth gently. Adjust your holds to move your pressure up the sheet and up her body, repeating the gentle rocking.

Traditional Birth Practices:

The Baby Blues

*P*ostpartum depression does not occur everywhere in the world. An emotionally and physically supported postpartum time seems invaluable for helping women recover from birth without experiencing the blues.[16,17] In many traditional cultures, women and new babies were once provided continuous support services for weeks or months. This support included delivery of food, baby care, and regular massages for mother and baby. These practices are changing as the world grows smaller.

In the Solomon Islands, where postpartum depression was once thought to be unknown, the Tikopians recognized that a new mother's health, on all levels, was critical to the baby's health. In honor of the woman's effort to grow and bring forth this child, the community focused on the fact that a *mother had given birth*, rather than on a child being born. The mother was cared for as long as necessary until her full recovery.[18]

Malaysians may experience occasional depression after birth, but their perspective on what it means is different from ours. In their view, a new mother's emotions or physical weakness during postpartum makes her vulnerable to spiritual malaise, the symptoms of which are similar to what we call depression, such as loss of appetite, difficulty bonding with the child, and weepiness. The ailment is treated spiritually, with prayers and by inducing a trance in which the woman is helped to release her emotions and frustrations, regaining the balance in her spirit.[19]

- Acupressure utilizes specific points to help address and potentially ease symptoms of depression.
- Use techniques that help increase lung and respiratory capacity as well as encouraging aerobic exercise to stimulate the flow of oxygen and blood circulation.

Specific Techniques

In addition to the general treatments listed above, a number of specific techniques may be used to address this condition. These are presented below.

Breath Expansion
Benefits: Helps increase respiration, increasing energy and cleansing the mind. Gives client a sense of breaking through a cloud of heaviness and opening in her heart and lungs; helps her inhale deeply and create intention for getting what she wants; stretches pectoralis muscles and opens the chest as she expands her arms.

Technique: The client is supine. Stand at her side, facing her head.

1. Place your hands on her lower ribs below her breasts and sternum.
2. Encourage her to inhale fully while keeping your hands firmly in contact with the skin over her ribs.
3. On her exhalation, press into her ribs slightly, encouraging more breath to exit and giving a sensation of compression (Figure 12.14A).

Case Study 12.2
A CASE OF POSTPARTUM BLUES

After having her first baby at age 38, Letty became what she considered to be mildly depressed. She described her relation to her baby as similar to her relationship with wild baby raccoons that she had raised in the past. Her own baby seemed like a wild creature to whom she was not related. She felt distant and disconnected as she cared for this totally dependent and very cranky creature that seemed to be sucking the life out of her. Sometimes, in moments of desperation, when he was screaming and unappeasable, she would put him in another room and shut the door, trying to escape from the noise of his screams, which made her feel an unfamiliar violent impulse inside her. She sometimes worried that she was "going insane." Yet she never acted on her urges and was always able to talk about how she felt.

Letty received occasional massages during this time period. She stated that the massages gave her an opportunity to connect with a deeper part of herself, and allowed her to relax and process the fact that she had become a mother and that her life would never be the same again. The touch gave her a brief interlude where she was nurtured and not expected to emotionally or physically feed someone else (her child). Eventually, this period of difficulty eased, and she finally bonded with and cared more easily for her child. This type of experience is not uncommon in our society but some feel it is taboo for women to discuss or admit it.

4. Continue holding as she breathes in and out several times. Then release.
5. As she inhales, lighten your hand contact as she pushes your hands out with her breath, giving a sensation of freeing restriction.
6. Slide your hand around her ribs and under her back to her spine, lifting up into the spinae erector muscles next to her spine. Use oil if you are directly on her skin. Then pull back around to the front while sliding your fingers through the intercostal spaces between her ribs (Figure 12.14B).
7. Encourage full breath and opening in her emotional heart as well as in her chest, both of which tend to collapse with depression.
8. Place the client's arms over her chest, but not crossed over each other. Stand at her head.
9. Place your hands on her forearms and ask her to push open her arms out to the side while inhaling deeply (Figure 12.14C).
10. Apply some resistance to her pushing, but do not prevent her from opening her arms; just give her a sense of pushing against some force as she opens.
11. As you repeat this, you may suggest to her to envision or express that which she would like to make space for in her life.

General Breast Concerns

Many American women nurse their baby for the first few weeks after birth, but most do not continue past a few months (only 14% exclusively breastfeed for the first 6 months, the time recommended by the American Academy of Pediatrics).[22] Physical challenges that occasionally accompany breastfeeding include the following:

- Engorged breasts are painful and tight.
- Clogged ducts can become infected, in a condition called **mastitis**.
- Women may believe they have too little milk, or occasionally feel they have excessive production.
- Many must cope with frequently leaking breast milk. (Be aware of this during massage).
- Nipples can become painfully sore and cracked.
- Breastfeeding difficulties can lead to emotional issues related to the strong symbolism embedded in a mother's ability to nourish her young from her own body.

Fortunately, with education, support, and touch, most of these issues can be prevented or solved, sometimes with the use of massage. La Leche League is a national organization that supports breastfeeding and is available for assistance to all women with breastfeeding concerns. One condition, which can be at least partially addressed with bodywork, is **engorgement**, or the swelling of the breasts with blood, lymph, and milk in preparation for the mature milk to be produced. This is covered in a separate section.

General Treatment

- Self-breast massage and healthy posture while nursing helps reduce mastitis, clogged ducts, and painful breasts. To help move energy through the breast and support lymph and milk flow, breast massage can be offered or taught for self-care.
- Specific acupressure techniques can be learned to stimulate lactation or reduce the risk of mastitis.

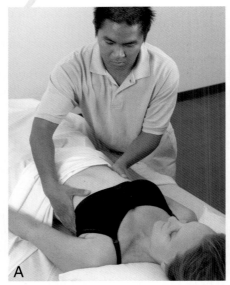
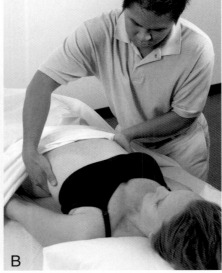
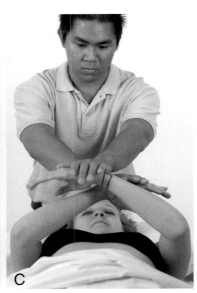

FIGURE 12.14   Enhancing inspiration.

(A) On the client's exhalation, press into her ribs slightly, helping encourage a more full breath out. As she inhales, maintain lighter hand contact as she pushes your hands out with her breath. (B) Slide your hands under her back, to her spine, pressing and lifting up into the spinae erector muscles, then pulling back around to the front while sliding fingers through the intercostal spaces between the ribs. (C) Place your hands on the client's forearms and ask her to push open her arms out to the side while inhaling deeply. Apply some resistance to her pushing, but do not prevent her from opening her arms; just give her a sense of pushing against a force as she expands.

- Muscular and emotional stress and tension inhibit the milk "let-down" response; exercise along with deep relaxation, yoga, and massage can help reduce this stress.
- If your client is having lactation issues, she may have underlying emotions related to these problems. These emotions may emerge during bodywork sessions. Support her by encouraging relaxation breathing along with visualizations that foster imagery of abundance and an unlimited ability to nurture.
- Help her practice tension relaxation (as discussed below) to foster and reinforce relaxation, which will improve her nursing capacity.
- Release the muscles of the chest, neck, shoulders, and arms with effleurage, petrissage, deep tissue massage, or trigger point work to free lymph and blood circulation and increase milk flow.

Breast Massage
Benefits: Stimulates the breasts and supports milk flow.

 CAUTION: Read all precautions for breast massage in Chapter 6 as well as the following precautions.

- Avoid breast massage when the client has a breast infection.
- The nipple area can have micro-abrasions that can transmit bacteria easily to the breast. Practice and teach good hand-washing technique before touching the breasts.
- Certain essential oils are contraindicated for breastfeeding women, and anything applied to the breast tissue can affect the baby if absorbed into the milk or not washed off thoroughly from the skin prior to nursing. Avoid the use of scented or essential oils unless you are trained in their use for postpartum.

Technique: Any of the techniques in Chapter 6 support lactation and breast care, in addition to the following techniques. These can be taught to the mother if it is not appropriate for the therapist to do the technique.

1. First apply a warm compress for 5 minutes to the breasts.
2. Remove the compress. Hold on either side of the base of the breast with the fingers and the thumb of one hand. Twist and slide with a moderate-light pressure, toward the nipple.
3. Repeat 3 to 5 times.

Self Care Tips FOR MOTHERS:

Breathing Practices

*C*onscious breathing oxygenates the blood and mind and circulates new energy through the body. Particular types of breathing practices can renew thoughts and rebalance glandular processes, helping to mediate mild depression. The following are breathing techniques that can be specifically helpful. Serious depression that is preventing a mother from caring for her infant or herself should be attended to by a medical professional.

Alternate Nostril Breathing

Benefits: Connects and balances the two sides of the brain; brings mental clarity; calms and sedates; relieves anxiety and headaches; helps clear sinuses; reduces blood pressure.

Technique: The client is in any comfortable sitting position.

1. Instruct the client to place her index and middle fingers on her "third eye," between her eyebrows, and lightly rest the thumb on one side of her nose and the little finger and ring finger on the other side, outside the nostrils (Figure 12.15).
2. With her eyes closed, instruct her to shut the right nostril with the thumb and inhale slowly through her left nostril.
3. Have her exhale more slowly through the left nostril.
4. At the end of the exhalation, ask her to close her left nostril with her little finger and inhale through her right nostril.
5. Repeat steps 2 through 4 for 5 to 15 minutes, or as long as desired.
6. Alternatively, she can breathe in through the right nostril and exhale through the *left*, then inhale through the left, and exhale through the right.

Note: The nostril of a person's dominant side is considered to be the active nostril and breathing through it will energize the body and mind (i.e., if one is right-handed, that is the dominant side). Breathing through the opposite side has more yin qualities and relaxes the body. To energize the body fully, one can do single nostril breathing—breathing in and out only through the dominant nostril, keeping the other closed off. To relax the body and decrease insomnia, one can breathe solely through the non-dominant side.

Breathing into the Earth

Benefits: Helps a mother connect with and receive the support of the Earth.

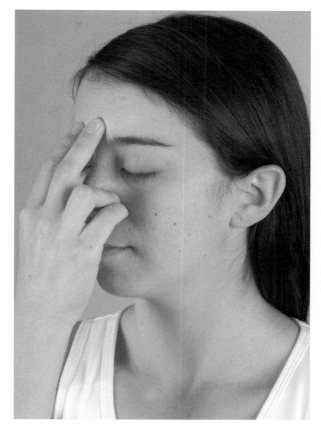

FIGURE 12.15   Hand position for alternate nostril breathing.

Technique: If the client finds a safe, quiet earth-space where she can lie directly on the ground, she can dig a small hole to put her face into, or she can just rest her head on her hands close to the ground. Inhaling, she breathes into her belly, then expands her ribs, breathing in the scent and power of earth. As she exhales, she can imagine releasing any darkness, sadness, or confusion through her breath and it being absorbed into the earth.

Aerobics and Walking

Any exercise a new mother can do will help refresh the mind, cleanse the circulatory system of cellular waste, and give her a new outlook on life. Walking in fresh air, in the company of trees, sunlight, and sky is especially helpful. The function of body and mind will improve with 20 minutes per day. Yoga postures can also help renew the body, rebalance hormones, and heal the mind.

4. Slide your fingertips sequentially from below the clavicle down toward the nipple, from the sternum laterally toward the nipple, and from the armpit region toward the nipple.

5. Cup the breast in the palm of the hand, with the fingers on the lateral side of the breast. Shake the breast gently, pushing with the fingertips into the breast tissue toward the sternum.

6. Replace the warm compress for 5 minutes.

Belly Palming

Benefits: Important acupressure meridians that affect the breasts and reproductive organs are located on a woman's anterior torso. Even without a background in acupressure, using palming on the belly can help reduce stress tension that may be related to breast and lactation concerns.

Technique: The client is supine. Stand or sit at her side.

1. Place one palm on or just superior to the client's pubic bone.

2. Keep that hand there as a grounding hand while moving your other palm, one hand width at a time, from just proximal to the first hand all the way up the belly and sternum to the sternoclavicular junction.

3. Hold each spot for up to 30 to 60 seconds until you feel energy filling that area below your hands.

4. Between the breasts, move your hand vertically if necessary to avoid pressing directly on the breasts.

Contraction–Relaxation Visualization

Benefits: All types of full-body relaxation are beneficial to reducing stress and fatigue that may affect nursing and milk production.

Technique: The client is in any relaxing position. Stand at her feet.

1. Place your hands on the client's feet. Ask her to inhale while contracting her feet and toes against your hand, dorsiflexing and pressing into the heels. Have her hold the tension and her breath for 5 to 7 seconds, then relax totally with the exhalation. Massage the feet gently as she relaxes.

2. Move to the hips, perineal area, and abdomen. Place one hand on the client's belly and slide the other underneath her belly at her lumbar area. Ask your client to inhale and then to tighten her gluteals, abdominals, and pelvic floor and hold that tension with her breath, then totally relax the muscles with the exhalation. Massage the belly gently to encourage relaxation after the exhalation.

3. Continue this practice, moving up to the upper chest and back, then to the neck and face, having her exaggerate whatever tightness is already there: shrugging her shoulders, grimacing on her face, opening her mouth. Place your hands on each area as she inhales and tenses, helping increase the sensations of tension.

4. Each time she exhales, ask her to imagine totally relaxing her tight muscles. As she

---

Self Care Tips FOR MOTHERS:

Arm Movement

*M*ovement of the arms helps stimulate the lymphatic and blood circulation and improve milk production. Teach your client to practice the following exercises several times each day.

Dynamic Arm Exercise

Teach the mother to rotate the arms in circles—lifting them forward, up over her head, around behind, and back down to the side. Inhale on the upswing, exhale on the downswing. Then have her reverse direction and repeat. Ask her then to lift just the shoulder and roll it backward, down, and forward at least 5 times. Repeat in the reverse

direction. Instruct her to do this at least 5 to 10 times, 1 to 3 times per day.

Chest Isometrics

Instruct your client to sit or stand, placing her hands together in a prayer-like position at her chest. Have her keep her elbows out to the side and forearms parallel with the elbows and the floor. Instruct her to press her palms together, feeling the pectoralis tighten. She should then breathe slowly into the abdomen while holding the isometric toner. Encourage her to hold for 15 seconds, then release, repeating 3 times.

Among the Mayan and Aztec, a hot steam lodge called the temazcal was an important part of the postpartum recovery used within the first month, often between 3 and 6 days after birth, depending on a woman's recovery and strength. It was considered a cleansing of her pregnancy and birth, as well as a rite of finality with this pregnancy cycle. This helped cleanse, heal, and tonify the uterus and perineum, bring warmth and healing to a depleted pelvic area, and renew and renourish the womb.

The temazcal was also a means of transforming a mother's milk from what was considered "raw" milk into milk that was healthier for her infant. Traditionally, the woman would enter a small, covered space with rocks heated on a fire. Water, steeped with special herbs, was poured onto the hot rocks to make steam as she sweated inside the lodge for 15 to 20 minutes. Protected from cold air and drafts afterward for 24 hours, she was then assimilated into the life of a new mother. Her breasts were massaged to help stimulate milk production, and a shawl or *rebozo* was squeezed around her from head to feet to help close her body; this was followed by long massage strokes down the entire body.

In the North Pacific, other communities called the technique of squatting over the steaming rocks "cooking the milk."[1]

In contemporary Japan, a special technique of breast massage is considered a critical part of postpartum care in order to increase milk production and to improve the quality and energy content of the milk. This treatment was developed by Oketani, a Japanese midwife who based it on traditional methods as well as current experience. Women are seen by trained midwives who practice this type of breast massage to successfully address a variety of breastfeeding concerns, including mastitis, clogged ducts, engorgement, and insufficient lactation.[23,24]

contracts and relaxes, underlying tension can begin to dissipate and her awareness will more clearly be focused on that particular spot.

Engorgement and Breast Tenderness

As milk production increases and the breasts fill, lymph and venous circulation may decrease, causing engorgement and pain. A woman with engorged breasts might experience breast heaviness; distention; tight, shiny skin; warmth or redness; more visible veins and tenderness; throbbing; and hardness in areas of the breasts. This normally occurs between the second and sixth postpartum day and can last for up to 48 hours. Even without engorgement, women's breasts may have times of soreness or tenderness with increases in milk production as the baby grows.

General Treatment

The best treatment and prevention for engorgement is to nurse the baby frequently and to use breast massage to support lactation. Warm or cold therapies to the breast may also help. For general tenderness, breast massage and hydrotherapies can ease discomfort and help a mother feel more comfortable with her changing breasts.

Specific Techniques

If it is appropriate for you to do so, teach or perform the following breast massage on your client to address her engorgement.

Benefits: To help release blocked ducts and stagnant energy.

 CAUTION: Do not massage if infection or fever is present, as this can damage the tissue and spread the infection.

Technique: Massage the breasts after nursing. (See "Breast Massage" in Chapter 6.)

1. First apply a cool compress to the breasts for 5 to 20 minutes.
2. Feel the breast for the sore area and massage carefully with the flats of the fingers or thumb.
3. Slide from above that area toward the nipple, staying in a small area until it begins to soften, then move to a new area. Never force any movement of a lump or clogged area; have patience and allow it to slowly and gradually dissolve under your touch. The massage should not be painful, though there may be discomfort in a swollen area.

 CAUTION: For many women, warmth used on engorged breasts may increase swelling and discomfort.[25] Keep heat applications to 3- to 5-minute durations or try using cool applications first.

Complementary Modalities:
Acupressure for Lactation

*A*cupressure and acupuncture have been used to help stimulate or support lactation. The acupressure points Small Intestine 1 and 2, located on the ulnar side of the pinky finger (A), are used to move qi, activate blood, and free the flow of milk. Since it is such a tiny spot to press on, some women activate Small Intestine 1 by carefully biting on the side of their little finger with their teeth. Gall Bladder 21 on the top of the shoulders and Lung 1 (B) just below the clavicle are both strong points for stimulating the milk let-down reflex.

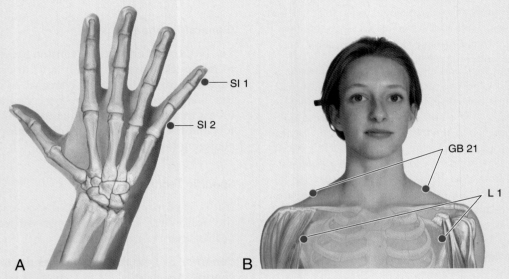

FIGURE 12.16   Acupressure for lactation.
(A) Small Intestine 1 and 2 are on the ulnar side of the pinky. (B) Lung 1, just below the clavicle, is a strong point for stimulating the milk let-down reflex. Gall bladder 21 on the shoulders moves energy downward. (From Clay JH, Pounds DM, Basic Clinical Massage Therapy. 2nd Ed. Philadelphia: Lippincott Williams & Wilkins, 2008.)

Self Care Tips FOR MOTHERS:

Breast Massage

*S*elf-breast massage can decrease engorgement. A mother might massage her breasts with her fingertips, making small circles from the top of her breast toward the nipple while the baby is nursing. If the baby is unable to nurse enough, the mother can also massage her breasts in the direction of the nipple to manually express the milk that is causing engorgement. If she nurses every 2 to 3 hours from both breasts, not just one side, engorgement issues generally decrease.

CHAPTER SUMMARY

Using techniques described earlier in this book, along with new ones in this chapter, you have a variety of tools to refer to when addressing the common complaints of your postpartum clientele. Remember that a client can be dealing with postpartum issues for a year or more after birth. Read Chapter 13 for details on caring for postpartum women who had birth by cesarean section.

CHAPTER REVIEW QUESTIONS

1. Discuss issues some women may have with abdominal work in general, and specifically during the postpartum period. Describe how you might suggest abdominal work to someone who has no experience with it and who might be hesitant about exposing her newly postpartum belly?

2. Describe methods you might use to encourage your client to relax her abdomen while receiving abdominal work. Describe two precautions you would use when doing postpartum abdominal work.

3. Explain the importance of a new mother's body mechanics and posture. Use specific examples of situations where improper body mechanics may lead to common postpartum muscular strains.

4. Describe bodywork precautions that should be in place for the first 6 weeks of postpartum recovery.

5. Explain why assessments of the spine, psoas, and abdomen might be appropriate for your postpartum clients.

6. Describe why sacroiliac pain can be a common complaint for postpartum women. Discuss the essence of the treatments described in this chapter for sacroiliac dysfunction.

7. Explain why a woman who has had more than one birth may experience an increase of postpartum cramps. Describe a bodywork technique that might help reduce cramping.

8. What is the first action a mother or massage therapist should take to help diminish the common complaint of nursing neck?

9. Explain what "closing the bones" might mean physically, emotionally, and spiritually in the postpartum period.

10. Describe in what ways bodywork may help a woman who is experiencing postpartum fatigue and depression or "the blues."

REFERENCES

1. Goldsmith J. Childbirth Wisdom From the World's Oldest Societies. Brookline, MA: East West Health Books, 1990.

2. Kitzinger S. Rediscovering Birth. New York: Pocket Books, 2000.

3. Jordan B. Birth in Four Cultures: A Cross-Cultural Investigation of Childbirth in Yucatan, Holland, Sweden, and the United States. Prospect Heights, IL: Waveland Press, 1993.

4. Herskovits MJ. Haitian birth customs. In: Meltzer D, ed. Birth: An Anthology of Ancient Texts, Songs, Prayers, and Stories. San Francisco: North Point Press, 1981:108–114.

5. Pukui MK. Hawaiian birth customs. In: Meltzer D, ed. Birth: An Anthology of Ancient Texts, Songs, Prayers, and Stories. San Francisco: North Point Press, 1981:129–136.

6. Jackson D. With Child: Wisdom and Traditions for Pregnancy, Birth and Motherhood. San Francisco: Chronicle Books, 1999.

7. Adewuya AO. The maternity blues in Western Nigerian women: prevalence and risk factors. Am J Obstet Gynecol 2005;193(4):1522–1525.

8. Hau FW, Levy VA. The maternity blues and Hong Kong Chinese women: an exploratory study. J Affect Disord 2003;75(2):197–203.

9. Gonidakis F, Rabavilas AD, Varsou E, et al. Maternity blues in Athens, Greece: a study during the first 3 days after delivery. J Affect Disord 2007; 99(1-3): 107–115.

10. O'Hara MW. Postpartum mental disorders. In: Drogeumeuller N, Sciarra J, eds. Gynecology and Obstetrics. Philadelphia, PA: Lippincott, Williams & Wilkins, 1991:1–13.

11. Mehta A, Sheeth S. Postpartum Depression: How to Recognize and Treat this Common Condition. Medscape Psychiatry Ment Health 2006;11(1).

12. O'Hara MW. Rates and risks of postpartum depression: A meta-analysis. Int Rev Psychiatry 1996;8:37–54.

13. Beck CT. Predictors of postpartum depression: an update. Nurs Res 2001;50(5):275–285.

14. Field T, Grizzle N, Scafidi F, Schanberg S. Massage and relaxation therapies' effects in depressed adolescent mothers. Adolescence, 1996;31(124) 903–911.

15. Jones N, Field T. Right frontal EEG asymmetry is attenuated by massage and music therapy. Adolescence. 1999;34(135): 529–534.

16. Murata A, Nadaoka T, Morioka Y, et al. Prevalence and background factors of maternity blues. Gynecol Obstet Invest 1998;46(2):99–104.

17. Heh SS, Coombes L, Bartlett H. The association between depressive symptoms and social support in Taiwanese women during the month. Int J Nurs Stud 2004;41(5):573–579.

18. Priya JV. Birth Traditions and Modern Pregnancy Care. Rockport, MA: Element Books, 1992.

19. Dunham C. Mamatoto: A Celebration of Birth. New York: Penguin Books, 1991.

20. Field T, Hernandez-Reif M, Diego M, et al. Cortisol decreases and serotonin and dopamine increase following massage therapy. J Neurosci 2005;115(10): 1397–1413.

21. Lund I, Yu L-C, Uvnas-Moberg K, et al. Repeated massage-like stimulation induces long-term effects on

nociception: contribution of oxytocinergic mechanisms. Eur J Neurosci 2002;16:330–338.

22. US Department of Health and Human Services, Health Resources and Services Administration. Women's Health USA 2005. Rockville, MD: US Department of Health and Human Services, 2005. (Heath Status: Maternal Health—Breastfeeding.) Available online at : http://www.mchb.hrsa.gov/whusa_05/pages/0428br eastfeed.htm.

23. Hongo H. The issue of breast massage and milk quality in Japan: when cultural perspectives differ. Leaven 2007;43(1):10–12.

24. Wakabayashi L. Massage helps women overcome breast-feeding difficulties. The Japan Times, Online. July 27, 2000. http://search.japantimes.co.jp/cgi-bin/fl20000727a1.html.

25. Walker M. Breastfeeding and engorgement. Breastfeeding Abstracts 2000;20(2):11–12.

CHAPTER 13

MASSAGE AFTER BIRTH-RELATED SURGERY

LEARNING OBJECTIVES

After reading this chapter, you should be able to:

- List 11 common reasons that a cesarean birth might be done.

- Describe what to expect and how to support your client with bodywork if you are with her during and after surgery.

- List six benefits and five precautions for bodywork after a cesarean section and five conditions that indicate the need for a medical release before offering bodywork.

- Describe three common complaints after birth-related surgery, and both general and specific bodywork techniques to address them.

- Determine appropriate assessment questions related to surgery that should be incorporated into a postpartum health intake-form.

- Describe when it is appropriate to begin working with new scars, as well as bodywork techniques for addressing scar tissue and adhesions.

*I*f your client had a birth-related surgery, she will have special needs in addition to those already discussed in the previous chapters. A careful health intake is required and a doctor's release is necessary if you have any uncertainty about whether your style of massage is appropriate at her current stage of her recovery. This chapter discusses reasons for cesarean sections, what to expect if your client should have one while you are with her, and ways of supporting her with bodywork in the recovery period. Many techniques discussed earlier in the book will be appropriate at some point in her recovery, but adaptations may be required initially if your client has difficulty lying prone or receiving touch on her abdomen after her surgery. Three postsurgical concerns are discussed: fatigue, back pain related to epidural anesthesia, and scars and adhesions.

BIRTH-RELATED SURGERIES

Besides the typical pains and discomforts of birth, women who undergo birth-related surgeries face additional issues in recovery. Two such surgeries, cesarean section and postpartum tubal ligation, along with recovery from them, are discussed here.

Cesarean Section

A **cesarean section** (C-section) is the delivery of a baby through a surgical incision in the mother's abdomen and uterus. It is the birth of choice in particular situations in which a vaginal birth may be too dangerous, when the mother or baby is in a life-endangering situation and a rapid delivery is necessary. It is also done for the convenience of the doctor or patient or, in some hospitals, for twin deliveries and for women with previous cesarean sections.

Cesarean section is one of the most common surgeries in the world.[1] According to the Centers for Disease Control and Prevention, 2005 statistics indicate that 30.2% of all births in this country are now by cesarean section—the highest rate it has ever been.[2] Although cesarean sections have their benefits, they also have inherent risks and adverse complications, as exist with any major surgery.

For some women, a cesarean birth can be a very traumatic experience, particularly if it was an unexpected emergency surgery due to problems with the mother or baby. Massage therapists can help a woman who has had a birth-related surgery with her emotional and physical recovery.

Therapeutic bodywork can also be beneficial for a variety of postsurgical conditions, including reducing adhesion formation and related discomfort, decreasing the experience of postoperative pain, and helping a woman overcome emotional stress related to surgery. These benefits and others are discussed throughout the chapter. See Box 13.1 for a general list of benefits of bodywork after surgery.

Indications for Cesarean Section

You do not need to know every detail about cesarean sections, but acquiring some knowledge about the reasons they are done will give you clues to potential emotional stress lodged in a mother's tissues, which may begin to release during a massage session. While receiving massage, some women may discuss their surgical experiences. The more knowledge you have, the more support you can lend.

Maternal Reasons for Cesarean Section
- Failure to Progress: If a mother who is in active labor does not continue dilating and becomes too exhausted to continue, a cesarean section may be performed. Medically, "failure to progress" is often defined as progress of less than 1 cm of dilation per hour for two hours.
- Previous Cesarean Section: Women who have experienced a previous cesarean section have a small but increased risk in subsequent pregnancies for a uterine rupture. Many facilities now require that a woman with a previous cesarean section have a repeat cesarean delivery without attempting labor.
- Preeclampsia: This is one condition that can lead to cesarean birth. If the preeclampsia is progressing dangerously or is uncontrolled, a speedy delivery to reduce the risk of eclampsia may be necessary. If a medical induction of labor is not successful, a cesarean section may be done.
- Maternal Infection: Women who have active genital herpes or are HIV positive at the time of birth typically will have a cesarean section birth to avoid transmitting the virus to the infant.
- Uterine Rupture: On rare occasions, the uterus may have a weakness in one area that causes it to rupture under the stress of contractions. This is more likely to occur if a woman had a previous uterine surgery or cesarean section. This condition requires an emergency cesarean section and possibly a hysterectomy, as it is a life-threatening condition for the mother and baby.
- Doctor or Mother's Convenience or Preference: There are situations in which, for convenience or preference, a cesarean birth is chosen by the doctor or patient.

BOX 13.1 | Benefits of Massage After Cesarean Section

Any client you have seen through pregnancy could end up with an unplanned cesarean section. For these clients, nurturing and therapeutic bodywork can be of aid by having the following effects:

- Reducing formation of scar tissue and adhesions[5,6]
- Encouraging respiration and increasing circulation, thereby decreasing risk of respiratory problems such as pneumonia, and complications of venous stasis, such as blood clots
- Relieving backaches sometimes related to epidural anesthesia or positioning during surgery

- Decreasing discomfort from bloating, gas distention, or constipation
- Decreasing postoperative nausea, vomiting, anxiety, and pain
- Helping the mother connect with her body and baby after a possible disassociation related to anesthesia and a lack of active participation in the delivery
- Encouraging awareness of healthy posture for the postpartum period and generating body awareness through touch

Fetal Reasons for Cesarean Section

- Large Baby: If the size of the baby relative to the size of a mother's pelvis does not allow for the passage of the baby through the pelvic outlet, a cesarean section is necessary.
- Malpositioned Baby: The baby's position sometimes prevents her or him from descending easily into the pelvis or from being able to fit easily through the pelvic outlet. An example of this is if the baby is positioned sideways or transverse.
- Fetal Distress or Umbilical Cord Prolapse: During labor, it is possible for the baby to experience distress: examples of this include fetal infection, a knot that tightens in the umbilical cord with each contraction, or compression of the umbilical cord for other reasons. A drop in the mother's blood pressure after an epidural or a change of position affects the flow of blood to the baby, sometimes causing fetal stress. Usually this is resolved quickly with IV fluids or another change of position, but if not, a cesarean section may be indicated.

  When the umbilical cord prolapses or comes through the vaginal canal before the baby, an emergency cesarean section is necessary, as the cord will be compressed when the baby is in the birth canal, cutting off its oxygen supply.
- Twins/Multiple Babies: Twins can be born vaginally, but if one or both are positioned sideways or in a position too difficult for vaginal delivery, a cesarean section may be necessary.
- Placental Concerns: Conditions in which the placenta has grown over the opening of the uterus (called a previa) or in which it pulls partly or totally away from the wall of the uterus (abruption) require cesarean delivery. An abruption will require emergency surgery, as it is a life-threatening situation for the mother and baby.

Cesarean Section Procedure

When the decision to perform a cesarean section is made, there are some standard procedures performed. A urinary catheter will be placed in the mother's bladder to keep her bladder empty during and after surgery. Her belly and pubic hair will be shaved to below the area of the incision line. Intravenous fluids will be given quickly. All who enter the surgical room, including you or other support team members, must wear protective hair and shoe coverings and a mask. Most frequently, a spinal or epidural anesthesia will be used for a nonemergency cesarean section. In a life-threatening emergency, general anesthesia (gas) is used, as it is faster.

Once a woman is comfortable and has no sensations in her abdomen, a low transverse or "bikini" cut will be made through the abdomen, the muscles will be pulled apart, and uterus will be incised to remove the baby. Delivery occurs within minutes after preparations have been made and anesthesia is in place.

Immediate Postsurgical Complications

If you are with a woman during a labor that progresses into a cesarean section or ends with a tubal ligation, you might be in the position of being with her during the immediate recovery period as well. During the first hours after surgery, medical personnel will assess her for a few risks. You can help to decrease the risk for several of these complications by encouraging particular activities for healing.

- *Respiratory Depression*: After abdominal surgery and anesthesia, a patient's respiratory capacity is temporarily decreased, increasing the risk of complications such as pneumonia and fluid in the lungs. Many massage therapists incorporate deep breathing with their bodywork. This along with muscle mobilizations and encouraging expansion of the ribs can help the newly postoperative client avoid risks associated with diminished breathing after surgery.[3]

  If you are supporting a woman in the first hours after a cesarean section, remind her every 15 to 30 minutes, with gentle touch to her head, neck, chest, or upper back, to take several deep inhalations. Use some of the techniques for shortness of breath from Chapter 9 during this time.
- *Blood Clots*: The development of DVT is increased during and after surgery.[4-6] Encourage a woman in the first hours after recovery to roll her legs externally and internally, bend the knees up and press them down against the bed, and generally contract and release her leg muscles. In the first hours after surgery, these activities along with massage (if approved by her PCP) can improve blood circulation[7] and prevent the development of clots.

 CAUTION: Obtain permission from the PCP before massaging the legs in the immediate postsurgical recovery time. Always maintain blood clot precautions as discussed earlier in this book.

- *Nausea/Vomiting*: Occasionally, after general anesthesia, nausea or vomiting can occur. Encourage a woman to brace her abdomen with a pillow if she does vomit, to reduce pain and stress to the incision. In addition, Pericardium 6 is a powerful acupressure point located on the inner wrist (Figure 13.1) that has proven to be very useful in reducing postcesarean nausea.[8-10]
- *Gas Cramping*: After abdominal surgery, intestinal activity may slow or stop temporarily. Once a new postsurgical mother begins to drink fluids and eat solid food (which may be the same or next day after surgery), she may experience bloating and painful gas cramps if her intestines are not operating at their normal efficiency. Massage can help relieve some of this discomfort with simple hands-on energy work and gentle effleurage to the upper abdomen, avoiding direct pressure on or near the incision. Reflexology, massage, and applications of warmth can also be effective in promoting peristalsis and releasing gas.[11-15]
- *Pain*: Massage can help decrease the experience of postoperative pain.[16-20] If the anesthesia is wearing off and a woman is not adequately medicated, she may begin to feel pain in her incision area. Until she has received another dose of medication and is experiencing relief of pain from it, try holding the soles of her feet or squeezing and massaging her toes. This can help her to feel more grounded and can relieve pain through the stimulation of sensory corpuscles in the feet.

Other residual effects related to cesarean sections and of concern to a bodyworker include the following:

- *Adhesion formation*: After surgery, scar tissue begins to form immediately, and adhesions may develop around the uterus or intestines. Numbness will exist around the incision for years or a lifetime. Scar tissue massage impedes the development of restricting and painful adhesions and speeds healing.[21-24]
- *Epidural-Related Back Pain*: If a mother had an epidural or spinal anesthesia, she may have short-term back pain related to positioning issues during the surgery, or specifically related to the anesthesia needle insertion.[25,26] Massage can be effective in reducing this back pain.
- *Physiological Stress:* Along with caring for a new baby, a client is also recovering from major abdominal surgery. The potential for muscular and ligamentous strains is increased as the pregnancy-stressed abdominals are further weakened by surgical incision and manual separation of the muscles. A massage therapist can help to speed recovery by stimulating lymphatic flow, increasing healing energy to the incision, instructing postural correction and encouraging the pursuit of abdominal strengthening.
- *Emotional Stress:* If she had a sudden, unexpected, or emergency cesarean section, a mother may need a recovery period from emotional trauma, as well as from general anesthesia (if she had that). A sense of confusion, ambivalence, disappointment, and fear, or a disassociation from the baby can be associated with an unplanned cesarean section. Massage provides nurturing care that can support a client's efforts to process her experience. It also increases circulation, thereby speeding the body's cellular release of anesthesia chemicals and enhancing recovery.

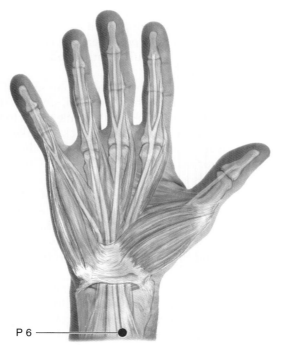

FIGURE 13.1   Pericardium 6: Acupressure point for nausea.

This point is well-known for its efficacy in relieving nausea, including after a cesarean section. It is located on the inner wrist, 2-3 fingerwidths up from the wrist crease, between the tendons of palmaris longus and flexor carpi radialis.

Postpartum Tubal Ligation

A minor surgery that a woman may undergo after or during birth is a postpartum **tubal ligation**, or cutting of the fallopian tubes as a permanent form of birth control. Since the uterus is still quite large at this time, relative to a nonpregnant uterus, it is easy to locate the fallopian tubes. Normally a tubal ligation is done laparascopically, with small incisions on either side of the navel. The fallopian tubes are then cut and tied or cut and cauterized. Though quick and usually an out-patient procedure, a woman must still be given anesthesia. When she awakes, she may have some pain in the abdominal area. Women may also develop adhesions from this procedure, along with tenderness of the abdomen for a few weeks afterward. Be sure to include questions about surgery during your postpartum intake, to determine whether abdominal massage is appropriate. Wait until the incisions are healed and the mother is feeling comfortable enough to receive touch on her abdomen before beginning abdominal massage; this may be 2 to 3 weeks after a tubal ligation.

Recovery From Birth-Related Surgery

Recovery from any major abdominal surgery normally takes at least 6 to 8 weeks, but cesarean recovery is compounded by accompanying postpartum changes, including the shift in hormones, musculoskeletal and postural alterations, and the emotional reality of becoming a mother. While some women feel comfortable with their birth and have no sense of loss by having a cesarean section, others may feel a disconnect with the baby. For some there may be grief, a sense of failure, and confusion about having a cesarean section. Lack of bonding with the baby may have developed out of the mother's emotional issues related to surgical birth as well as from the possibility that the baby was sleepy and less responsive if general anesthesia or other medications were used prior to birth. Skin-to-skin contact with the baby and frequent massage for both the mother and baby, as well as encouraging the mother to touch and massage her baby, may help to diminish these issues.[27]

PREPARING TO MASSAGE POSTSURGICAL CLIENTS

When working with women who have recently undergone birth-related surgery, learn about the nature of her surgery by asking appropriate health intake questions and recognizing key contraindications and precautions.

Health Intake for Postsurgical Clients

Always do a thorough health intake when beginning work with a new postpartum client to determine if there are any risk factors that would affect your work or require a medical release. See Box 13.2 for conditions requiring medical release.

Women who have had a cesarean section or tubal ligation may require additional intake questions beyond the standard postpartum ones. Questions one might ask, along with the reasons for asking them, include the following:

1. *Was the cesarean section an emergency surgery or planned?* The therapist may encounter emotional turmoil or trauma for either type of cesarean section, but for those for whom it was an emergency there can often be residual post-traumatic stress that could arise during a massage session. If the surgery was due to maternal or fetal complications, you will need to assess whether she is past all risks related to the condition. For instance, preeclampsia is a condition that can continue into the postpartum period for up to 6 weeks. A medical

---

BOX 13.2 | When to Obtain Medical Release After Surgery

A medical release for Type I massage is necessary for the following conditions after surgery:

- Less than 2 weeks postsurgery
- Less than 6 weeks postpartum with history of serious preeclampsia during pregnancy
- Surgery due to maternal complications that may still be problematic, such as hemorrhage after placenta abruption leading to anemia

- Client still on bedrest for high blood pressure or other issues
- Known thrombophlebitis or blood clot
- Pre-existing cardiac or circulatory conditions

release would be necessary before beginning work with this client. If the surgery was due to fetal problems, the baby could still be having difficulties adjusting to life outside the womb, causing increased stress for the mother.

2. *How is the baby?* If the surgery was related to fetal distress, the baby may be continuing to have problems now, or perhaps did for some time after birth, increasing anxiety and stress for the mother and family.

3. *Did she labor or push for hours before surgery occurred?* A woman who labored or pushed before a cesarean section will have all the same types of aches and pains that a woman with a vaginal birth might have. She has done all the work of labor, except for the actual delivery.

4. *How is she feeling now about her surgery?* Assessing her emotional status may help you identify how to support her physically or emotionally if feelings do arise.

5. *Is she having pain related to the surgery?* Her discomforts might indicate the need to position sidelying or semi-reclining.

Contraindications and Precautions for Postsurgical Massage

Review the contraindications and precautions for general postpartum clients, which will also apply to a woman who had a surgical birth. There are a few other specific precautions to follow when working with a woman who had a cesarean section.

- *Avoid deep pelvic work:* For 6 to 8 weeks postsurgery, deep pelvic abdominal work, such as work on the psoas, is contraindicated. This is due to the 3 to 5 times increased risk of clots related to surgery, and the healing required for the incision area of the abdomen and uterus. This risk is further compounded if the client is obese, older than 35, or has had several births already.[4-6]

- *Cautious stretching:* In the first month after surgery, it can be easy to strain the abdominals, potentially causing injury to the incision site or to the recovering muscles. Be cautious when doing passive or assisted stretches that may affect the incision area. To prevent straining her abdominals, instruct your client in proper body mechanics for sitting up from lying down on your table.

- *Positioning:* In the first 1 to 2 weeks after surgery, a mother may feel too tender in her belly to be comfortable lying prone. Use the sidelying position or a massage chair if that is comfortable, to access her back.

- *Infection:* Adhere to standard massage precautions and avoid massage to a client who is experiencing a uterine, bladder, or other infection, which sometimes develops after surgery. Symptoms of incision infection may include oozing, redness, heat to the area, increased swelling, or fever.

- *Incision:* Usually wound dressings are removed before a client leaves the hospital and staples are removed within the week. While you will not begin direct scar work before the incision is healed, be certain that any staples or dressings have been removed if you are doing any light abdominal work that moves the superficial tissues. Do not perform *deep* scar work until the tissues have healed and are well aligned.

General Postcesarean Section Treatment

In general, a woman who has had a cesarean section can benefit from any of the following practices:

- If your client had a cesarean section, hold lightly over the scar and envision warm healing light melting into the scar, mending and repairing the tissues.

- Warm hydrotherapy packs (not hot) or ice packs (whichever is more comfortable for her) to the incision site can help relieve some discomfort and increase healing of the wound. Apply these packs while massaging other parts of her body.

- Offer gentle superficial abdominal work.

- Position the client on the table with an awareness of potential abdominal discomforts and offer a small pillow to help her brace her abdomen if necessary when she is sitting up or shifting sides in the massage.

- Begin in the early postpartum period to address postural corrections. Women who have incision pain may find themselves hunched forward to protect their abdomen.

- Some women feel very uncomfortable touching the area of their incision, afraid to feel the physical or emotional sensations connected with the area. If appropriate and necessary, you can help increase their comfort by introducing gentle contact on the abdomen and incision area through the sheet. Instruct her to focus her breathing into the area, and envision softening and healing energy flowing in. Begin gentle rocking, vibration, and soft palpation, gradually feeling into the area superficially, then more deeply, noting where pains and lumps are.

COMMON COMPLAINTS AFTER BIRTH-RELATED SURGERY

A mother who has had a cesarean section will experience incision pain as opposed to perineal discomfort, but she could also have many of the other discomforts of a vaginal birth. She may also have additional low backache resulting from the spinal insertion of an epidural catheter and from the increased loss of muscle tone in the abdomen due to surgery. Gentle Type II bodywork, including reflexology and acupressure, is appropriate and helpful immediately after surgery. Moderate Type I techniques are useful on the head, neck, shoulders, and upper body beginning 1 to 2 days after surgery.

Depleted Energy

Many women who have had a cesarean section may appear to recover more quickly than those who have had other types of major abdominal surgery. There are at least two possible reasons for this. First, it is typically a quick surgery, without much manipulation of the organs besides the uterus. Second, the mother is typically so absorbed in the care of her new child that she may become more distracted from the discomfort from surgery.

However her surgical recovery transpires, the need for gentle rejuvenating care will be compounded by the generalized energy depletion that often accompanies the postpartum period. With the addition of a surgical invasion into a woman's interior world—a horizontal incision that cuts across the energetic acupressure meridians of her torso—and the consequent development of scar tissue in this area of multiple meridians, this energetic depletion can be significant.

Review the treatment for depleted energy during the postpartum period in Chapter 12, which can be applied to women who have had a cesarean section as well.

Epidural Back Pain

Epidural anesthesia is administered to the epidural space of the lumbar area of the spine. A large needle is used to puncture through the skin and muscles into this area, and then a tiny catheter is slid in, through which numbing medication will be continuously pumped, causing numbness from the waist down. Many women find that for weeks or sometimes months after receiving an epidural, they experience pain specifically at the site of the needle insertion.

General massage to this area, myofascial release, and deep tissue work can help to reduce some of this discomfort. While many anesthetists deny that an epidural is a cause of back pain, this author's personal experience along with the reported experiences of many bodywork clients, indicate otherwise.

Abdominal Scar Tissue

Surgery and scar tissue can cause long-term numbness from at least 1 inch above and below the incision due to the cutting of nerves during surgery. As the scar heals, a woman might experience sensations of itching, pulling, and tingling as some nerves regenerate. Adhesions develop in the scar area that can attach to the colon and intestines, causing pain with intestinal activity.

Benefits of Scar Tissue Massage

Proper attention to a new or older scar can have the following effects:

- Increase circulation to the scar area, hastening healing
- Reduce, eliminate, or prevent adhesions and alleviate discomfort associated with them[21-24]
- Desensitize the client to issues about the surgery and scar

When to Begin Scar Massage

Scar tissue and adhesions begin to form immediately after surgery, binding muscles and connective tissue and restricting movement in the abdomen and inner organs. If possible, address the scar soon after surgery, beginning with gentle superficial work within the first 7 to 14 days after the surgery.[28] The first 3 months after surgery is the optimum time to affect and influence the formation of a scar with massage, before the collagen becomes more set and rigid. Scars can be worked on years later, however, early work provides quicker and easier results. Light energy work can be done over the scar or in the surrounding area, without actually touching the scar, as soon as the staples are removed. Touch can be applied for 5 to 15 minutes per day, keeping the hands a couple of inches away from the incision and working the area around it. The client can also do this work to herself. Use her comfort level and sensations as your guide to depth, pressure, and movement. With a fresh scar of less than 3 months, there may be emotional discomfort, but there should not be significant pain associated with your work as the collagen fibers are still malleable, as opposed to stuck in place.

Once the staples are removed or absorbed, the incision is healed on the surface, the scab is gone, and there is no drainage or bleeding, you can begin superficial scar tissue work. This is usually within the first 7 to 14 days, a time when the scar is still quite malleable to the touch. Generally it will be 4 to 6 weeks after surgery before you may apply deeper, direct pressure to the scar. By this time, the incision should be well-healed externally and internally, and deeper work can be done without danger of disrupting the healing. Encourage your client to work on her scar herself, 2 to 4 times per week during these first months.

Assessing the Scar

Before beginning scar tissue work, determine how old the scar is and whether or not the client experiences any sort of pain in relation to it. Look at the incision to ascertain that there are no signs of infection, that the incision looks well-healed, and that there is no bleeding or oozing.

Feel the incision first superficially and gradually more deeply, determining its pliability and eventually moving into deeper work as the client tolerates. Always use good communication and touch slowly when approaching the abdomen and scar area.

Initial Scar Work

Benefits: When the superficial incision is healed and the client feels ready, this technique can be used every day to help speed healing and reduce adhesions.

Technique
1. With your fingertips, lightly vibrate the skin over the incision site. Increase the vibration to include the superficial fascia beneath.
2. Slide along the skin, elongating the scar in all directions. If the skin does not move or catches in a particular direction, work more on that area. As it frees up, you can work deeper and deeper into the fascia.

Sliding, Rolling, Stretching, Lifting

Benefits: Assesses the scar, breaks up adhesions, increases mobility of tissues

Technique
1. Place the flats of your fingers on the client's abdomen and gently move your fingers across the superficial layers of her abdomen close to and over the scar, moving skin across

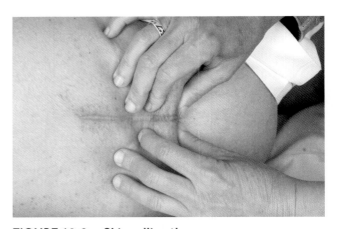

FIGURE 13.2   Skin rolling the scar.

Using your thumbs and fingertips, roll the skin of the scar gently from one side to the other, end to end as well as across the scar.

fascia, feeling for restrictions, and moving back and forth across areas that feel stuck.
2. Communicate with your client to ensure that she informs you about her comfort and pain levels. Emotional pain associated with a cesarean section can be manifested as physical pain and may arise during scar work.
3. Using your thumbs and fingertips, roll the skin of the scar gently from one side to the other, end to end as well as across the scar (Figure 13.2).
4. Place your fingertips of both hands directly on the scar. Press down into the tissue to a level appropriate to the client's comfort and for the age of the scar—lighter for new scars, deeper for old scars. Slide the fingers slowly along the direction of the scar, feeling for restrictions along the way, and focusing on the areas with restriction.
5. Return to one side of the scar and move your fingers up and down, pressing into and releasing from the scar, as if playing a flute (Figure 13.3).
6. Place your fingers or thumbs on either side of the scar. Press in gently to the superficial fascia. Apply a stretching motion to the tissue, pulling diagonally across the scar (Figure 13.4). Hold the stretch for 30 seconds, then release slowly and move to another section. Work this way stretching in all directions, helping the fascia to realign itself.
7. Place your hands on either side of the client's abdomen, grasping hold of the abdominal tissue on either side of the midline.
8. Lift up, creating space in the abdomen as you hold the belly tissue, as described in Figure 12.5B.

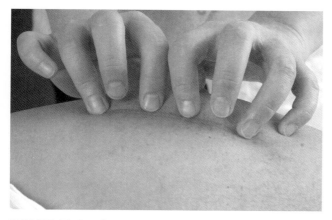

FIGURE 13.3   Pressing on the scar.

Move your fingers up and down, pressing and releasing on the scar, as if playing a flute.

Cross-Fiber Friction

Benefits: Reduces adhesions and fascial restriction.

This technique is used once you are able to go below the surface layers.

Technique

1. With your fingertips or thumbs, use gentle cross-fiber friction directly on the scar, feeling for lumps, restrictions, or tension .
2. Focus on these areas for several minutes, warming the area with the friction. Imagine helping to realign fascia into an organized alignment, moving it out of any disjointed mazes it may have made on its own.

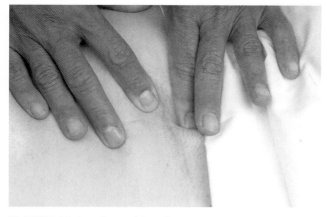

FIGURE 13.4   Stretching the scar.

Press in gently to the superficial fascia. Apply a stretching motion to the tissue, pulling diagonally across the scar.

CHAPTER SUMMARY

If you were with a client during a labor that progressed to a cesarean section, you may well be there with her in the immediate postoperative period. This is a perfect time to use therapeutic bodywork to support her recovery. More commonly, you will see a client several weeks or months after the experience, at which point scar tissue massage and attention to the potential emotional issues associated with the surgery will still be very effective and beneficial. Cultivate an understanding of the emotional and physical ramifications of this type of birth-related surgery to optimally support your client during the postsurgical/postpartum period. At any time along the journey, whether it is in the first hours after surgery, or a year or more later, a mother can benefit from nurturing touch by those educated in perinatal bodywork issues and skilled in the use of relevant techniques that can address them.

CHAPTER REVIEW QUESTIONS

1. Give six maternal-related reasons and five fetal-related reasons for a cesarean section.
2. Explain how a massage therapist can improve her or his ability to support postpartum clientele by understanding reasons for cesarean births.
3. Identify common postsurgical risks of the immediate recovery period from a cesarean section and how a massage therapist might be able to help with any of them, if he or she is still present with the client after the delivery.
4. Name five precautions to working with a postsurgical client.
5. Discuss four assessment questions you would ask a postsurgical mother and incorporate into a health intake-form. How would this information help you with your work?
6. Describe what techniques or positioning would be appropriate if your client has difficulty lying prone or receiving touch on her abdomen after her surgery.
7. Describe three ways a massage therapist can improve a client's immediate physical or emotional experience during a cesarean section recovery.
8. Discuss criteria that must be met before working directly on fresh scars. Describe two bodywork techniques for addressing scar tissue.
9. Describe the general approach to beginning abdominal scar tissue work. Discuss elements of your communication, your way of touching, and your way of helping a client feel comfortable.

What kind of issues might arise for a woman during the course of abdominal scar tissue treatment?

10. Your client who is 3 weeks postpartum pushed for 3 hours, and finally delivered her baby with an epidural and cesarean section. She has 2 children at home. She is experiencing general fatigue, low back pain, and some pain around her incision area. She saw her PCP 1 week ago, while having the same symptoms and was told her recovery was normal. What questions would you ask to assess her current condition and history and what might you suspect as causes of her complaints?

REFERENCES

1. Romero R, Tarca AL, Tromp G. Insights into the physiology of childbirth using transcriptomics. PLoS Med 2006;3(6):e276. Published online 2006 June 13. doi: 10.1371/journal.pmed.0030276.
2. Hamilton BE, Martin JA, Ventura SJ. Births: Preliminary Data for 2005. National vital statistics reports. Vol 55. Hyattsville, MD: National Center for Health Statistics. Forthcoming.
3. Scheidegger D, Bentz L, Piolino G, et al. Influence of early mobilization on pulmonary function in surgical patients. Intensive Care Med March 1976;2(1):35–40.
4. Richter ON, Rath W. [Thromboembolic diseases in pregnancy.] [Article in German] Ann Med Interne (Paris) 2003;154(5-6):301–309.
5. Geburtshilfe Z. [The risk of maternal venous thromboembolism disease. synopsis and definition of high-risk groups][Article in French] Neonatol 2007;211(1):1–7.
6. Palareti G. Pregnancy and venous thrombosis. [haematologica reports] 2005;1(10):13–17.
7. Beck MF. Theory and Practice of Therapeutic Massage. Clifton Park, NY: Thomson Delmar Learning, 1999.
8. Agarwal A, Bose N, Gaur A, et al. Acupressure and ondansetron for postoperative nausea and vomiting after laparoscopic cholecystectomy. Can J Anaesth 2002;49:554–560.
9. Alkaissi A, Stålnert M, Kalman S. Effect and placebo effect of acupressure (P6) on nausea and vomiting after outpatient gynaecological surgery. Acta Anaesthesiol Scand 1999;43(3):270–274.
10. Chen HM, Chang FY, Hsu CT. Effect of acupressure on nausea, vomiting, anxiety and pain among post-cesarean section women in Taiwan. Kaohsiung J Med Sci 2005;21(8):341–350.
11. Ayas A, Leblebici B, Sözay S, et al. The effect of abdominal massage on bowel function in patients with spinal cord injury. Am J Phys Med Rehabil 2006;85(12):951–956.
12. Albers B, Cramer H, Fischer A, et al. [Abdominal massage as intervention for patients with paraplegia caused by spinal cord injury—a pilot study] [Article in German] Pflege Z 2006;59(3):2–8.
13. Ernst E. Abdominal massage therapy for chronic constipation: A systematic review of controlled clinical trials. Forsch Komplementarmed. 1999;6(3):149–151.
14. Yang Y, Chao L, Meng, G, et al. Exploring the Application of Foot Reflexology to the Prevention and Treatment of Functional Constipation. 1994 China Reflexology Symposium Report, Beijing: China Reflexology Association: 62–65.
15. Eriksen L. Using Reflexology to Relieve Chronic Constipation. The Danish Journal of Nursing, Sugeplejersken 1992;June 24.
16. Silva MA. The effects of relaxation touch on the recovery level of post anesthesia abdominal hysterectomy patients. Virginia Henderson International Nursing Library;1992. Last accessed online Aug13, 2007 at: http://nursinglibrary.org/Portal/main.aspx?pageid=4024&sid=647.
17. Piotrowski MM, Paterson C, Mitchinson A, et al. Massage as adjuvant therapy in the management of acute postoperative pain: a preliminary study in men. J Am Coll Surg Dec 2003;197(6):1037–1046.
18. Taylor AG, Galper DI, Taylor P, et al. Effects of adjunctive Swedish massage and vibration therapy on short-term postoperative outcomes: a randomized, controlled trial. J Altern Complement Med 2003;9(1):77–89.
19. Field T, Hernandez-Reif M, Miguel D, et al. Cortisol decreases and serotonin and dopamine increase following massage therapy. Int J Dev Neurosci 2005;115(10):1397–1413.
20. Nixon M, Teschendorff J, Finney J, et al. Expanding the nursing repertoire: the effect of massage on postoperative pain. Aust J Adv Nurs 1997;14:21–26.
21. LaFrano C. Scar-tissue massage. Massage Magazine May/June 2001:151–160.
22. Whitridge P. The role of massage in scar healing. Massage Magazine, March 2007:91–96.
23. Archer P. Three clinical sports massage approaches for treating injured athletes. Athletic Ther Today 2001;6(3):14–20.
24. Sefton J. Myofascial release for athletic trainers, Part 3: Specific techniques. Athletic Ther Today. 2004;9(3)40–41.
25. MacArthur C, Lewis M, Knox EG, Crawford JS. Epidural anaesthesia and long term backache after childbirth. Brit Med J 1990;301(6742):9–12.
26. Butler R, Fuller J. Back pain following epidural anaesthesia in labour. Can J Anaesth 1998;45(8):724–728.
27. Onozawa K, Glover V, Adams D, et al. Infant massage improves mother-infant interaction for mothers with postnatal depression. J Affect Disord 2001;63(1–3):201–207.
28. Witte MB, Barbul A. General principles of wound healing. Surg Clin North Am 1997;77(3):509–528.

Abdominal support binders Elastic or cloth support for the abdomen that wrap around the belly and support its weight during the later stages of pregnancy.

Active labor The phase of labor in which cervical dilation is from 4 to 8 cm or so and contractions average a rate of every 3 to 5 minutes and last 60 to 90 seconds.

Amniotic sac The membranous bag that holds intact the developing fetus, placenta, and amniotic fluid in utero; also known as the "bag of waters."

Back labor A condition when a laboring mother feels contractions primarily in her back, rather than in her abdomen or pelvis; often caused by a posteriorly positioned baby.

Bloody show A brownish, reddish discharge as the cervix begins to dilate. The blood may have occurred as a result of cervical exams by a PCP.

Braxton-Hicks contractions Irregular "practice contractions" that are generally mild and do not cause the cervix to dilate. Women in their first pregnancy tend to have fewer Braxton-Hicks contractions than those in subsequent pregnancies. Braxton-Hicks contractions are *not* the same as preterm labor contractions which tend to be more regular and consistent, may sometimes be feel crampy in the low pelvis, and which can cause an early delivery of the baby. If the client has more than 4 contractions in 1 hour and it is unclear what type of contractions they are, she should be referred to her prenatal care provider.

Breech When the baby is positioned in utero with the buttocks in the mother's pelvis and head up toward her ribs. The normal vertex position for birth is with the baby's head down in the mother's pelvis.

Broad ligament Wide and thin uterine ligament that spreads out like a sheet from the lateral aspects of the uterus and sinks into the iliac fossa area in the anterior hip, the walls of the pelvic cavity, and the connective tissue of the pelvic floor. The ovaries and round ligament are suspended within the broad ligament.

Cardinal ligament A band of ligamentous tissue, also known as the *ligamentum transversalis colli*, that supports the cervix and uterus and attaches to the lateral vagina.

Catecholamines Chemicals produced by the adrenal medulla, such as epinephrine, that act as hormones and neurotransmitters. They stimulate the sympathetic nervous system, cause an increase in heart rate, blood pressure, and respirations, and divert blood away from digestion. They also relax smooth muscle, which, during pregnancy, results in slowing or stalling labor.

Cervix The bottom neck of the uterus that joins with the vagina.

Cesarean section (c-section) The surgical delivery of a baby through a mother's abdomen.

Chakra Sanskrit word referring to a spinning vortex of energy located in specific areas of the body.

Chloasma Darkening of the skin like a mask on the face, caused by estrogen effects during pregnancy; it resolves after pregnancy.

Contractions Rhythmic uterine cramping that helps move the baby down and out and dilates the cervix.

Corpuscles Special tactile receptors found in different layers of the skin and sensitive to specific types of touch, such as continuous pressure, vibration, cold, and deep pressure.

Crowning The point during birth when the widest part of baby's head fills the vagina, expanding the perineum and causing the tissues to stretch.

Deep vein thrombosis Development of a clot in the deep veins, usually in the legs.

Diastasis recti Thinning of the fascial linea alba so that the rectus abdominus muscles separate, reducing anterior support of the torso and often leading to back pain.

Diastasis symphysis pubis Separation of the symphysis pubis due to postural imbalance and/or relaxin's softening effects. This condition can be very painful, especially with hip abduction.

Dilate/dilation The process of cervical opening during labor that allows the baby to enter the vaginal vault. This process of opening is called dilation.

Doula An Ancient Greek term for the handmaidens and birth companions to the upper echelon women, now used to describe professional birth and postpartum supporters. Many studies have been done indicating that doulas, or continuous birth supporters have a powerful and beneficial influence on the process and outcome of birth.

Due date A date when labor is expected to begin. It is determined by adding 40 weeks to the first day of the last menstrual period (LMP), (assuming a woman has a regular 28 day menstrual cycle), or adding 38 weeks to the known day of conception. Alternatively, 3 months can be subtracted from the LMP, and 7 days added onto that. Only 10% of births actually occur on the due date. The due date is often written in medical notes as EDC or expected date of confinement. This is a relic of days when women were kept separated from her family or community during birth. It is also sometimes called the EDD (estimated date of delivery).

Early labor The early part of labor, when the cervix begins to dilate from 0 to 4 cm or so.

Eclampsia Seizures during pregnancy, often following preeclampsia.

Efface/effacement The thinning or shortening of the uterine cervix that occurs before or in the process of labor. The cervix is normally 1.5 to 2 inches long. As it thins, or shortens, it is measured in percentages. Fifty percent effaced means it is about 1 inch long. The cervix must normally be 100% effaced and fully dilated before pushing begins.

Embolus Blood clot that becomes dislodged from the venous wall and travels through the circulation with the potential of becoming lodged in a vessel in the lungs, brain, or heart, often with devastating consequences. When it obstructs a blood vessel, it is called an *embolus* (plural: emboli).

Endorphins Neurotransmitters that help reduce painful sensations or affect pain perception. They are also related to mood, feelings of euphoria, memory retention, and the release of sex hormones.

Engaged The state in which the widest diameter of the baby's head settles into the mother's pelvis in preparation for or during birth.

Engorgement The swelling of the breast tissue with lymph, blood, and milk during the second to fifth postpartum day in preparation for mature milk production. Until this time, the baby has been drinking the pre-milk or colostrum, which contains primary antibodies that build a baby's immune system. Nursing stimulates the production of milk, and engorgement may follow as the milk "comes in." For some women, engorgement can be very painful.

Epidural anesthesia Anesthesia often used during labor to numb sensations from the waist down. A thin catheter is placed in the epidural space of the spine, and medications are injected which cause the numbing.

Episiotomy Cutting of the perineal tissues to help the baby to be born faster.

Estrogen Normally produced by the ovaries and adrenal cortex, estrogen is produced in early pregnancy first by the corpus luteum and then the placenta. Estrogen has multiple influences in the pregnant body, including softening connective tissue and preparing the endometrium for caring for the fertilized egg, embryo, and fetus. It also increases breast size, vascularity, and the number and size of milk-producing ducts and lobes. It contributes to the development of darker skin on the abdomen and face with the linea negra and chloasma. Estrogen contributes to extra blood flow to the nasal mucosa, causing swelling, stuffiness, and sometimes bloody noses.

Fibrolytic activity This is the clotting mechanism of the blood—the blood clots faster than normal during pregnancy to help prevent excessive blood loss by hemorrhage at birth.

First stage of labor The first of three stages of labor involves dilation and effacement of the cervix from 0 to 10 cm, until pushing. The phases of pre-labor, early, and active labor and transition are all part of the first stage.

Gestational diabetes A type of diabetes, different from the common diabetes mellitus, that only occurs during pregnancy and resolves after delivery. When controlled, it generally does not require the use of insulin but does demand attention to diet to prevent excessive blood sugar level. Excess maternal blood sugar level will cause the baby to grow larger, thereby causing size-related difficulties at delivery.

Gestational hypertension High blood pressure that develops during pregnancy, usually beginning between 20 weeks' gestation and 1 week postpartum.

HELLP syndrome An acronym for Hemolysis, Elevated Liver enzymes, and Low Platelets. An insidious syndrome considered by some to be a variation of advanced preeclampsia. It is characterized by pain in the epigastric area or right upper quadrant of the abdomen, often accompanied by general malaise, nausea, vomiting, headache.[1]

High-risk pregnancies Pregnancies in which the woman has conditions that put her more at risk for complications. While these conditions place a woman at a higher *risk* for developing problems, they *are not necessarily a problem in and of themselves.*

Interstitial fluid Fluid located between cells with the functions of bathing and protecting the cells, filtering and removing waste. Lymph fluid originates as interstitial fluid. When excessive interstitial fluid builds up in the tissues, it manifests as edema. This is not uncommon in the hands or feet during the third trimester of pregnancy due to extra blood volume and more sluggish circulation in the extremities.

Intrauterine growth restriction The fetus is small for its estimated gestational age, as indicated by measurements and ultrasound. This condition may indicate it has fetal anomalies or other problems.

Involute To involute, or the process of involution is, in this case, the act of the postpartum uterus contracting back down to a nonpregnant size.

Kegel exercises Exercises that tone the perineal muscles.

Labor Commonly defined as the time when uterine contractions last 60 to 90 seconds, have been occurring consistently every 3 to 5 minutes for at least a couple hours, and are causing cervical changes.

Lightening In the late third trimester, the baby will usually "drop" down into the pelvis, engaging more fully into position for labor. The mother will feel relief of pressure in her diaphragm, be able to breathe more easily, and will suddenly have more pressure on her bladder. This shift of the baby's position is normally very obvious, as a mother's posture and appearance visibly change.

Linea alba Fascial line where abdominal muscles insert in centerline of abdomen.

Linea negra Skin in the area of the linea alba that darkens in pregnancy.

Mastitis Inflammation of the breast, often caused by a blocked milk duct or bacteria entering the breast through cracked nipples. Symptoms usually involve heat, hardness, and red streaking from the site of infection or inflammation, and maternal fever. Heat, massage, and frequent nursing will help to heal mastitis, along with antibiotics when needed.

Meconium The baby's first bowel movement, which is usually green or black and tarry.

Medical release A form signed by client's PCP which indicates approval for massage during the pregnancy, based on an obstetrical point of view. It can indicate restrictions or concerns applicable to bodywork according to the type of risk factors or complications the client has.

Milk ejection reflex Response to prolactin release from the pituitary gland when the baby nurses on the breast. The prolactin stimulates the release of oxytocin. Oxytocin, which causes the uterus to contract, also triggers the milk glands to contract, squeezing milk through the ducts to the nipple, to the baby. The sensation when the hormones trigger this response is often described by women as tingling, filling, and sensual, and often the breasts will begin to leak when the milk "lets down." Often this occurs in response to baby crying, or close to regular feeding times.

Miscarriage Birth before week 20 of gestation. The vast majority of miscarriages occur in the first trimester as a healthy response to the early abnormal development of an embryo. However, other known associations with miscarriage include maternal issues, such as problems with the cervix or uterus or conditions such as diabetes, infection, or virus. Miscarriage is also associated with maternal drug use, including tobacco and alcohol use.

Mucous plug Thick mucous in the cervical opening that prevents the intrusion of bacteria into the uterus. It is discharged during labor.

Oligohydramnios Condition in which too little amniotic fluid is produced. It is associated with placental dysfunctions, fetal anomalies, or fetal death.

Orthostatic hypotension Due to extra blood and fluctuations in blood pressure, some women will experience a sudden drop in blood pressure when shifting from lying down to standing or sitting, resulting in sudden dizziness, nausea, blurred vision, headache, or fatigue.

Oxytocin Hormone released from the posterior pituitary gland that causes the uterus to rhythmically contract during labor and stimulates the "let down" reflex during lactation.

Pelvic floor The group of muscles located between and below the lower bones of the pelvis, also called the *perineum* or *perineal muscles*. These provide vital support for all the internal organs. When weak, multiple pelvic floor dysfunctions develop, including urinary incontinence and uterine, rectal, and bladder prolapse.

Pitocin A synthetic oxytocin used to stimulate or augment contractions during labor, as well as used in the immediate postpartum period to decrease the risk of postpartum hemorrhage.

Pitting edema Tissue swelling in which an indentation is left for more than a brief moment after pressing a finger pad into the tissue for 5 seconds and then lifting the finger up. It can vary from mild to extreme and may indicate potential problems, such as preeclampsia.

Placenta previa In this condition, the placenta has implanted itself partially or completely over the opening of the cervix, increasing risks for bleeding and preventing vaginal delivery.

Placental abruption A condition of pregnancy where the placenta begins to separate from the wall of the uterus before the delivery of the baby. It may separate only partially, or there may be a complete abruption, where the placenta detaches entirely. It occurs in an average of 1 out of 150 to 200 pregnancies.

Polyhydramnios A condition in which excessive amniotic fluid is produced in the uterus. It is associated with maternal shortness of breath, diabetes, preterm labor, and fetal anomalies. With the increased fluid, there is an increased intrauterine pressure and impaired perfusion of blood between the uterus and placenta.

Posterior position The position in which the baby in utero is head down, with the occiput toward the mother's sacrum, and the face looking toward the mother's abdomen.

Postpartum "blues" Normal fluctuation of mood and emotions in the first few days after birth, and peaking around postpartum day 5. Symptoms may involve labile moods, teariness, fatigue, difficulty sleeping, and irritability. Typically resolves within 2 weeks.

Postpartum period Also known as *puerperium*, this is the period of time after the birth of a child until anywhere from 6 weeks to 1 year later. Minimally, it is considered the period of time until the uterus involutes as much as possible to its prepregnant state. But many new mothers find themselves in a period of emotional, physical, and psychological adjustments for at least 1 year after birth, that can still be considered the *postpartum period*.

Preeclampsia A condition of pregnancy and postpartum, characterized by changes to the organ systems, blood chemistry, and by a rise in blood pressure. It has the potential to lead to the dangerous complications of eclampsia or convulsions. Some of the common symptoms a woman might experience include headache, visual changes, epigastric pain, and pitting edema. Blood pressures causing alarm may range from slightly high (140/90 to 150/100 mm Hg) to moderately high (150/90 to 180/110 mm Hg)

Pre-labor The earliest start of labor. Also called *prodromal* or *latent* labor. The mother may be having contractions, but they are gentle and having little effect on dilating her cervix.

Premature birth A birth that occurs between gestational weeks 20 and 37.

Preterm labor Also known as premature labor, onset of contractions with changes to the cervix (dilation, shortening, and effacing) before 37 weeks' gestation and with risk of the baby being born early. Preterm contractions do not always lead to preterm *labor*. Also known as *premature labor*.

Preterm labor contractions Uterine contractions that begin after 20 weeks' and before 37 weeks gestation and promote birth before fetal development is completed. They may be felt as mild aching in the pubic area or low back, pelvic pressure, or as intermittent abdominal pains. Alternatively, they may not be noticed at all by the mother. They may be accompanied with diarrhea or watery or bloody vaginal discharge. Contractions are usually at least 4 per hour, and may grow in frequency or strength. To positively diagnose the situation as preterm labor, the client would need a cervical exam to determine if she had dilated. A uterine monitor would also be used to validate the presence of contractions. Treatment is often bedrest, hydration, and/or the use of medications to stop contractions.

Progesterone A hormone produced by the corpus luteum during the first 2 to 3 months of embryonic development until the placenta is formed and functioning, at which point the placenta takes over. Progesterone thickens the uterine lining and prepares it for implantation, then relaxes smooth muscles to prevent uterine contractility.

Prolactin Hormone released by anterior pituitary gland which stimulates milk production and may increase general immune function.

Prolapse The sagging or dropping of the bladder or uterus. The level of prolapse can range from partial, where the organ is just slightly lower in the pelvis than normal, or complete, where the organ is suspended mostly outside of the vagina between the thighs.

Pulmonary embolism Occurrence of a blood clot traveling through the circulation and becoming lodged in an artery of the lung. Symptoms include shortness of breath and chest pain, and can lead to death.

Quickening First fetal felt movements by mother.

Relaxin Hormone produced by the ovaries beginning in week 10 of pregnancy that relaxes and loosens connective tissues and ligaments, including the cervix and the pelvic joints, to create more space for the baby's birth.

Ring of fire Sensations of burning or tearing of the perineum as it stretches and as the baby's head is crowning and being born.

Round ligament An anterior cord-like uterine ligament held within the broad ligament and connecting to the pubic mons, the inguinal area of the pelvis, and the labia of the vagina.

Sciatica Pain caused by compression of the sciatic nerve. The majority of "sciatica" during pregnancy is rarely true nerve compression, but more often a referred pain from psoas tightness and uterine broad ligament pain. However, the sensations of sharp shooting pain, vague numbness, or dull aching discomfort down the back, front, or sides of the leg or in the buttocks feel similar to sciatica. SI joint hypermobility can also lead to radiating pain in the gluteals and leg.

Second stage of labor The second of three stages of labor, this stage involves pushing the baby out after complete dilation of the cervix.

Spider angioma Also called telangiectasias, sunburst varicosities, or spider veins. These are thin, tiny blood vessels visible near the surface of the skin. They may have a dark or red dot in the center and wavy tiny vessels radiating out from it, or they may be linear, especially around the inner knee. These are not the same as the troublesome varicose veins, which are larger, darker, and are a contraindicated condition for massage.

Striae gravidarum Commonly called stretch marks, these are lines on the skin which develop on the abdomen during pregnancy and seem to be caused by changes in the collagen deposits and rapid stretching of the abdomen. There is no known effective and reasonable treatment for the reduction of stretch marks once they have developed, although two creams were studied that were associated with a decrease in of the development of stretch marks.[2] Stretch marks will often become less noticeable or change to a silvery color, within a year postpartum.

Superficial thrombophlebitis Development of clots in the superficial veins of the extremities, most often the calf. Emboli do occur originating in the superficial veins, but are more common from the deeper veins.

Third stage of labor The third of three stages, this stage involves the delivery of the placenta.

Transition The final stage of cervical dilation from 8 to 10 cm.

Transverse lie The position in which the baby in utero is sideways to the pelvic opening.

Trimester One of three 13-week periods into which pregnancy is divided as a way of measuring dates and changes.

Tubal ligation Surgical birth control method in which the fallopian tubes are cut or tied or otherwise blocked off to prevent future pregnancies.

Urinary tract infection (UTI) A common infection during pregnancy. It increases the risks of preterm labor, kidney infection, and premature rupture of the membranes.

Uterine fundus The top part of the uterus.

Uterosacral ligament A uterine ligament that attaches from the posterior uterus to the anterior sacrum and pelvic cavity.

Vertex Fetal position with the baby's head down in the mother's pelvis, and the buttocks up toward her ribs. This is the most common and optimal position for a baby to be in for a vaginal birth.

REFERENCES

1. Wolf J. Liver disease in pregnancy. Med Clin North Am 1996;80:1167–1187
2. Young GL, Jewell D. Creams for preventing stretch marks in pregnancy. The Cochrane Database of Systematic Reviews. 1996, issue 1.

INDEX

Page numbers followed by "f" indicate figures; those followed by "t" indicate tables.

A

Abdominal bodywork, 58–59, 85. See also
    Belly rubs
  after cesarean section, 240
  in first trimester, 58, 105
  during labor, 160
  postpartum, 212–216
  precautions and contraindications to,
    54–57, 245
  in second trimester, 58, 60
Abdominal effleurage warm-up, 214
Abdominal energizing, 213–214
Abdominal muscles, 32, 35, 41–44
  cloth support for, 42
  diastasis recti of, 32, 39, 41–44, 42f, 45f, 257
  postpartum, 199
Abdominal myofascial release, 215, 216f
Abdominal scar tissue, 241–243
  assessment of, 242
  benefits of massage for, 241
  cross-fiber friction for, 243
  initial work for, 242
  sliding, rolling, stretching, and lifting of,
    242, 242f–243f
  when to begin massage for, 241–242
Abdominal support binders, 33, 33f, 38, 257
Abdominal tenderness, 56
Abdominal trigger point and tension release,
  214
Abdominal/perineal connection, 211
Acupressure, 9, 10, 52, 60–62, 61f, 84
  in ankle region, 63, 63f
  for back release, 99f
  for breech baby, 118
  to increase pain threshold in labor, 146
  during labor, 137, 149, 163, 165
  for lactation, 232f
  on Large Intestine 4, 193
  precautions and contraindications to,
    60–62, 61f, 245
  in preparation for birth, 132, 134, 137
  prohibited acupoints, 60–62, 61f, 99–100
  turning a baby with, 191
Acupuncture, 60
Adductor resistance, 135
Adhesion formation, postsurgical, 238, 241
Adrenaline, 146
Aerobic exercise, 229
Affirmations, 132, 133, 134, 149, 158, 161–162
Alcohol use, xi, 68
Ambivalence about pregnancy, 15, 18
American College of Obstetrics and
  Gynecology, 49
Amniotic fluid, 154–155
Amniotic sac, 154
  rupture during massage, 156
Anemia, 19
Ankle massage, 63, 63f
Ankle squeeze, for back labor, 192, 192f
Ankle swelling, 19, 23, 24
Anticoagulants, 65
Anxiety, 6, 7, 15. See also Fear
  during labor, 181–183, 182f
Arm exercise, dynamic, 230
Arm massage, 98–100
Arm mobilization, 219
Arm raise, 129
Arm stretch, 78
Aromatherapy, 62, 83, 131, 136
  postpartum, 204

precautions and contraindications to, 62,
  246
Artificial insemination, 13
Arvigo, Rosita, 85, 118
Assessment of client
  addressing client health information with
    sensitivity, 54
  health history intake form for, 52, 53f
  for postpartum bodywork, 209–210
  questions for, 53–54
  symptoms of discomfort, 54–57
  trimester considerations for, 86t
Assisted psoas stretch, 111, 112f
Asthma, 68, 246

B

Baby in utero
  descent and position of, 5, 153–154, 154f
  development of, 14–23
  effects of massage on, 1
  effects of maternal stress on, 6
  identifying position of, 189
  postural effects of size and position of, 33
  turning with acupressure, 191
Back labor, 153, 189–193, 257
  ankle squeeze for, 192, 192f
  belly lifts for, 190, 190f
  due to posterior baby, 187–189, 188f
    belly rubs for, 188–189
    general treatment for, 187–188
    hot and cold therapy for, 188, 189f
    positions for massage in client with,
      187–188
  general treatment of, 189–190
  hip pull for, 193, 193f
  hot or cold therapy for, 191
  sacral foramen stimulation for, 191–192
  sacroiliac relief for, 192f, 192–193
  techniques for, 190
Back massage, 6, 97, 98f
Back pain, 6, 7, 18, 19, 29, 32, 38, 46, 107–114
  epidural, 238, 241
  low, 107–111, 113
    assisted psoas stretch for, 111, 112f
    causes of, 108
    diastasis recti and, 41, 108
    duration of, 107
    full body stretch for, 110–111, 111f
    general treatment of, 108
    postpartum, 199
    quadratus lumborum compression
      points for, 108–110, 109f
    quadratus lumborum extension for, 110,
      111f
    quadratus lumborum release for, 110,
      110f
    risk factors for, 107–108
    sacral rub for, 111
    self-care tips for mothers to decrease,
      113, 113f
  mid and upper, 111–115
    causes of, 112
    chest opening for, 114
    general treatment of, 112
    pectoralis stretch and resistance for, 114f,
      114–115
    postural awareness and, 114
    subscapularis stretch for, 115, 115f
  postpartum, 107, 219–223

  mid and lower, 219–223
  upper, 219
  potential problems indicated by, 55
Back release
  acupressure for, 99f
  postpartum, 208–209
Bed rest, 77
  bodywork precautions for client restricted
    to, 77, 246–247
  health intake for client on, 77–78
  for preterm labor, 75
  stress relief for client restricted to, 78
Belly breathing, 18, 94
Belly lifts, 190, 190f
Belly palming, 230
Belly rubs, 102–105
  for back pain due to posterior baby,
    188–189
  benefits of, 102
  choosing position for, 104
  for contractions, 170, 170f
  duration of, 102
  oils for, 136, 170
  in preparation for birth, 134, 136
  in semi-reclining position, 104–105, 105f
  in sidelying position, 102–103, 102f–103f,
    104
Bicycle riding, supine, 224
Birth, 177–178
  creating satisfying experience of, 2, 146
  environment for, 145, 146, 157
  fear of, 146, 148
  massage for (See Labor/birth massage)
  nurturing support for, 146, 146t
  respecting role of client's partner during,
    157, 158
  role of massage therapist during, 144–145,
    155–159
Birth ball, 174
Birth preparation, 132–140. See also Labor
  acupressure for, 132, 134
  adductor resistance for, 135
  belly rub for, 134, 136
  case study of, 134
  cupping for, 135–136
  emotional space for, 139–140
  full-body relaxation massage for, 133, 134
  jaw release for, 133, 135, 135f
  sacral releases for, 135, 137f
  squatting practice for, 136f
  visualizations and affirmations for, 132,
    133, 134, 149
Birth-related surgeries, 235–244
  bodywork after, 239–243
    for abdominal scar tissue, 241–243,
      242f–243f
    for depleted energy, 241
    for epidural back pain, 241
    health intake for, 239–240
    medical release for, 239–240
    postcesarean section treatment, 240–241
    precautions and contraindications to, 240
  cesarean section, 235–238
  common complaints after, 241–243
  postpartum tubal ligation, 238–239
  recovery from, 239
Bladder infection, 23, 24, 27–29
Blankets, electric, 64, 246
Blastocyst, 14

Bleeding, 247
  postpartum, 198, 205
Blood clots, ix, 27, 50, 56, 62, 68–70, 69f, 258, 247
  assessment for, 69–70
  case studies of, 65, 76
  after cesarean section, 237
  incidence of, 69
  nonsymptomatic, 62
  postpartum, 204–205
  risk factors for, 64, 69
Blood pressure, 27. *See also* Hypertension; Hypotension
Blood type, 18
Blood volume, 26, 27, 28
Bloody show, 154, 257
"Blues," postpartum, 225–227, 259
Body fluids, 83, 156, 205–206
Body image, 7–8
Body mechanics, 83, 84
Body memories, 9
Body temperature, 24, 29
Body-awareness, 7
bodyCushion, 90
Bony pressure, 83
Brachial plexus syndrome, 32
Braxton-Hicks contractions, 19, 21, 24, 56, 154, 257
Breast drape, 84
Breast massage, x, 2, 62, 115–116, 116f–117f
  after nursing, 231
  postpartum, 228
  precautions and contraindications to, 62, 115–116, 246
  self-massage, 227, 232
Breast tenderness, 115–117
  breast massage for, 115–116, 116f–117f
  cause of, 114
  general treatment of, 114
  lymph pump for, 116–117, 117f
  postpartum, 231
Breastfeeding, 7, 227–231
Breasts
  compression in prone position, 93
  engorgement of, x, 227, 231, 258
  estrogen effects on, 24
  inflammation of, 258
  mastitis, 206, 227, 258
  postpartum concerns related to, 227–231
Breath attunement, 83
Breath expansion, 226–227, 228f
Breathing, 25–26, 82
  abdominal, 161
  alternate nostril, 229, 229f
  belly, 18, 94
  cleansing breaths, 161
  conscious, 78, 93–94, 229
  deep abdominal, 78
  into the earth, 229
  ineffective patterns of, 161
  intentional, for anxiety, 183
  intuitive patterns of, 161
  during labor, 158, 160–161
  light breath, 94
  during massage, 93–94
  observation of, 161
  self-care tips for, 229, 229f
  shortness of breath, 19, 26, 32, 127–130
  sipping breaths, 161
  stretches to increase respiratory capacity, 129, 129f
  Ujjayi victorious, 161
  visualization and, 94
  whale, 161
Breech baby, 117–118, 153, 154f, 257
Broad ligament, 37f, 38
  spasm of, 38
Bulbospongiosus muscle, 38, 40f

C
Cardinal ligament, 38, 257
Cardiovascular system during pregnancy, 27

Carpal tunnel syndrome, 98
Catecholamines, 146, 152, 257
Cervix, 257
  dilation of, 149, 153, 167–168, 257
  effacement of, 153, 167, 257–258
Cesarean section, x, 235–238, 257, 236
  benefits of massage after, 236
  fetal reasons for, 237
  general treatment after, 240–241
  immediate postsurgical complications of, 237–238
  maternal reasons for, 236
  procedure for, 237
Chakra massage, 183, 257
Chest isometrics, 230
Chest opening, 78, 97, 98f, 114
  yoga chest opener, 129, 129f
Chloasma, 24, 29, 257
Circular massage, 182–183
Circulatory massage to legs, 122
"Closing the bones," 224, 225f
Cold application
  after cesarean section, 240
  during labor, 162–163
    for back pain due to posterior baby, 188, 189f
    for general back pain, 191
Comadrona, 4
Comfort of client, 29, 30
  in sidelying position, 89–91
Common complaints after birth-related surgeries, 241–243
  abdominal scar tissue, 241–243, 242f–243f
  depleted energy, 241
  epidural back pain, 241
Common complaints during labor, 181–194
  anxiety/fear, 181–183, 182f
  back pain due to posterior baby, 187–189, 188f
  exhaustion, 183–184
  general back pain, 189–193, 190f–193f
  general labor pain, 194
  stalled or slow labor, 184–186
Common complaints during pregnancy, 107–131
  assessment of, 54–57
  breast tenderness, 115–117
  breech baby, 117–118
  edema, 118–119
  groin pain and round ligament pain, 119–121
  leg cramps, 121–123
  low back pain, 107–111, 113
  mid and upper back pain, 111–115
  sciatica and sacroiliac pain, 123–127
  shortness of breath, 127–130
Common complaints in postpartum period, 210–231
  breast engorgement and tenderness, 231
  edema, 212, 213
  fatigue, 223–225, 225f, 226f
  general breast concerns, 227–231
  low and mid back pain, 219–223, 221f–223f
  nursing neck, 217–219, 218f
  pelvic misalignment and sacral-iliac pain, 210–212, 212f
  postpartum "blues," 225–227
  upper back pain, 219, 220f
  uterine and abdominal concerns, 212–217, 213f, 215f, 216f
Compression and cross-fiber friction, for groin pain, 120–121, 121f
Conception, 13–14
Constipation, 19, 23, 24, 26, 108
Contraction/dilation imagery, 162
Contraction–relaxation, 162
Contraction–relaxation visualization, 230–231
Contractions. See Uterine contractions
Contraindications to massage.
    See Precautions and contraindications
Cooper's ligaments, 116
Corpus luteum, 14, 18, 23

Corpuscles, 147, 257
Cradle rock, 224–225, 226f
Craniosacral therapy, 52, 153
Creative power, 5–6, 8
Crowning, 176, 257
Culture. See Traditional birth practices
Cupping, 135–136

D
"Dai," 4
Deep tissue massage, 51
Deep vein thrombosis, 27, 28f, 50, 64, 68–70, 69f, 84257. *See also* Blood clots
  after cesarean section, 237
  postpartum, 204–205
Depression, 7
  postpartum, 225
Diabetes, gestational, 72–73, 258
Diastasis recti, 32, 39, 41–44, 42f, 46, 257
  assessment for, 43–44, 45f
  postpartum, 209
  bodywork considerations for, 43
  case study of, 44
  low back pain due to, 41, 108
  occurrence and symptoms of, 43
  postpartum management of, 199
  risk factors for, 42–43
Diastasis symphysis pubis, 25, 205, 248, 257
Dilation of cervix, 149, 153, 167–168, 257
Doctors, education for, 9
Doula, 4, 6, 145, 146, 158, 257
Draping, 88–89
  of back, 89, 89f
  of breasts, 84
  to expose gluteals and superior leg, 89, 90f
  to expose inferior leg, 89
  in sidelying position, 88–89
Drawing energy down, 182
Dreams, 18, 19
Drug use, 68
Due date, 14, 152–153, 257
  pregnancy past, 21, 23, 24t, 132
    labor induction for, 132, 137
    massage and, 137

E
Eclampsia, 76–77, 247, 257
Edema, 118–119
  ankle/foot, 19, 23, 24, 118
  edema reduction technique for, 119, 119f
  general treatment of, 118
  hand, 24, 98–99, 118
  myofascial hip opening for, 119, 120f
  nonpitting, 118
  pitting, 54, 65, 66f, 259, 118
  postpartum, 212, 213
  third-trimester, essential oils for, 121
  tips for mothers for circulation improvement and reduction of, 120
Education
  for doctors, 9
  for massage therapists, 9
  for mothers, 9
Efface/effacement, 153, 168, 257–258
Effleurage, 62, 63
Egg, 13–14
Ejaculation, 13
Electric blankets, 64, 246
Electromagnetic field exposure, 64, 246
Embolus, 69, 258
  postpartum, 204–205
  pulmonary, 62, 69, 260
Emotional changes, postpartum, 199
  "blues," 225–227
Emotional grounding, 181–182
Emotional space, 139–140
Emotional wellbeing, 7
Endocrine organs, 23
Endopelvic fascia, 37
Endorphins, 147, 152, 179, 258
Energizing the abdomen, 213–214

Energy, 7
  drawing energy down, 182
  exhaustion during labor, 183–184
    relaxing and renewing energy, 183–184
    stimulating energy, 184
  postpartum, 198, 199
  postsurgical depletion of, 241
Energy work, 52
Engaged, 153, 258
Engelmann, George, 6
Engorgement of breasts, x, 227, 231, 258
Environment for massage, 83–84
Epidural anesthesia, 160, 258
Epidural back pain, 238, 241
Episiotomy, 176, 258
Erector spinae muscles, 32, 97
Erector spinae/bladder meridian acupressure
    points, 99f
Estimated date of delivery, 14, 257. *See also*
    Due date
Estrogen, 13, 14, 18, 23, 24–25, 258
Excretory system during pregnancy, 27–29
Exercise(s), 35, 46
  aerobics and walking, 229
  chest isometrics, 230
  for client restricted to bed rest, 78
  dynamic arm exercise, 230
  isometric stretches, 64–65
  Kegel, 40–41, 42, 78
  for postpartum strengthening, 224
Exhaustion during labor, 183–184
  relaxing and renewing energy for, 183–184
  stimulating energy for, 184
Expected date of confinement, 152–153. *See
    also* Due date

F
Fallopian tubes, 13
Fanning trochanter attachments, 97, 100f
Fans, 83
Fatigue, 15, 18, 38, 84
  during labor, 183–184
  postpartum, 223–225
Fear. *See also* Anxiety
  of childbirth, 146, 148
  during labor, 181–183, 182f
  of miscarriage, 8, 9, 71
Femur traction and mobility, 127, 127f
Fetal development, 14–23
  in first trimester, 14–15, 15f, 16t–17t
  past the due date, 21, 23, 23t
  in second trimester, 17–18, 19f–20t
  in third trimester, 19–21, 21f, 22t
Fetal distress, 237
Fetal ejection reflex, 176
Fetal genetic disorders, 72, 247
Fibrolytic activity, 27, 258
Field, Tiffany, 6
Fifth or subsequent pregnancy, 72
First trimester
  bodywork during, 10, 16t–17t, 84, 85, 86t
  abdominal massage, 58, 105
  fetal development during, 14–15, 15f,
    16t–17t
  maternal sensations during, 15, 16t–17t
  miscarriage in, 14–15, 58, 70,
    84, 85, 105
  precautions for mother during, 14
Foot circles, 78
Foot massage, 63, 65, 101–102
  during labor, 163, 164f, 165
  precautions and contraindications to, 65,
    66f, 246
  for slow labor, 185
Foot swelling, 118
Full body stretch, 110–111, 111f

G
Gait assessment, 34
Gas cramping, after cesarean section, 238
Gastrointestinal system during pregnancy,
    26–27

Gate control theory of pain, 147
Genetic disorders, fetal, 72, 247
Gestational diabetes, 72–73, 258
Gestational hypertension, 75, 205, 258
Glossary, 257–260
Gluteal muscles, 32
  massage of lateral hip rotators and, 97–98,
    100f
Goddess Khamakya, 5, 5f
Groin pain, 55, 119–121
  cause of, 120
  compression and cross-fiber friction for,
    120–121, 121f
  general treatment of, 120
  lifting effleurage for, 120
  tips for mothers for relief of, 122
Grounding
  emotional, 181–182
  the feet, 182, 182f

H
Hamstring muscles, 32
Hand edema, 24, 98–99, 118
Hand massage, 98–100
  during labor, 165–166, 166f
  for slow labor, 185
Hand pressure, for anxiety, 182, 182f
Hand stretches, 78
Head and neck relaxation techniques, 95–97,
    96f, 97f
Headaches, 32, 54, 55
Health factors that increase risk during
    pregnancy, 67–78, 246–248
  client restricted to bed rest, 77–78, 246–247
  conditions requiring special precautions,
    67–71
  high-risk complications, 71–77
Health intake, 52, 53f, 84, 239–240
  after birth-related surgery, 239–240
  for client on bed rest, 77–78
  for postpartum massage, 203
Heart murmurs, 27
Heartburn, 19, 24, 26–27, 83
Heat application, 66–67
  after cesarean section, 240
  contraindications to, 246
  during labor, 162–163
    for back pain due to posterior baby, 188,
      189f
    for general back pain, 191
Heating pads, 64, 246
HELLP syndrome, 75–76, 247, 258
Hemorrhage, postpartum, 205
High-risk complications of pregnancy, 71–77
  eclampsia, 76–77
  gestational hypertension, preeclampsia,
    and HELLP syndrome, 75–76
  as indication for medical release, 71
  placenta previa, 73–74, 74f
  placental abruption, 73
  polyhydramnios, 74–75
  preterm labor, 75
High-risk pregnancy, 49, 50, 51, 258
  medical release for bodywork in, 57–58
Hip adductors, 32
  adductor resistance technique, 135
  massage to inner thigh and, 62, 64, 64f
Hip flexors, 32
Hip pull, for back labor, 193, 193f
Hip rotators, 32
  hamstring and lateral hip rotator releases,
    124
  lateral hip rotator anchor and stretch, 222f,
    222–223
  lateral hip rotator attachments for sciatica,
    125
  massage of lateral hip rotators and
    gluteals, 97–98, 100f
Hip soreness
  positioning client with, 94
  related to sidelying, 89
Homan's sign, 69–70

Home birth, 144, 176
Hormones
  changes during pregnancy, 23–25
  contractions induced by, 152
  to increase fertility, 72
  low back pain and, 108
  poor posture and, 32–33
Hot tub, 65–66
Hydration
  during labor, 185
  after massage, 10, 29, 83
Hydrotherapy
  after cesarean section, 240
  during labor, 162–163, 163f
  for postpartum renewal, 217
Hypertension
  chronic, 68, 247
  gestational, 75, 205, 258
Hypotension, orthostatic, 27, 29, 30, 130, 259

I
Iliacus muscle, 32
Iliopsoas muscle, 32, 45
Iliotibial band compression, 101, 101f
Immunity, 7
Implantation, 14
Indigestion, 15, 19
Infection
  bladder, 23, 24, 27–29
  as indication for cesarean section, 236
  kidney, 28, 29, 108
  urinary tract, 27–29, 73, 248, 260
  uterine, 206, 247
Infertility, 72, 247
Interstitial fluid, 27, 258
Intimacy during pregnancy, 8
Intrauterine growth restriction, 72, 247, 258
Intrauterine pressure, 93
Involute/involution of uterus, 198, 258
Isometric stretches, 64–65

J
Japanese pregnancy massage, 6
Jaw release, 133, 135, 135f
  for slow labor, 186
Jin Shin Jytsu, 52
Joint instability, postpartum, 205

K
Kegel exercises, 40–41, 42, 258
  benefits of, 40
  for client restricted to bed rest, 78
  instructions for, 41
  perineal massage and, 139
  in postpartum period, 197, 198
Kidney infection, 28, 29, 108
Kidneys, 27–29

L
Labor, ix, 132, 143–150, 258. *See also* Birth;
    Birth preparation
  active, 153, 155, 171–174, 178, 257
  acupressure during, 163, 165
  affirmations and visualizations during,
    157, 158, 161–162
  back, 153, 189–193, 257
  beginning of, 153
  breathing during, 158, 160–161
  common complaints during, 181–194
  descent and position of baby during,
    153–154
  early, 155, 169–171, 257
  effects of stress on, 145–146
  facilitating relaxation during, 1–2, 7,
    132–133, 159
  failure to progress, 236
  first stage of, 155, 258, 167–176
  hydrotherapy during, 162–163, 163f
  impending, signs of, 154
  induction of, 132, 137
  latent, 168
  length of, 153, 155

Labor (*continued*)
lull in, 175–176
overview of, 152–155
pain of, 147–148, 194
back pain due to posterior baby, 187–189, 188f, 189f
gate control theory of, 147
general back pain, 189–193, 190f–193f
management of, 155–156
phases of, 155
positions for, 171–174, 172t, 173f–174f, 185
pre-labor, 155, 168–169, 259
preterm, 75, 247, 259
prodromal, 168
pushing phase of, 176–177
questions for mother regarding, 156–157
recognizing, 155
reflexology during, 163, 164f
second stage of, 155, 260, 176–178
stalled or slow, 184–186
support tools for, 159
third stage of, 155, 260, 178–179
transition phase of, 155, 174–175, 260
without touch, 148
Labor/birth massage, 144f, 144–145, 155–180
acupressure, 137, 149
amniotic sac rupture during, 156
for back pain due to posterior baby, 187–189
benefits of, 145
of client unknowingly in active labor, 178
by client's partner, 186
contraindications to, 160
in early labor, 170–171
to encourage contractions, 149
hand and foot massage, 165–166, 166f
long strokes for, 166
in lull, 175–176
pain threshold increased by, 146–147
petrissage, 165
for placental delivery, 179
precautions for, 159–160
in pushing phase, 177
rebozo massage for, 167, 169f
sacral counterpressure for, 167, 168f
for slow labor, 185–186
traditional practices of, 184
in transition phase, 175
two-person grounding stroke for, 166f, 166–167
Lactation, 7, 227–231
acupressure for, 232f
traditional practices for improvement of, 231
Lateral hip rotator anchor and stretch, 222f, 222–223
Lateral hip rotator attachments, for sciatica, 125
Lateral hip rotator massage, 97–98, 100f
Left tilt positioning, 92
Leg cramps, 6, 18, 19, 32, 55, 62, 100, 121–123
causes of, 121–122
circulatory massage for, 122
general treatment of, 122
inversion, eversion, and dorsiflexion stretch-resistance for, 122–123
tips for mothers for prevention of, 123
Leg massage, 50, 62, 76, 100–101, 100f–101f
contraindications to, 246
Leg press, 78
Leg roll, 78
Leg swelling, 18, 62
Levator ani muscle, 38, 40f
Lifting effleurage, 120
Ligaments
postpartum changes in, 38, 197, 198–199
posture and, 32–33
relaxin effects on, 25, 32–33
uterine, 37f, 37–38
bodywork considerations related to, 38, 39f
preventing strain of, 38, 39f
spasm of, 19, 38

Ligamentum transversalis colli, 38
Light breath, 94
Lightening, 19, 21f, 128, 153, 258
Linea alba, 24, 41, 258
Linea negra, 24, 258
Lomi lomi, 51
Lull, 175–176
Lumbar lordosis, 32, 47, 93
Lymph pump, 116–117, 117f

M
Massage therapist
education for, 9
resources for, 249–255
scope of practice of, x–xi, 7, 138
unique role of, 4
Massage therapist tips, x
addressing client health information with sensitivity, 54
choosing position for belly rub, 104
fatigue, 18
have partner massage client during labor, 186
heartburn, 26
identifying baby's position, 189
is medical release necessary?, 60
labor without touch, 148
making your table comfortable for pregnancy, 91
maternal respiratory changes, 26
positioning for client with hip pain, 94
postural awareness, 114
postural checklist, 36
reminders about birth, 149
respecting role of client's partner, 157, 158
strengthening the pelvic floor, 42
stretch marks, 131
supporting your hands during labor, 193
working with your scope of comfort, knowledge, and skill, 77
Mastitis, 206, 227, 258
Meconium, 155, 258
Medical release, ix, 57–58, 59f, 258
for client being treated for blood clot, 62
for client with high-risk complications of pregnancy, 71
necessity of, 60
for postsurgical clients, 239–240
Meissner's corpuscles, 147
Melzack, Ronald, 147
Menstrual cycle, 5
Merkel's disks, 147
Midwives, 4, 144, 148, 149
Milk ejection reflex, 25, 228, 259
Miscarriage, 70, 259
fear of, 8, 9, 71
in first trimester, 14–15, 58, 70, 84, 85, 105
massage and, 10, 58, 71, 85, 105
prevalence of, 14–15
repeat, 70–71, 247
Mother(s)
education for, 9
self-care tips for, x
arm movement, 230
belly lifts, 190, 190f
breast massage, 232
breathing practices, 229, 229f
to decrease low back pain, 113, 113f
improving circulation and reducing edema, 120
to prevent leg cramps, 123
preventing abdominal and uterine ligament strain, 39
to reduce sacroiliac joint pain, 125
to relieve groin spasm, 122
re-stabilizing after birth, 211
squatting practice, 136f
stress relief for client restricted to bed rest, 78
stretches to increase respiratory capacity, 129, 129f
therapeutic strengthening exercises, 224

two important reminders for labor, 185
words in various languages for, 5, 5t
Mucous plug, 154, 259
Multifidus muscle, 32
Multiple gestation, 14, 70, 70f, 247, 237
Muscle tension, 33
Muscle tone, 33
Musculoskeletal pain reduction, 6, 7
Musculoskeletal system. *See also* specific muscles
assessing symptoms of discomfort related to, 54–56
effects of weight gain on, 31–32
lumbar lordosis and, 32
muscles supporting abdomen, 32
muscular areas stressed by pregnancy, 37–47
Music, 83
Myofascial hip opening, 119, 120f
Myths about pregnancy massage, ix, x, 10, 85, 93, 105, 137

N
Napropath, 85, 118
Nasal congestion, 18, 24, 29, 30, 83, 93
Nausea/vomiting, 10, 15, 24, 26–27, 64, 85, 247
after cesarean section, 238
Neck pain, 32
nursing neck, x.217–219
positioning for relief of, 88
Neck release, 218, 218f
Neck rolls, 78
Neck traction, 218–219
Nightmares, 19
Nipple contact, 116
Nosebleeds, 18, 24
Nursing neck, x, 217–219, 218f
Nurturance, 7, 82, 146, 146t

O
Obesity, 68
Oblique abdominal muscles, 41
Occipital traction, 96, 96f
Occiput and eyebrow points, 96–97, 97f
Odent, Michel, 176
Office setup, 83–84
Office temperature, 84
Oils, 84
for belly rubs, 136, 170
for circular massage of anxious laboring woman, 182–183
for perineal massage, 138
for postpartum massage, 203–204
for stretch marks, 131
for third-trimester edema, 121
Oligohydramnios, 72, 247, 259
Organ system adaptations during pregnancy, 25–29
Orthostatic hypotension, 27, 29, 30, 130, 259
Ovulation, 14
Oxytocin, 25, 116, 132, 146, 152, 259

P
Pacinian corpuscles, 147
Pain. *See also* specific types
attention to, 147
back, 6, 7, 18, 19, 29, 32, 38, 46, 107–114
after cesarean section, 238
dysfunctional, 148
effect of touch on threshold for, 146–147
emotional, 148, 150
functional, 148, 150
gate control theory of, 147
groin, 55, 119–121
of labor, 147–148, 194
back pain due to posterior baby, 187–189, 188f, 189f
gate control theory of, 147
general back pain, 189–193, 190f–193f
management of, 155–156
neck, 32, 88

sacroiliac, 32, 123–127
shoulder, 32, 88
traditional cultures and, 148
Paraspinal muscles, 32
Partners of pregnant women, x
  belly rubs for contractions, 170, 170f
  help with postural support, 36
  help with sacral compression and
    unwinding, 95
  perineal massage by, 138–139
  reactions to her body changes, 8
  respecting role of, 157, 158
Passive range of motion, 64–65, 246
Pectoralis stretch, 219
Pectoralis stretch and resistance, 114f,
    114–115
Pelvic alignment rock, 223, 223f
Pelvic floor muscles, 32, 38, 40f, 40–41, 259
  Kegel exercises for strengthening of, 40–41,
    42
  problems associated with weakness of, 38,
    40
Pelvic heaviness, 19
Pelvic misalignment, postpartum, 210–212
Pelvic rebalancing, postpartum, 209, 211
Pelvic tilt, 32, 35, 41, 45
  to decrease low back pain, 113
  to relieve groin spasm, 122
"Peri Life Events Scale," 21
Perineum
  massage of, 7, 138–139
  muscles of (See Pelvic floor muscles)
  postpartum changes in, 198
  softening of, 177
  stretching of, 176
  tears of, 138, 176, 179
Personal boundary violations, 7, 8
Petrissage, during labor, 165
Physiological effects of massage in
    pregnancy, 6–7
Pillows and supports, 1, 84, 87f, 88, 90, 91
Piriformis muscle, 40f
Pitocin, 132, 259
Pitting edema, 54, 65, 66f, 259, 118
Placenta, 14, 17–18
  delivery of, 178–179
  traditional birth practices and, 177
Placenta previa, 73–74, 74f, 237, 248, 259
Placental abruption, 73, 237, 248, 259
Polarity therapy, 52
Polyhydramnios, 74–75, 247, 259
Positioning for bodywork, 1, 21, 50, 87–92
  for belly rub, 104
  after cesarean section, 240
  for client with hip pain, 94
  left tilt, 92
  from lying down to sitting, 39f
  postpartum, 201
  when baby accompanies mother, 201–202,
    203f, 204
  prone, 93
  to relieve pain, 88
  semi-reclining, 91–92, 92f
  sidelying position, 1, 38, 87–91
  supine, 65–66, 67f, 85, 92
  trimester considerations for, 84–85
Positions for labor, 171–174, 185
  to allay anxiety, 183
  for back pain due to posterior baby,
    187–188, 188f
  benefits of, 172t
  birth ball, 174
  hands and knees, kneeling leaning
    forward, or leaning over a counter or
    chair, 174, 186
  sidelying, supine, or semi-reclining, 174
  sitting in a chair, 173–174, 174f
  for slow labor, 186
  squatting OM, 186
  straddling a chair, 171, 173, 173f
  supported squatting in front of a chair, 173,
    173f

Positions of baby in utero, 153–154, 154f
  breech, 117–118, 153, 154f, 257
  posterior, 153, 154f, 259
    back pain due to, 187–189, 188f, 189f
    transverse lie, 153–154, 154f, 260
    turning baby with acupressure, 191
    vertex, 153, 154f, 260
Posterior position, 153, 154f, 259
  back pain due to, 187–189, 188f, 189f
  general treatment for, 187–188
Postpartum "blues," 225–227, 259
Postpartum bodywork, 200–206, 208–233
  assessments for, 209–210
    diastasis recti, 209
    psoas, 209–210, 210f
    spinal, 209
  attending to client for, 201
  for back pain, 219–223
    low and mid back, 219–223, 221f–223f
    upper back, 219, 220f
  benefits of, 200, 201t
  birth history and, 202
  for breast engorgement and tenderness, 231
  client positioning for, 201
    when baby accompanies mother,
      201–202, 203f, 204
  for edema, 212, 213
  for fatigue, 223–225, 225f, 226f
  five "Bs" for, 202t
  for general breast concerns, 227–231
  health intake questions for, 203
  house calls for, 202
  hydrotherapy, 217
  in immediate postpartum period, 208–209
    low-back release, 208–209
    sacroiliac and pelvic rebalancing, 209
  for nursing neck, 217–219, 218f
  for pelvic misalignment and sacral-iliac
    pain, 210–212, 212f
  for postpartum "blues," 225–227
  precautions for, 203–206
    body fluids, 205–206
    embolism and varicose veins, 204–205
    gestational hypertension/preeclampsia,
      205
    hemorrhage, 205
    mastitis, 206
    separated symphysis pubis and unstable
      joints, 205
    surgical incision, 205
    use of oils, 203–204
    uterine infection, 206
  preparation for, 202–203
  therapeutic strengthening exercises, 224
  for uterine and abdominal concerns,
    212–217, 213f, 215f, 216f
  when to begin, 202
Postpartum period, ix–x, 197–200, 259
  bleeding in, 198
  common complaints in, 210–231
  emotional changes in, 199
  energy in, 199
  Kegel exercises in, 197, 198
  low back pain in, 107
  physical changes in, 197–199
    abdomen, 199
    ligaments, low back, and pelvis, 198–199
    perineum, 198
    uterus, 198
  traditional practices for care in, 200
Postpartum tubal ligation, 238–239
Postural awareness, 114
Posture, 7, 31–37
  adjustment of, 34, 35f, 35–36
  assessment of, 33–35, 34f, 46, 82–83
  baby's size and position and, 33
  discomforts related to, 32, 34–35
  effects of tight psoas on, 45, 47f
  factors contributing to, 32–33
  gravity and, 32, 34
  healthy, 34f
  hormones and, 32

low back pain related to, 108
  muscle tension and, 33
  muscle tone and, 33
  partner's help with, 36
  poor, 32–33, 34f
  self-esteem and, 33
  sitting, 36–37
  weight gain and adjustments in, 31–32
Precautions and contraindications, ix, x,
    49–79, 82, 107, 245–248
  for abdominal bodywork, 54–57, 245
  for acupressure, 60–62, 61f, 245
  for ankle massage, 63, 63f
  for aromatherapy, 62, 246
  assessing symptoms of discomfort, 54–57
  assessment questions, 52–54
  for breast massage, 62, 115–116, 246
  for electromagnetic field exposure, 64, 246
  for foot massage, 65, 66f, 246
  health factors that increase risk during
    pregnancy, 67–78, 246–248
    client restricted to bed rest, 77–78,
      246–247
    conditions requiring special precautions,
      67–71, 246–248
    high-risk complications, 71–77
  health history intake form, 52, 53f
  in high-risk pregnancy, 49, 50, 51, 71–77, 258
  for labor massage, 159–160
  for leg massage, 246
  for massage to adductors and inner thigh,
    62, 64, 64f
  medical releasee, 57–58, 59f, 60
  for passive range of motion, 64–65, 246
  for perineal massage, 138
  for postpartum massage, 203–206, 246
  for postsurgical massage, 240
  primary considerations for pregnancy
    massage, 50–51
  standard precautions, 51, 51t
  for supine positioning, 65–66, 67f, 246
  symptoms requiring referral to prenatal
    care provider, 49, 50, 54–56
  for thermal therapies, 246
    saunas and hot tubs, 66–67
  trimester considerations for, 84–85, 86t
  for Type I and Type II touch, 51–52
  working with your scope of comfort,
    knowledge, and skill, 77
Preeclampsia, 75, 207, 236, 247, 259
Pregnancy, 1–11
  changes noted by massage therapist
    during, 1, 13
  common complaints during, 107–131
  culture and tradition of respect
    surrounding, 5
  fetal development during, 14–23
  fifth or subsequent, 72
  high-risk, 49, 50, 51, 71–77, 258
  hormonal changes during, 23–25
  intimacy during, 8
  length of, 152
  organ system adaptations during, 25–29
  partner's reactions to woman's body
    changes in, 8
  weight gain in, 7–8, 31–32
Pregnancy massage, 82–106
  avoiding bony pressure during, 83
  avoiding heartburn during, 83
  baby activity during, 83
  benefits of, 6–7
  breath attunement for, 83
  client comfort during, 29, 30
  client expectations for, 82
  client positioning for, 1, 21, 50, 83, 87–92
  considerations specific to, 83
  to create length and space in woman's
    body, 82
  dangers of, 10
  dispelling myths about, ix, x, 10, 85, 93,
    105, 137
  effects on baby in utero, 1

Pregnancy massage (*continued*)
in first trimester, 10, 16t–17t, 58, 84, 85, 86t
functions of, 5
hydration after, 10, 29, 83
issues with, 7–9
body image, 7–8
body memories, 9
education for doctors, 9
education for massage therapists, 9
education for mothers, 9
fear of miscarriage, 8, 9, 71
violation of personal boundaries, 8–9
labor induction and, 137
nurturance and, 82
office setup for, 83–84
precautions and contraindications to, ix, x, 49–79
preparation for, 83–84
primary considerations for, 50–51
proper body mechanics for, 83, 84
safety of, 1, 8, 10
techniques for, 92–105
arms and hands, 98–100
back, 97, 98f
belly rubs, 102f–103f, 102–105, 105f
breathing and connecting, 93–94
feet, 101–102
head and neck, 95–97, 96f, 97f
lateral hip rotators and gluteals, 97–98, 100f
legs, 100–101, 100f–101f
sacral compression and unwinding, 94–95, 95f
shoulders and chest, 97, 98f
traditions of, 4f, 4–6
trimester considerations for, 84–85, 86t
use of relaxing touch for, 83
"Pregnancy waddle," 34
Pre-labor, 155, 168–169, 259
Premature birth, 259
precautions for client with history of, 71–72, 248
Prenatal care provider, symptoms requiring referral to, 49, 50, 54–56
Preterm labor, 75, 247, 259
Preterm labor contractions, 21, 75, 259
Progesterone, 14, 18, 23–24, 28, 260
Prolactin, 7, 25, 152, 260
Prolapse, 40, 260
Prone positioning, 93
Psoas assessment, postpartum, 209–210, 210f
Psoas muscle, 45, 47, 47f
Psoas release, 220–221, 221f
Psoas stretch, 113, 122
assisted, 111, 112f
Pulmonary embolism, 62, 69, 260
Pushing phase, 176–177

Q
Quadratus lumborum compression points, 108–110, 109f
Quadratus lumborum extension, 110, 111f
Quadratus lumborum muscle, 32, 47
Quadratus lumborum release, 110, 110f
Quadratus lumborum stretch, 113, 113f
Quadratus lumborum work, postpartum, 222
Quadriceps muscle, 32
Quadriceps work, postpartum, 222
Quickening, 18, 260

R
Rebozo massage during labor, 167, 169f
rebozo friction, 167
rebozo hip jiggle, 167
Rectus abdominis muscle, 32, 41, 42f
Rectus femoris muscle, 32
Reflexology, 63, 65, 149. *See also* Foot massage during labor, 163, 164f
Reiki, 52
Relaxation skills, 1–2, 7
Relaxin, 19, 23, 25, 32, 108, 197, 260
postpartum, 198–199

Relaxing and renewing energy, 183–184
Relaxing touch, 83
Resources, x, 249–255
Respiratory system
during pregnancy, 25–26
respiratory depression after cesarean section, 237
stretches to increase respiratory capacity, 129, 129f
Re-stabilizing after birth, 211
Restroom facilities, 83
Revisioning, 183
Rib raking and trigger point release, 128–129, 128f–129f
Ring of fire, 176, 260
Rolfing, 51
Round ligament, 37f, 38, 260
spasm/pain of, 38, 119–121
cause of, 120
compression and cross-fiber friction for, 120–121, 121f
general treatment of, 120
lifting effleurage for, 120
tips for mothers for relief of, 122

S
Sacral compression and unwinding, 94–95, 95f
Sacral counterpressure, during labor, 167, 168f
Sacral foramen stimulation
for back labor, 191–192
for slow labor, 186
Sacral palming, 186
Sacral push, 211–212, 212f
Sacral releases, 135, 137f
Sacral rub, 111
Sacroiliac and pelvic rebalancing, 125–127, 127f
postpartum, 209, 211
Sacroiliac pain, 32, 123–127
cause of, 123
femur traction and mobility for, 127, 127f
general treatment of, 123–124
postpartum, 210–212, 212f
sacroiliac and pelvic rebalancing for, 125–127, 127f, 209, 211
tips for mothers for reduction of, 125
trochanter and sacroiliac joint traction for, 125, 126f
Sacroiliac relief, for back labor, 192f, 192–193
Safety concerns, 1, 8, 10, 51. *See also* Precautions and contraindications
Sartorius muscle, 32
Sauna, 65–66
Scents, 83–84. *See also* Aromatherapy
Sciatica, 123, 260
cause of, 123
general treatment of, 123
hamstring and lateral hip rotator releases for, 124
lateral hip rotator attachments for, 125
Scope of practice, x–xi, 7, 138
Second trimester
bodywork in, 84–85, 86t
abdominal massage, 58, 60
fetal development during, 17–18, 19f, 20t
maternal sensations during, 18, 20t
Self-esteem, 33
Semi-reclining position, 1, 91–92, 92f
belly rub in, 104–105, 105f
comfortable positioning in, 92
indications for, 91–92
table height for, 92
Serotonin, 7
Sheets, 84
Shiatsu, 51
Shortness of breath, 19, 26, 32, 127–130
cause of, 127–128
general treatment of, 128
rib raking and trigger point release for, 128–129, 128f–129f

shoulder mobilization for, 128
stretches to increase respiratory capacity, 129, 129f
Shoulder compression, related to sidelying, 90
Shoulder mobilization, 128
Shoulder pain, 32
positioning for relief of, 88
Shoulder pressure resistance, 218
Shoulder relaxation techniques, 97
Shoulder rolls, 78
Shoulder shrugging, 78
Sidelying position, 1, 38, 87–91
belly rub in, 102–103, 102f–103f, 104
changing sides for, 91
client comfort in, 89–91
client positioning in, 87–88
draping in, 88–89, 89f
indications for, 87
instability during, 90
practitioner comfort and, 90–91
support for, 87f, 87–88
table height and, 87
Sitting
in a chair during labor, 173–174, 174f
posture for, 36–37
repositioning from lying down to, 39f
Skin rolling/fascial lift, postpartum, 214–215, 215f
Sleep, 6
Smoking, xi, 68
Social Readjustment Rating Scale, 21
Sperm, 13–14
Spider angioma, 24, 260
Spinal assessment, postpartum, 209
Spinal curvature, 32
Spirituality, 139, 143
Sports massage, 51
Squatting practice, 136f
Standing arm raise, 129
Stepstool, 84
Stimulating energy, 184
Stress, 6, 21
after cesarean section, 238
effects on labor, 145–146
relief of, 6, 7
for client on bed rest, 78
Stress hormones, 6, 7
Striae gravidarum (stretch marks), 19, 131, 199, 260
Subscapularis massage, 219, 220f
Subscapularis stretch, 115, 115f, 219
Superficial thrombophlebitis, 68–69, 260
Supine bicycle riding, 224
Supine pelvic unwinding, 212, 213f
Supine positioning, 65–66, 67f, 85, 92
precautions and contraindications to, 65–66, 67f, 246
Surgical incision, 205
Swedish massage, 51–52, 63
Symphysis pubis, 25, 40f
separation of, 25, 205, 248, 257

T
Tensor fasciae latae, 32
Terminology, 49, 51–52
Therapeutic benefits of touch, 2
Thigh
compressing iliotibial band and, 101, 101f
kneading of, 100f, 100–101
Third trimester
bodywork in, 85, 86t
essential oils for edema in, 121
fetal development in, 19–21, 21f, 22t, 23f
maternal sensations during, 18–19, 22t
Thromboembolic disorders, 68–70, 69f. *See also* Blood clots; Deep vein thrombosis; Pulmonary embolism
Time requirements, 84

Tobacco use, xi, 68
Toe hold, 186
Traditional birth practices, 4–6, 5f
    baby blues, 226
    breech baby, 118
    improving lactation, 231
    Japanese pregnancy massage, 6
    keeping mother and baby safe, 68
    massage for birth across cultures,
        144, 144f
    mysteries of creation, 14
    postpartum care, 200
    power of the placenta, 177
    recognizing labor, 155
    softening the perineum, 177
    soothing the womb, 214
    support for the belly, 42
    touch for labor, 184
    traditional cultures and pain, 148
    uterine massage, 85
Trager bodywork, 64
Transition phase, 155, 174–175, 260
Transverse abdominis muscle, 32, 41
    strengthening exercises for, 224
Transverse lie, 153–154, 154f, 260
Transverse perineal muscle, 38, 40f
Trigger point massage, 51
Trimesters of pregnancy, 14, 260
    first, 14–15, 15f, 16t–17t
    second, 17–18, 19f, 20t
    third, 18–21, 21f, 22t
Trochanter and sacroiliac joint traction, 125,
    126f
Tubal ligation, 260
    postpartum, 238–239
Twins, 14, 70, 70f, 149, 247, 237

Two-person grounding stroke, 166f, 166–167
Type I and Type II touch, 49, 51–52

U
Umbilical cord prolapse, 237
Universal precautions, 83, 156
Urinary incontinence, 38
Urinary tract infection, 27–29, 73, 248, 260
Urinary urgency/frequency, 19, 29
Uterine contractions, 56, 153, 167, 257
    in active labor, 171
    belly rubs for, 170, 170f
    Braxton-Hicks, 19, 21, 24, 56, 154, 257
    duration and frequency of, 153, 169
    in early labor, 169
    felt as low back pain, 108
    preterm labor, 21, 75, 259
    sensation of, 150, 153
    supportive touch for encouragement of,
        149
    in transition phase, 175
Uterine fundus, 153, 260
Uterine infection, 206, 247
Uterine ligaments, 37f, 37–38
    preventing strain of, 38, 39f
    spasm of, 19, 38
    strain in prone position, 93
Uterine massage, 85
    postpartum, 215–217, 216f
        to relieve uterine cramping, 216–217
        traditional practices of, 214
    self-massage, 4
Uterine rupture, 2326
Uterosacral ligament, 37f, 38, 260
    spasm of, 38
Uterus

changes during pregnancy, 37
    in first trimester, 10
    involution of, 198, 258
    muscle cells of, 37
    postpartum changes in, 198
    in second trimester, 18
    weight of, 37

V
Vaginal discharge, 18
Varicose veins, ix, 18, 24, 62, 64f, 84, 205
Vertex position, 153, 154f, 260
Visualization, 94, 132, 133, 134, 149, 157,
    161–162
    contraction–relaxation, 230–231
for slow labor, 186

W
Walking, 229
    "pregnancy waddle," 34
Wall, Patrick, 147
Water drinking after massage, 10,
    29, 83
Water immersion, during labor, 162–163, 163f
Weight gain in pregnancy, 7–8, 31–32
Womb massage, postpartum, 215–217, 216f
    contraindications to, 246
    to relieve uterine cramping, 216–217
    traditional practices of, 214

Y
Yates, Suzanne, 94
Yoga chest opener, 129, 129f

Z
Zygote, 14